THE GLOBAL PAIN CRISIS

WHAT EVERYONE NEEDS TO KNOW®

THE GLOBAL PAIN CRISIS

WHAT EVERYONE NEEDS TO KNOW®

JUDY FOREMAN

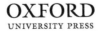

OXFORD
UNIVERSITY PRESS

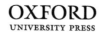

OXFORD
UNIVERSITY PRESS

Oxford University Press is a department of the University of Oxford. It furthers
the University's objective of excellence in research, scholarship, and education
by publishing worldwide. Oxford is a registered trade mark of Oxford University
Press in the UK and certain other countries.

"What Everyone Needs to Know" is a registered trademark of
Oxford University Press.

Published in the United States of America by Oxford University Press
198 Madison Avenue, New York, NY 10016, United States of America.

© Oxford University Press 2017

Library of Congress Cataloging-in-Publication Data
Names: Foreman, Judy, author.
Title: The global pain crisis : what everyone needs to know / Judy Foreman.
Description: New York, NY : Oxford University Press, [2017] |
Series: What everyone needs to know
Identifiers: LCCN 2016032534 | ISBN 9780190259235 (pbk. : alk. paper) |
ISBN 9780190259242 (hardback : alk. paper)
Subjects: LCSH: Chronic pain. | Chronic pain—Treatment. |
Opioid abuse—History.
Classification: LCC RB127 .F673 2017 | DDC 616/.0472—dc23
LC record available at https://lccn.loc.gov/2016032534

CONTENTS

2 Who Is Hardest Hit by Chronic Pain?   31

4 The Opioid Mess Worldwide   **93**

5 Marijuana 111

6 Western Medicine Treatments for Chronic Pain   137

7 Complementary and Alternative Medicine Treatments for Chronic Pain 165

8 The Way Forward   **203**

INTRODUCTION

In the United States alone, 100 million Americans—40 percent of adults—live in chronic pain, according to the Institute of Medicine. This is clearly an underestimate because the report does not count children, people in the military, or people in nursing homes or prisons. In fact, chronic pain is a bigger problem than heart disease, cancer, and diabetes *combined*, costing the United States $560 billion to $635 billion a year in direct medical costs and lost productivity.[1]

Yet the US government allocates almost nothing to pain research.[2,3,4] The National Institutes of Health's own calculations show that out of a recent budget of slightly over $30 billion, only 1.6 percent was targeted for pain research.[5,6,7] Outside analysts put the figure at closer to 0.63 percent.[8] Put even more starkly, while the government spends $2,562 on research for every person with HIV/AIDS, it spends only $4 for every person with pain.[9]

This, even though pain is the main reason Americans go on disability.[10]

Even at the end of life, when palliation of pain should be virtually guaranteed, one-third of Americans *in hospice care* still die in pain.[11,12,13]

And that's the good news.

Pain is ubiquitous. It spares no nation on the planet. All around the world, in both developed and developing countries, roughly 40 percent of people (most of them, women) live in chronic pain.[14]

As bad as the chronic pain situation is in the United States, it is even worse in the rest of the world. Indeed, of all the health inequalities, the gap between rich countries and poor in access to morphine and other prescription pain relievers is the widest gap of all, according to researchers from the Harvard Global Equity Initiative.[15]

In one study of 21 eastern European and 20 western European countries, researchers found huge problems in access to pain medicine. In Lithuania, Tajikistan, Albania, Georgia, and Ukraine, some essential opioid medications were virtually unavailable, creating what researchers called "a public health catastrophe."[16]

Overall, tens of millions of people around the world suffer in pain because of lack of access to controlled medicines, according to the World Health Organization—not just one million end-stage HIV/AIDS patients, 5.5 million terminal cancer patients, and nearly a million people who have had accidents or been the victims of violence but also people with chronic illnesses, people recovering from surgery, children, and women in labor.[17]

The global pain crisis is perhaps most tragic at the end of life.

In 2011, Human Rights Watch, an independent, nonpolitical organization that tracks human rights abuses, reported that tens of millions of people worldwide face death in agony because they have little or no access to morphine, an opioid (narcotic) that is both cheap and effective. This is probably an underestimate because Human Rights Watch tracked only pain at the end of life, not people in living in pain for extended periods, and it tracked only people dying from two diseases, cancer and AIDS.[18]

Another international organization, Treat the Pain, part of the American Cancer Society, confirms this dismal picture. In Ethiopia, a country of 90 million people, there is only one ward (with 10 beds) offering morphine in the entire country.[19] In Nigeria, with about 174 million people, basically no one is receiving pain relief, even though morphine costs only pennies a dose.[20,21] Every year, 173,000 Nigerians die from cancer or AIDS, yet there are only enough opioids to treat 274 of them.[22]

In some places, it's even worse. By one 2012 estimate, 2.4 million people around the world died with no pain treatment whatsoever.[23]

It was not supposed to be this way.

Back in 1961, the world community adopted an international agreement called the Single Convention on Narcotic Drugs, officially launched in 1968. The agreement says that the manufacture, import and export, distribution, prescription, and dispensation of narcotics (opioids) must occur with government authorization and be overseen by the body created by the Single Convention, the International Narcotics Control Board.

The Single Convention is supposed to address two problems—drug abuse *and* access to opioid drugs for pain. In fact, the Single Convention makes quite clear that narcotic drugs are "indispensable for the relief of pain and suffering and that adequate provision must be made to ensure the availability of narcotic drugs for such purposes."[24]

But today, 50 years later, the promise of this agreement remains largely unfulfilled. In fact, the International Narcotics Control Board has acknowledged that the needs of pain patients are being ignored. A special report from the board in 2010 admitted that "equal attention has not been given to the other objective of the treaties—ensuring the adequate availability of controlled substances," a view with which palliative care specialists emphatically agree.[25,26]

There are many reasons for this tragic state of affairs.

One is that in many, if not most, countries, including the United States, there are two colliding epidemics, though only one receives public attention. The abuse of opioids, which killed 16,235 Americans in 2013, grabs headlines almost every day, with news reports focusing on overdose, addiction, and criminal activity.[27] The larger epidemic of chronic pain is rarely mentioned.

The result of this lopsided reporting, according to a blue-ribbon panel convened by the National Institutes of Health in 2014, is that pain patients are stigmatized,[28] and thus opioids for legitimate patients become harder to obtain.

Another reason for the chronic pain tragedy is inconsistent and often-excessive regulation of pain medications. In one survey, 33 of 40 countries were found to impose restrictions on morphine prescribing that were actually more severe than and *not even required* by international drug conventions.[29]

Yet another reason is that, while pain scientists are gaining a sophisticated understanding of what happens to the body in chronic pain, doctors on the front lines, both in the United States and around the world, know almost nothing about chronic pain because medical schools barely teach it. In 2011, researchers from Johns Hopkins University reported on their survey of 117 medical schools in the United States and Canada.[30] During four years of medical school, they found, American medical students receive a median of only 9 hours of pain education, Canadian students, 14. Other studies show that even veterinary students receive more—on average, 87 hours.[31]

It is the same in other developed countries. In 2011, British researchers from King's College in London reported on their survey of 19 professional schools of dentistry, medicine, midwifery, nursing, occupational therapy, pharmacy, physiotherapy, and veterinary science.[32] They found that, on average, students received 12 hours of pain education, with physical therapists and veterinary students obtaining the most.

And in less developed nations? Training in pain management is often nonexistent. In a dozen countries surveyed in Africa and the Middle East, nearly half offered no training in pain management to postgraduate medical students.[33]

Even in the United States, an estimated 40 to 70 percent of people with chronic pain are not receiving proper medical treatment.[34] Few doctors offer an individualized, integrated approach that could include acupuncture, massage, physical therapy, exercise, psychotherapy, and other treatments, even marijuana, whose potential for pain reduction is increasingly recognized.

In short, the global pain crisis amounts to nothing less than "torture by omission." In this book, I offer ways out of this crisis. There is no need in the twenty-first century for millions of people around the world to live—and die—in pain.

Judy Foreman
Cambridge, MA
October 2016

1

WHAT IS CHRONIC PAIN?

What is pain?

The official definition of pain is "an unpleasant sensory and emotional experience associated with actual or potential tissue damage, or described in terms of such damage." This comes from the International Association for the Study of Pain, the world's top pain research group comprised of about 7,000 scientists in more than 130 countries. The organization adds—and this is crucial—that "the inability to communicate verbally does not negate the possibility that an individual is experiencing pain and is in need of appropriate pain-relieving treatment."[1] In people with chronic pain, nerve cells can keep on sending pain signals to the brain even in the absence of injury.[2]

What is chronic pain?

Chronic pain is usually defined as pain lasting more than three to six months; it is not just acute pain that does not go away but can be a transformation of the nervous system itself. When this happens, chronic pain is not just a symptom of something else but a disease of the nervous system in its own right.

Are there different kinds of pain?

Yes. Pain comes in four basic "flavors"—nociceptive, inflammatory, dysfunctional, and neuropathic. Sometimes, chronic pain can involve several types. Cancer pain, for instance, is often a combination of nociceptive, inflammatory, and/or neuropathic pain.

What is nociceptive pain?

Nociceptive pain is that instant, intense reaction you get when you hit your thumb hard with a hammer. The word "nociception" means the perception of a noxious, or unpleasant, stimulus. Nociceptive pain is relatively simple—essentially an on/off switch. To trigger nociceptive pain, it takes a pretty big (i.e., high intensity) wallop. If you just touch your hand lightly with a hammer, you won't feel pain.

The usual stimuli for nociceptive pain are mechanical forces, like the hammer, too much heat or cold, and chemicals, including acids.[3,4] Less obviously, nociceptive pain also happens when some part of the body is subject to unusual mechanical force, like the grinding of bone on bone in osteoarthritis or injury to an organ like the heart when it is deprived of oxygen. Nociceptive pain is basically "good," or adaptive, because it serves a biological purpose, alerting people to danger.

What is inflammatory pain?

Inflammatory pain is different. Both big wallops and smaller ones can trigger inflammatory pain; once that sore thumb swells up and gets red, even the slightest touch can hurt. Inflammatory pain persists as long as the tissue remains damaged and swollen. Inflammatory pain can be "bad," or nonadaptive, because body-made chemicals called proinflammatory cytokines amplify, or rev up, the transmission of pain signals along nerves, sometimes to the point where people end up with more pain than they started with.[5]

What is dysfunctional pain?

The third type of pain, dysfunctional pain, is really nasty and, as its name implies, is totally maladaptive. In dysfunctional pain conditions like fibromyalgia, irritable bowel syndrome, and some types of headache, pain can be triggered without any obvious external pain stimulus at all. With dysfunctional pain, there is no damage to the nervous system and no inflammation. As with inflammatory pain, though, there *is* sensory amplification, or revving up, of pain signals in both the peripheral and central nervous systems.[6]

What is neuropathic pain?

Worst of all, in many ways, is the fourth type of pain, neuropathic pain.[7,8] Neuropathic pain is caused by damage to the nervous system itself—an alteration in the way nerves function that results in an insult to the very system that is supposed to deal with pain. While nociceptive pain, that simple kind, is all over when it's over, neuropathic pain goes on and on—long after the initial trigger, if there was an obvious one, is history.

Like dysfunctional pain, neuropathic pain is amplified and revved up in both the peripheral and the central nervous system. It can occur in conjunction with many diseases and different types of damage to the nervous system, including trauma to nerves (as in surgery), pressure on nerves (as from a herniated disc in the neck or back), injury from toxic chemicals landing on nerves (as in chemotherapy), neurotropic viruses like herpes zoster, and so on.

A dramatic demonstration of the differences between neuropathic and inflammatory pain was reported in late spring 2012 by University of California, San Francisco pain researchers Allan Basbaum and Joao Braz.[9] Their team transplanted fetal cells that make a chemical pain-inhibitor called GABA into mice with neuropathic pain. The cells dampened neuropathic pain but did not affect inflammatory pain.

How does the nervous system work?

Researchers and physicians use a lot of jargon when they talk about the nervous system, but the concepts are fairly simple.

The central nervous system consists of the brain and spinal cord and is chock-full of nerve cells. Interestingly, scientists have recently discovered that other cells called microglial cells—which are part of the immune system—also live amidst the nerve cells and contribute significantly to the processing of pain signals.

Basically, electrical signals travel along sensory nerves from the periphery—our limbs—to a structure in the spinal cord called the dorsal horn. There, the nerves release chemicals that communicate with a second nerve cell that runs all the way to the brain, where a third nerve cell takes the stimulatory message to various regions of the brain where we feel what we interpret as pain.

The most impressive thing about nerve cells is their sheer number. In the adult human brain alone, there are an estimated 100 billion neurons with perhaps 100 trillion connections.[10] And then there's the peripheral nervous system—all the nerves *outside* the brain and spinal cord.

The peripheral nervous system is divided into the *somatic* nervous system, the nerves just under the skin, and the *autonomic* nervous system, the nerves everywhere else. The autonomic nervous system is further subdivided into the *sympathetic* and *parasympathetic*. The sympathetic system is in charge of the famous fight-or-flight response, the body's instantaneous reaction to stress via the hormone adrenaline. Well-known signs of the sympathetic response are increased heart rate and blood pressure, constricted blood vessels, and sweating. The parasympathetic system is the quieter partner, dominating things while the body is at rest. Normally, the two systems act in concert to produce homeostasis.

What is the purpose of the nervous system?

The raison d'être of the entire nervous system, of course, is to convey information from the outside world to the brain or from one part of the body to the brain, all of which is accomplished by translating a huge variety of incoming information into bite-sized electrical and chemical signals. Nerve cells, also called neurons, are electrically excitable and come in three basic types: sensory neurons, which respond to light, touch, sound, chemicals, and other stimuli and are the most important nerve cells for pain; motor neurons, which act on signals from the brain and spinal cord to make muscles contract; and interneurons, neurons in the central nervous system that "talk" only to other nearby neurons. Scientists also use the word "nociceptor," which refers to a subcategory of sensory nerves that respond to the noxious, tissue-damaging stimuli that cause pain.

What are the component parts of a nerve cell?

Each nerve cell consists of a cell body, where the nucleus of the cell resides, one axon, and a bunch of filaments called dendrites that look like the messy split ends of a strand of hair and function as receiving centers for incoming information.

Axons are incredibly long filaments that can extend a meter or more. When bundled together into fibers and further bundled into cables, they're called "nerves." The sciatic nerve, the longest nerve in the body (and famous for the leg pain it causes), has one long axon that runs from the base of the spine down to the foot.

Interestingly, nerve fibers carry information at different speeds. The so-called A-delta fibers, which are relatively large in diameter and are covered with myelin, convey information very fast and are major players in pain transmission. C-fibers, which are skinnier, conduct pain information 15 times more slowly because they are not coated with myelin. A-beta fibers, which carry information from the skin about touch and pressure but not pain, are the biggest and fastest fibers.

What is small fiber neuropathy?

Small fiber neuropathy involves damage to peripheral nerves, specifically small, myelinated A fibers and unmyelinated C fibers. A number of diseases can lead to small fiber neuropathy, including diabetes, thyroid dysfunction, and some chemotherapy drugs, though often the original cause is never found.[11] Small fiber neuropathies can lead to profound pain and autonomic dysfunction.[12] Some cases of small fiber neuropathy are linked to genetic mutations that make nerves hyper-excitable.[13,14]

How specialized are nerves for processing pain signals?

Nerves are amazingly specialized for receiving different types of information—from mechanical, chemical, thermal, or other stimuli.[15,16]

In fact, the specialization of these nerves is so fine-tuned that there are different thermal receptors that have evolved to respond to fairly small differences in temperature. For instance, a receptor called TRPV1 on the tip of certain nerves is programmed to detect heat at more than 109 degrees Fahrenheit. A closely related receptor, TRPV2, detects hotter temperatures—above 126 degrees Fahrenheit. Yet a different receptor, TRPA1, detects cold temperatures—less than 63 degrees Fahrenheit.[17]

What happens after an incoming stimulus hits a nerve cell receptor?

Once the incoming sensory information is collected by the receptors, the next task of the nervous system is to transport it to the brain, a problem for which evolution has come up with a remarkably elegant solution: pass information *along* a nerve cell electrically and *between* one nerve and the next chemically.[18]

Incoming information enters the system through dendrites (those "split ends") and exits at the other end of the nerve cell through an axon. When information reaches the far end of the axon, the axon releases chemical messengers that float into a narrow gap called a synapse. In the synapse, waiting dendrites from the *next* nerve cell in the chain pick up the chemical signal, convert it to an electrical message that travels through the second nerve to *its* axon, which in turn pumps out *its* chemical messengers into the synapse for the dendrites from the third nerve in the chain to pick up, and so on. Electrically, the passage of information works through impulses called "action potentials" that act like on/off switches, giving a nerve a simple message: to fire or not. It is an all-or-nothing, yes/no, binary system.

Like other cells, nerve cells are encased in an insulating membrane. It is in this fatty membrane that the receptors, also known as ion channels, lie. Some ion channels are "voltage-gated," which means they are activated by electrically charged ions that flow back and forth across the membrane in and out of the cell. Others are chemically gated, which means they are activated by chemicals—neurotransmitters—floating around outside the cell. In its normal, resting state, the interior of the nerve cell has a negative charge compared to the outside. It's a big difference. There are 10 times more sodium ions outside the cell than inside. (With other charged particles, such as potassium, it's the other way around—the concentration of potassium ions is 20 times higher inside the cell than outside.)

When the nerve receives a signal—say, mechanical pressure on one's thumb or an acid on an acid-sensitive dendrite—sodium from the outside rushes into the cell through sodium channels. (There are now nine known genes that code for sodium channels.[19]) The sudden influx of sodium "depolarizes," or reverses, the electrical charge. Now the outside of the cell has the negative charge and the inside the positive. The cell "thinks" of this as an unnatural state and immediately seeks to correct it by having potassium ions rush outside. Once this happens, the electrical balance returns to normal.

Sodium channels, in other words, act as molecular amplifiers, turning small electrical signals into action potentials that can conduct for long distances along an axon.[20] The short-lived change in the electrical charge—just milliseconds long—is passed step by step from one little section of the axon to the next. In many axons, these sections are covered with myelin, but there are tiny gaps (called nodes) between the sections, and it's actually in these gaps that the sodium channels lie. So when sodium rushes in through these channels, the change in electrical charge literally "jumps" across the gap with enough electrical energy to depolarize the next section of the axon, then the next and the next, all along the axon. In technical jargon, this is called a "wave of depolarization." (In nerve cells that don't have a myelin sheath, there's no gap for energy to jump across, so transmission of the signal is slower.)

When the wave of depolarization reaches the end of the axon, the mode of information transfer changes from electrical to chemical, with the release of a chemical—a neurotransmitter—that lands on receptors in the dendrites on the other side of the synapse to keep the signal going, nerve after nerve. But the chemical—neurotransmitter—signals can carry different messages. If the neurotransmitter is "excitatory," as happens with the chemical glutamate, the result is an increase in nerve activity and, ultimately, continued transmission of the pain signal. On the other hand, if the neurotransmitter is inhibitory, or calming, like the neurotransmitter GABA, the result is a damp-ening of pain.

Granted, this is pretty esoteric stuff, but it matters. Think of this—with gratitude—the next time you go to the dentist. It's only because scientists have unraveled these basic mech-anisms that they were able to come up with excellent local anesthetics such as lidocaine that work by blocking sodium channels. With sodium channels blocked, the wave of depo-larization never happens and pain signals—from a dentist's drill—never get going. (Researchers are working on new ways to block sodium channels, including with a paralytic shellfish toxin that is showing promise in an early human trial.[21])

How are pain signals transmitted to the brain?

For pain actually to be "felt," pain signals must travel upward from the dorsal horn in the spinal cord to the brain, specifically to the brainstem and also to the thalamus (the so-called "spi-nothalamic tract") and finally to the rest of the brain, where perception of the pain finally occurs.

As pain signals pass through the spinal cord, cells in the dorsal horn act like a "gate," either sending the signal straight on up or modifying it.

Once pain signals reach the brainstem, the brainstem begins sending electrochemical signals downward (so-called "descending modulation") to try to block incoming pain signals.[22] In fact, some of the drugs that help control pain—anticonvulsants, opioids, and antidepressants—work in part by enhancing this descending modulation.

But even as the brainstem "tries" to dampen pain, some pain signals manage to keep going upward, eventually reach-ing the thalamus.[23] Here, they are passed on to three main areas of the brain: the somatosensory cortex in the parietal lobe, which tries to figure out where in the body the pain is coming from; the limbic system, which adds emotional impor-tance to the pain; and the frontal cortex, the part of the brain behind the forehead that governs thinking and gives meaning to the pain. And meaning really counts. For instance, severely injured soldiers, brimming with feelings of heroism and nobility, have long been known to report significantly less pain than similarly injured civilians, whose pain has no lofty meaning.[24] Similarly, childbirth hurts like hell—but we see it as beautiful, at least afterward, because we get a lovely new baby for our efforts.

Why does the brain feel "phantom" pain from a missing limb?

The somatosensory cortex—and a fascinating little site inside it called the "homunculus" (Latin for "little man")—have been the site of some of the most profound discoveries in science.[25]

In the 1940s, pioneering neurosurgeon Wilder Penfield operated on epileptic patients who were awake and could talk. (The brain itself does not have receptors to detect noxious stimuli, so an acute injury to the brain is not painful.[26]) He applied mild electrical currents to different areas on the surface of the brain and asked patients where in their bodies they felt a tingling or movement. From this information, he was able to create a map that showed where sensations from different parts of the body are processed in the somatosensory cortex.[27,28]

The homunculus is a grotesque-looking but kind of adorable little thing, essentially a very distorted map of the body. The first thing we notice about this map is that a hugely disproportionate amount of brain tissue is devoted to sensations coming from the mouth, tongue, lips, face, and hands. Obviously, this suggests that information coming from these areas is extremely important for survival.

Like other parts of the nervous system, the homunculus is also quite plastic, or changeable. For instance, the homunculus hand of a concert pianist would look quite different from that of a newborn baby. The homunculus plays a key role in the mysterious problem of phantom limb pain. Many, though not all, people who by accident or surgery wind up with an amputated arm, leg, breast, or other body part often feel pain in the missing body part, and sometimes it's excruciating. Someone with a missing arm, for instance, may feel as though the fist on that limb is tightly clenched, with the fingernails digging painfully into the palm.

Interestingly, in the homunculus, the area that maps sensations coming in from the face is located very close to the area for incoming information from the hands, as University of California researchers have dramatically demonstrated with a person whose left arm was lost in a car crash. As an experiment, they touched the patient's cheek with a Q-tip, then asked him what he felt. The man said he felt his cheek being touched—but his phantom thumb as well. Perhaps, the researchers speculated, the somatosensory cortex "noticed" that it was not getting any more information from the left arm (because it was missing), and somehow the space in the homunculus that *had been* allocated to the arm was taken over by nerves from the face.[29]

They then found a way to help some people with phantom limb pain. Using a box with two armholes cut in the side and a mirror placed inside, they asked the patient to place his good arm and his stump through the holes then look inside. What the person "saw," because of the mirror, was the illusion that he had both arms. The researchers then asked the person to clench and unclench his good fist. Because of the mirror, the person actually "saw" both fists clenching and unclenching. By unclenching the "good" fist, it felt to him as if both fists opened, which, over time, relieved the pain in the phantom limb.

How does the body turn acute pain into chronic pain?

In a sizeable percentage of people, a series of unhappy events conspires to turn acute pain into chronic pain, which is not just acute pain that doesn't go away but the result of fundamental changes in the nervous system itself. When pain becomes chronic, it quite literally changes the brain, in some cases causing a loss of gray matter equivalent to 20 years of aging, as Northwestern University neuroscientist Vania Apkarian showed dramatically with brain scans in 2004.[30,31]

How does this change happen?

The transformation of pain involves "neural plasticity," or the changeability of the nervous system, and "sensitization," which means nerve cells become more and more responsive to weaker and weaker pain signals, as if, like good students, they "learned" to get better and better at transmitting pain.

This results in a kind of runaway hyper-arousal of the nervous system that is also called "wind-up." In fact, the properties of nerve cells can be altered so much that the pain is no longer coupled to the presence, intensity, or duration of noxious stimuli.[32] It is now physically transformed from short-term, acute pain into a long-term, *self-perpetuating* phenomenon.[33,34,35,36,37] This "learned" hypersensitivity occurs in both peripheral and central nerves.

Nerves that used to be responsive only to nasty—noxious—stimuli "learn" to react to benign substances as if they were noxious, too. Nerves also become hyper-responsive to the original noxious stimulus. It's almost as if the system becomes addicted to all the excitement, craving more and more stimulation. Scientists call this ugly new state of affairs "allodynia." The system is so over-revved that the brain now responds to the most benign of stimuli—like a feather stroking the skin—as if it were a burning blowtorch. Mere touch now triggers excruciating pain.[38]

Consider what happens in inflammatory pain. In inflammation, immune cells begin secreting chemicals called cytokines, among them tumor necrosis factor-alpha (TNFα), interleukin 1B, specific pain messengers like bradykinin and prostaglandin E2, and even the normally benign nerve growth factor. Together, these chemical messengers act on the tips of nerve cells in the periphery, making them increasingly sensitive to pain signals. Inflammatory diseases such as rheumatoid arthritis are prime examples of the cycle of misery caused by this revved-up process.

But sensitization doesn't just occur in the periphery; it happens in the central nervous system too, starting in the first signal relay station in the spinal cord, the dorsal horn. That's the place where axons from peripheral nerves spurt out their chemical signals to waiting dendrites of nerve cells across the synapse, spurring the transmission of pain signals up to the brain.

A key player in this process is the excitatory neurotransmitter glutamate. When glutamate is released by the axon of a C-fiber, it floats across the synapse and lands on several different types of receptors, mostly important, receptors called NMDA. When triggered by glutamate, ion channels—in this case, for calcium—open up in the receiving cell. This triggers a cascade of chemical steps inside the cell, the net result of which is the cell puts even more NMDA receptors on its surface. This, of course, makes the cell extra sensitive to pain, allowing even more pain signals to get through.

Researchers from the University of Texas have recently shown that an important chemical messenger in the brain, dopamine, may also be involved in the transformation of acute to chronic pain. In mice, the researchers used a toxin to destroy a clump of neurons called A11 that contain dopamine. Afterward, acute pain signals were still normal, but chronic pain was gone.[39]

Once this hypersensitivity process is started in the central nervous system, it takes less and less stimulation from peripheral nerves to keep it going.

This has huge potential implications. To keep central sensitization to a minimum, it helps to "keep ahead of the pain." In one study, for instance, when doctors gave prostate surgery patients spinal injections of painkillers *before* surgery, the patients had less pain afterward than those treated conventionally.[40]

But it's not just that the nervous system learns to react to a benign stimulus as if it were a blast from a blowtorch.

In some kinds of pain, particularly neuropathic pain, once a nerve is injured and gets revved up, the firing of electrical impulses can keep going *without any trigger* at all from the periphery.

It's as if the nerves get on a roll, turned on by having been turned on before, eventually becoming free of the need for a triggering event. Worse yet, it's not just the nerves that once *were* triggered that gallop away with all these spontaneous signals. Nearby nerve cells get caught up in the process as well, just like the flu spreading from person to person. At the most basic, neurological level, pain becomes contagious, spreading from one nerve to the next. Adding significantly to the changeover from acute to chronic pain is the fact that nerves that are injured can actually change the activity of their genes, in many cases, *increasing* the activity of genes that pump out substance P, BDNF, and other pain-producing molecules.

And even all this, unfortunately, is only half the story—immune cells called glial cells that live inside the nervous system also get into the act.

What are glial cells?

Years ago, early neuroanatomists dubbed these cells "glia," Greek and Latin for glue.[41] Shocking as it may seem, glial cells outnumber nerve cells in the central nervous system by 10 to 1. Glial cells come in three basic types—astrocytes, oligodendro-cytes, and microglia.

Astrocytes, which look a bit like stars, carry nutrients and waste to and from blood vessels and mediate communication among neurons.[42] Although they come from nerve cell progenitors, they act like immune cells, pumping out proinflammatory substances called cytokines. (Researchers first began to suspect that glial cells were involved with pain more than 20 years ago when they administered a poison to animals in whom pain had been induced. The poison was designed to selectively kill astrocytes. With their astrocytes knocked out, the animals exhibited far less chronic pain.[43])

Oligodendrocytes also come from nerve cell progenitors; their job is to coat axons with myelin, that protective, fatty insulation that increases the speed at which pain signals travel along neurons.

The third type of glial cells, and the most important for pain, is the microglia, which come from—and are—genuine immune cells. They fight infection and help repair damaged cells and are crucial to brain functioning.[44]

How do glial cells increase pain?

Like many things in biology, glial cells have a Jekyll and Hyde personality—a good side and a dark side. Normally, glial cells are benign and quiescent. But if they become activated by pain signals from nerves, they send out chemical signals that end up *increasing* pain.[45,46]

When a pain signal lands on a glial cell receptor called TLR-4, the glial cell swings into action, pumping out a swarm of chemicals, most important the cytokines interleukin 1 (IL-1), interleukin 6 (IL-6), and TNF. These cytokines are "good" in the sense that they boost the body's immune response during infections, but they are "bad" because they also act as "neuro-excitatory" molecules, which rev up nerve cells. Nerve cells wind up firing faster and faster, generating ever more pain signals headed for the brain. What started out as short-term, acute pain turns into long-term, chronic pain.[47]

The good news is that more than 200 animal studies have shown that *preventing* this glial activation can reduce pain.[48,49] In people, too, researchers have shown that blocking TLR-4 (with a drug called naloxone) and stopping microglial cells from pumping out cytokines can reduce pain.[50,51,52] Using a new brain scanning technology, neuroscientists have recently produced dramatic images of glial cell activation in chronic pain patients.[53]

How can brain scans help assess pain?

Brain scanning technology is a major step forward, not just because it adds significantly to our understanding of how chronic pain affects different parts of the brain but because it makes real, explicit, and *visible* a phenomenon that, until now, has been totally subjective.[54]

In the fall of 2011, Stanford University researchers showed that they could use functional magnetic resonance imaging (fMRI) scans to detect specific patterns of brain activity and, in essence, to tentatively diagnose pain.[55]

In the study, the researchers took volunteers, put them in the brain scanner, then applied heat to their forearms, producing moderate pain.[56] Brain patterns with and without pain were then recorded and analyzed to create a computerized model of what thermal pain looks like in the brain. The computer was then asked to look at the brain scans of other volunteers to see if it could detect when they had thermal pain. The computer got it right 81 percent of the time. In 2012, the Stanford team used a different kind of MRI scan to detect a distinctive pattern of brain activity linked to chronic back pain.

At the University of Colorado, neuroscientists have also found that fMRI scans show a clear "neurologic signature," further evidence of how pain is registered in the brain.[57] Indeed, brain scans have documented specific areas of damage with different types of pain.[58,59,60]

These fMRI scans are not quite ready to be used to diagnose—and confirm a patient's report of—pain.[61] But it is a major first step—with enormous legal, as well as clinical, implications.[62] (Hundreds of thousands of legal cases every year depend on "proving" the existence of pain.[63])

Just as important, brain scans are making it abundantly clear that chronic pain literally ages the brain. About a decade ago, neuroscientists at Northwestern University showed that people with chronic back pain have 5 to 11 percent less gray matter in their brains than healthy people.[64] Normally, it would take 20 years of aging to lose this much brain volume.

Moreover, the researchers showed that the decrease in tissue in the prefrontal cortex and thalamus was linked to how long a person had been in chronic pain. Researchers have since found similar losses of brain tissue in people with fibromyalgia, irritable bowel syndrome, tension headaches, the facial pain of trigeminal neuralgia, and other chronic pain problems.[65,66,67,68] Even phantom pain and spinal cord injury can trigger losses of gray matter.[69,70]

Somewhat to scientists' surprise, brain scans are also showing that if the underlying pain problem is resolved, some brain volume loss may be restored. German researchers, for instance, studied people with osteoarthritis who were scheduled for total hip replacement surgery. Before the surgery, the researchers used brain scans to document decreases in gray matter in several parts of the brain. After the surgery, which eliminated the hip pain, the researchers did more scans and found good news—an *increase* in gray matter in previously affected brain areas.[71] In England, researchers at Oxford did a similar study and came to similar conclusions.[72] In Canada, too, McGill University researchers have shown that effective treatment of low back pain restores normal brain function.[73]

Functional MRIs are also beginning to document precisely where in the brain opioid drugs like morphine—and drugs like naloxone that block morphine—work, according to Harvard Medical School researchers.[74] Just as one would expect, when the researchers map the actions of morphine and naloxone, the two drugs show opposite brain activation patterns. This suggests that brain scanning will increasingly be useful not just to document chronic pain but to test which drugs might be most effective in which people with pain.[75,76,77]

Brain scans may also be used to predict which patients would still have pain a year later and which will be pain-free.[78,79,80] In one Northwestern University study, half of the patients with acute back pain had chronic pain a year later and half did not. The researchers were able to predict which patients would have chronic pain by analyzing activity in two brain areas—the medial prefrontal cortex and the nucleus accumbens. Interestingly, brain activity shifts from areas associated with classical pain to areas involved with emotion.[81]

Recently, researchers at Massachusetts General Hospital in Boston used a new brain scanning technology to document activation of glial cells in people with chronic back pain.[82,83]

Can pain be assessed without brain scans?

Yes, but it's tricky.

Because pain is such a subjective phenomenon, and because reliable diagnostic tests such as fMRIs are still in their infancy, other methods are still used to assess pain.

These include looking at the faces of people in pain; asking people to rate their pain on numerical, linear, or pictorial scales; asking them to keep track of their pain on iPads or other personal digital devices; or, as doctors have done for generations, simply asking people to describe their pain verbally. More recently, doctors have been combining a few well-chosen questions with a very specific physical exam that takes less than 15 minutes.

The attempt to capture pain in some sort of orderly fashion began decades ago with what's now known as the McGill Pain Questionnaire.[84] The questionnaire divides pain into different types by the words people use to describe it. For instance, to determine the temporal qualities of pain, the questionnaire asks people to pick one of the following words: "flickering," "quivering," "pulsing," "throbbing," "beating," or "pounding." To discover the spatial aspects of pain, the questionnaire asks people to say if their pain is "jumping," "flashing," or "shooting." The questionnaire also asks whether the pain feels like "pricking" or "stabbing." It asks about thermal features of the pain, from "hot" to "searing"; about the "dullness" of pain, from "dull" to "heavy"; and about the overall pain, from "annoying" to "unbearable."

Although some pain clinics still use the McGill Questionnaire, many now use other methods. For young children, many doctors use the "faces" scale in which the child picks the one picture out of six that most closely matches his or her pain. These scales show a range of faces from a happy face showing no pain to a scrunched-up face grimacing in agony. Partly because the faces scales have so few gradations, they're not very reliable scientifically.[85]

A bit better is the simple zero (no pain) to 10 (the worst pain imaginable) numerical scale, and even better is a numerical scale with finer gradations, from zero to 100. Somewhat better than these linear scales are scales, such as the visual analog scale, that use ratios that measure more subtle factors such as the amount of improvement that a certain drug or treatment provides.[86]

Even more important than just giving pain a number is to gauge how it is affecting a person's ability to function and participate in the activities of daily life.[87] Online pain tracking programs use what psychologists call "ecological momentary assessment." A handheld device beeps at random times during the day, prompting people to plug in their current pain rating, functioning, and mood. This is more reliable than asking people to remember—at the end of the day or in a doctor's office a month later—what the pain has been like. Indeed, research shows that when patients show these factual "e-diaries" to their doctors, doctors are more likely to change medications to improve pain control.[88,89]

There's also another way for doctors to determine the "phenotype" of a person's pain—by combining a short physical exam with the patient's verbal descriptions. The approach, called StEP (Standardized Evaluation of Pain), involves just six questions and 10 physical tests, takes only 15 minutes, and can determine, for instance, whether a person's back pain is neuropathic (i.e., caused by damage to the nervous system itself) or not.[90]

In one study of 137 people in pain, STeP was able to distinguish "axial" back pain (nonspecific pain that does not travel to the buttocks, legs, or feet) from "radicular" back pain (also known as sciatica), which is neuropathic pain caused by inflammation of the nerve root, bulging discs, or bone spurs. This difference matters. If the pain is axial, the best treatment may be plain old nonsteroidal anti-inflammatory drugs). But if it's radicular, the best choices may be gabapentin (Neurontin) or duloxetine (Cymbalta).

What about just looking at a person's face to assess pain?

Facial cues do convey pain, but there's debate over how well observers can decipher these signals, in part because it is possible to fake pain expression.[91]

It turns out that health-care professionals—the very people we would hope would be most attuned to facial pain cues—routinely *underestimate* their patients' pain. And if the doctor in question has reason to suspect—as doctors are trained to do—that the person is just seeking drugs, the tendency to misread and underestimate facial cues becomes even worse.[92,93,94,95] Indeed, study after study shows that health-care professionals minimize patients' pain far more than non-health-care professionals looking at the same patient.[96]

In one demonstration, researchers took videotapes of people with shoulder pain being asked to move their shoulders in a painful way. The videotapes were then shown to 120 health-care professionals, who were divided into three different groups and told to rate the patients' pain.[97] One group saw only the videotaped faces. The second group saw the videotaped faces and was also given the patients' numerical pain ratings. The third group was given the same information as the second group but was also told that the patients were faking their expressions of pain to seek narcotics.

All the health-care professionals underestimated the patients' pain. But those who also received the patients' own pain ratings gave estimates closer to the patients' own ratings. Those who were told the patients might be cheating underestimated pain just as badly as the group that saw only the faces.

But there *is* a way to tell if a person is faking facial cues, because these cues, after all, are subject to both voluntary and involuntary muscle movements. When a person is faking, he or she often times the winces and grimaces incorrectly. The muscle movements during faked pain are out of sync and typically exaggerated, almost like a caricature of pain expression.[98]

Interestingly, computers do a much better job of detecting fakers than people. In experiments at several universities, researchers asked 205 people to assess the authenticity of people's painful expressions—some of the "patients" were not in pain and some were undergoing painful stimulation in the lab. The human observers were poor at telling the difference. Computers were right 85 percent of the time, in part because they could detect changes that were too small or happened too quickly for the human eye to see.[99] One clue that the computers caught but people did not? People who are faking pain open their mouths too regularly and with less variation.

How do genes affect susceptibility to chronic pain?

We might be tempted to think—as many scientists did until recently—that it's pretty much of a crapshoot which people in acute pain would wind up in intense, even chronic pain and which would sail through. As Norwegian researchers have observed, "Among people with the same condition, pain ratings typically cover the entire scale from 'no pain' to 'the worst pain imaginable.'"[100]

The question is: Why? Why do only 1 in 10 people over 50 who contract shingles—the painful problem caused by the chickenpox virus—go on to develop another pain syndrome called post-herpetic neuralgia?[101,102,103] Why doesn't everyone get it? Millions of people have diabetes too, but only 60 to 70 percent develop a kind of nerve damage called neuropathy (usually tingling or numbness), and only 13 percent of these go on to develop persistent painful neuropathy.[104] Why don't they all wind up with this debilitating pain?

It's possible, of course, to explain some individual differences in the experience of chronic pain as psychological. But scientists know that genes—those 22,000 regions in our DNA that we all inherit from our parents—are especially crucial.[105]

Scientists now think that genes control 40 percent of susceptibility to chronic pain.[106] This is not just intellectually interesting; it means that knowing which genes predispose someone to chronic pain can in theory enable scientists to target drugs to enhance or suppress specific genes.

A small number of people, for instance, are born with a genetic mutation that runs in families and makes them feel severe pain much of the time, even driving some to suicide. The condition is called erythromelalgia, or "burning man" syndrome. On the other hand, a small number of people are born with a different mutation in the same gene that makes them unable to feel pain at all, a problem called "congenital pain insensitivity."[107] In both conditions, the mutations occur in a gene called *SCN9A*. (A gene mutation is a permanent change in the DNA sequence of a gene.)

In its normal, healthy form, the *SCN9A* gene helps the body make sodium channels. (This sodium channel is called Nav1.7—it's basically a little opening in nerve cells through which sodium ions flow in and out.)

The job of sodium channels is to transmit messages along a nerve. When a nerve cell receives a signal such as contact with a nasty acid, that signal is converted into an "action potential" that, like an electric current flowing through a copper wire, travels along the long axons of nerve cells. The end result is the firing of the nerve, which causes the pain signal to be passed along through the spinal cord to the brain. In congenital pain insensitivity, the sodium channels do not conduct sodium ions properly and so do not pass on pain signals. This is called a "loss-of-function" mutation.[108]

In the opposite problem, the constant pain comes from a "gain-of-function" mutation in the *SCN9A* gene, which means that instead of not working at all, the sodium channels work overtime, ramping up pain signals day and night.[109,110,111] More than a dozen families around the world are now known to have this "gain-of-function" mutation.[112]

Researchers are now working on drugs to control overactive sodium channels, including the common anesthetic drug lidocaine (plus its oral form, mexilitine) and carbamazepine.[113,114] The downside is that, so far, most existing sodium-channel blockers are nonspecific; that is, they block many sodium channels—not just those that cause pain but also "good" ones in our muscles, heart, and brain as well, which can have lethal results.[115,116,117,118,119]

How heritable is susceptibility to chronic pain?

In 1999, McGill University researchers picked 11 common laboratory mouse strains and ran all the mice through 12 common pain tests. They found that susceptibility to pain is quite heritable and ranges from 30 to 76 percent.[120,121] That spurred other researchers to study humans, especially identical twins who have the same genes but often manifest diseases—including chronic pain—differently because of different environmental exposures and experiences.

For instance, British researchers looked at 1,064 women, including 181 identical twin pairs and 351 fraternal twin pairs, and concluded that low back and neck pain were significantly heritable. For low back pain, there was a 52 to 68 percent chance that if one identical twin had the problem, the other did too. For neck pain, the figure was 35 to 58 percent.[122] Another British team looked at twins to study experimental, as opposed to clinical, pain.[123] They recruited 51 pairs of identical twins, as well as 47 pairs of fraternal twins, all of them women. They brought the women into the lab and put them through many of the same tests that the McGill researchers had used in mice. Just as in the mouse studies, the British researchers found sensitivity to pain was 22 to 55 percent heritable.

Norwegian researchers, too, have studied pain sensitivity in 53 pairs of identical twins and 39 pairs of fraternal twins, both male and female. In their research, they added an extra test—sensitivity to an extreme cold stimulus.[124] Intriguingly, the cold and heat pain stimuli produced different effects. With cold, there was a 60 percent chance that one twin would have the same response as the other; with heat, there was only a 26 percent chance. (Puzzling, isn't it? And a reminder of how careful researchers—and drug makers—need to be in the pain tests they choose to study.)

The Danes and Finns have also found significant heritability in pain susceptibility. A huge Danish study of 15,328 male and female twins found that inherited susceptibility explained 38 percent of lumbar (lower back) pain, 32 percent of thoracic (mid-back) pain, and 39 percent of neck pain.[125] A Finnish twin study of 10,608 twins found that susceptibility to fibromyalgia was 51 percent inherited.[126] Other studies have documented a strong hereditary link for migraines, menstrual cramps, back pain in general, and sciatica specifically, as well as osteoarthritis.[127] With osteoarthritis, twin studies have shown that heredity probably accounts for 39 to 65 percent of knee problems and 60 percent of hip problems—at least in women.[128]

In fact, a recent British study from King's College in London involving 8,564 twins found that common genetic risks appear to underlie several disparate pain conditions—chronic widespread pain, chronic pelvic pain, irritable bowel syndrome, and dry eye.[129,130] Curiously, in this research, migraine headaches did not appear to be part of this common genetic predisposition.

How do scientists look for pain genes?

In addition to the *SCN9A* gene, researchers are now deciphering dozens more pain susceptibility genes. Ultimately, the idea is to put together a "panel" of pain genes that could provide a genetic risk profile for each person. This way, for instance, doctors could identify *before surgery* which people would be likely to have intense pain afterward or to have acute post-surgical pain turn into chronic pain. Those people could have their pain treated more aggressively.

There are various ways to determine which genes contribute to pain susceptibility. One way is to "think backward." Once it's known which particular neurological mechanism transmits pain—such as a nerve receptor for heat or acid—scientists can look for the gene that makes that receptor. Another way to hunt for pain susceptibility and sensitivity genes is through "linkage analysis." Scientists take two or more strains of mice and run them through various tests of experimental pain. Some strains of mice turn out to be more sensitive to certain types of pain than others, while some strains are strikingly pain resistant. Scientists then look at the DNA—the whole genome—of the different strains and see where the genes differ. The implication is that the differences in genes may account for the differences in pain sensitivity.

In humans, scientists often do something similar, called genome-wide association studies. They start with two groups of people, one with a certain disease, like chronic pain, and the other without. They then compare the genomes of both groups in hopes of finding genes that have different forms (alleles) in the sick versus the healthy people. Again, at least in theory, the different genes might be responsible for the different "phenotypes" (e.g., having or not having chronic pain).

Yet another major approach to finding pain genes is to use a "microarray" (also called the "gene chip" method), which involves RNA, not DNA. (DNA is a long, double-stranded chain of molecules called nucleotide bases that is the master blueprint for our genes; DNA makes RNA, which is a single strand of nucleotides that carries the code for all the proteins in our cells. Think of it like recipes: DNA is the recipe book, while RNA is the individual recipe that is carried away from the book or library to the "kitchen," where the action really starts.[131])

In the gene chip technique, scientists compare mice that are in pain with mice that are not. (There are multiple ways— including a mouse "grimace scale"—to tell if a mouse is in pain.[132]) The scientists then sacrifice the mice and take samples from specific tissues such as the dorsal root ganglia looking for RNA. Since different genes are active, or "turned on," in animals with pain as opposed to those not in pain, finding the RNA produced by pain nerves is a step toward identifying the pain genes themselves.

Still another way to understand pain genes is to create special strains of mice in which a possible pain gene is "knocked out" (deleted altogether) or "knocked down" (made somewhat less active). Then these mice are tested for their sensitivity to pain.

How many pain genes have been discovered?

So far, researchers have identified roughly 418 potential pain genes, with new ones being discovered every couple of weeks.[133,134] Researchers at McGill University have established a databank to keep track of newly discovered pain genes.

In addition to the sodium channel genes, scientists are exploring genes that control other ion channels, particularly those for calcium and potassium. For instance, if just one tiny speck of DNA is changed in a potassium channel gene, people who inherit this mutation are at significantly higher risk for pain, as demonstrated by genetic studies of 1,359 patients.[135] Indeed, an estimated 18 to 22 percent of the population inherits two copies of this mutation—one from each parent—and thus is at significantly higher pain risk. An additional 50 percent of people inherit one copy of the mutation and are at somewhat higher risk. People who inherit no copies of the mutation are the lucky ones—they are at lowest risk. On the flip side, geneticists have found a mutation in a calcium channel gene that seems to *protect* against pain rather than raising the risk.[136]

Numerous genes are believed to raise the risk of migraine headaches, which afflict an estimated 20 percent of adults.[137] One type of migraine, called familial hemiplegic migraine, has been linked to problems in ion channels for both calcium and potassium.[138] (A different gene variant on chromosome 8 has been linked to an even more common form of migraine.[139])

What other genes are linked to pain?

It's not just genes for ion channels that pain geneticists are chasing. One of the other important genes is called *GCH1*.[140] This gene makes an enzyme that controls production of a molecule called BH4, which scientists joke could stand for "Big Hurt."[141,142] People who have high levels of BH4 have more pain, while people with less BH4 have less pain. It is now possible to predict which people are likely to be more or less sensitive to pain by screening for only three tiny bits of DNA.[143]

Another important pain gene is *COMT*. Everyone has some form of the *COMT* gene, but some people have a highly active version while others have a form with low activity.[144,145] High activity is better because it is associated with less pain sensitivity, while low *COMT* activity means higher pain. The luckiest 40 percent of Caucasians have the high activity form and are relatively *unsusceptible* to pain. In fact, these folks are only half as likely as normal to develop certain painful conditions such as temporomandibular joint disease (TMD).

There's already good news emerging from this research. A common blood pressure drug, propranolol, which blocks norepinephrine, blocks pain too. Genetic testing for *COMT* can help identify which people are most likely to benefit from the drug.[146,147]

There's another key finding emerging from the *COMT* research. The hormone estrogen decreases *COMT* activity. Because lower *COMT* means more pain, this may partly explain—though this is controversial—why women, who have more estrogen, have more pain than men, as we'll see in the next chapter.

Other genes generating excitement are the *PAP* gene, which boosts the body's production of a pain-killing substance called adenosine, and another gene that, when deleted in mice, reduced chronic pain.[148,149]

Less exciting, unfortunately, is the research on genes that control receptors for opioids (narcotics). There are three main opioid receptors—*mu, delta,* and *kappa*—each of which is produced by separate genes. The hope, still unfulfilled, is that studying mutations in opioid receptor genes might lead to better opioid drugs, including forms of the drugs that are less likely to lead to addiction.[150] So far, the best studied is the gene that makes the mu-opioid receptor. At least three subtypes of mu receptors, and perhaps as many as 10, can be made as the gene is chopped up and spliced in different ways by the body.[151] But, so far at least, the effort to link specific variants of opioid receptor genes to differences in susceptibility to pain and responsiveness to opioid drugs has been disappointing.[152]

One particularly exciting gene research project is the $25 million OPPERA project, funded by the federal government and based at the University of North Carolina.[153,154] The first part of the project was a prospective study in which 3,200 men and women, all healthy volunteers, were tested in the lab for sensitivity to various kinds of experimental pain. They were also administered psychological tests for anxiety and depression to see how those factors may influence development of pain, and they had blood drawn and saved for genetic testing. The idea is to follow them and see who develops TMD. Ultimately, the goal is to compare people with and without TMD to see which genes confer risk.

Is all this knowledge about pain reaching doctors?

No, and that's a major problem. Except for a few thousand physicians who specialize in pain management, doctors on the front lines know very little about pain for one obvious reason: medical schools barely teach it. This is not just an American problem. In 80 percent of the world, pain biology and modern principles of pain relief and palliative care still aren't taught to medical students.[155]

In 2009, researchers from the University of Toronto reported on a survey of 10 major Canadian universities that train doctors, nurses, dentists, pharmacists, and physical or occupational therapists. The team also surveyed four veterinary schools. The research design was hardly rocket science: researchers simply asked the schools how much pain education their students were receiving. The majority of schools *didn't even know.*[156] As for the schools that could answer the question, the responses were still dismal. Across all the years of medical training, students received an average of 13 to 41 hours of pain education. Even veterinary students received more than twice that—87 hours on average.

In 2011, British researchers from King's College in London found much the same thing.[157] They surveyed 19 professional schools of dentistry, medicine, midwifery, nursing, occupational therapy, pharmacy, physiotherapy, and veterinary science. On average, students received 12 hours of pain education, with physical therapists and veterinary students obtaining the most.

Johns Hopkins University researchers reported in 2011 on a study of 117 US and Canadian medical schools. They found that "pain education for North American medical students is limited, variable, and often fragmentary."[158] Over the course of four years in US medical schools, they found, the median number of pain teaching hours was nine. Canadian medical students received about twice that.

As the 2011 Institute of Medicine report put it: "Most people in pain are cared for by primary care physicians who likely received little initial training or experience in best practices in pain management. . . . Too many physicians harbor outmoded or unscientific attitudes toward pain and people with pain."[159]

2

WHO IS HARDEST HIT
BY CHRONIC PAIN?

The short answer is women, blacks and Hispanics, children, older people, and the poor.

We'll talk about the poor as part of the discussion about the global inequality of access to morphine and other opioids, especially at the end of life. In this chapter, we focus on the higher prevalence and greater severity of chronic pain in women, the undertreatment of children's pain, and the persistent social prejudices and other factors that influence higher pain prevalence and inadequate treatment of pain in older people, blacks, and Hispanics.

What is the evidence that women have more pain than men?

Beyond the obvious sex differences that everyone recognizes, the sexes differ at an even more basic level, that is, in the "expression" (activation) of genes. In fruit flies, for instance, males and females differ in the expression of a whopping 90 percent of all their genes, meaning that sex plays a significant role in how active a particular gene is and how much of a role it plays in the animal's physiology and behavior.[1,2] This has obvious implications for the genes that influence susceptibility to pain.

Clinically, women are both more likely to *have* painful conditions that can afflict both sexes and to report *greater pain* than men with the same chronic condition.[3,4] (Women also have more *acute* pain than men after the same surgeries, such as wisdom-tooth extraction, gall bladder removal, hernia repair, and hip and knee surgery.)[5,6]

In 2008, when researchers looked at 42,249 people in 10 developed and 7 developing countries, they discovered that the prevalence of any chronic pain condition was 45 percent among women versus 31 percent among men.[7] In a 2009 review, researchers found that, around the world, women have more irritable bowel syndrome, more fibromyalgia, more headaches (especially migraines), more neuropathic pain (from damage to the nervous system itself), more osteoarthritis and more jaw problems like temporomandibular joint disorder (TMD), as well as more musculoskeletal and back pain.[8]

A type of neuropathic pain called complex regional pain syndrome seems to stalk women almost everywhere.[9,10,11,12] Fibromyalgia, too, affects mostly women, as shown by studies from Sweden, the Netherlands, the United Kingdom, Israel, and the United States.[13] With osteoarthritis, the wear-and-tear joint disease of later life, both the prevalence and the severity are greater in women.[14,15,16] Jaw pain—better known as TMD—is also far more common in women, as are other types of facial pain, according to studies in Finland, Germany, Sweden, Turkey, the United States, Nigeria, and Brazil.[17,18]

Irritable bowel syndrome, a condition that causes abdominal pain and abnormal bowel movements, is 3.2 times more common in women[19] (except, curiously enough, in India and a few other places where the ratio is inverted[20]). With headaches in general and migraines in particular, women are also much more likely to be afflicted. Over the course of a given year, for instance, the prevalence of migraine ranges from 3 to 33 percent in women but from 1 to 16 percent in men.[21]

Overall, in a study of 11,000 patients, Stanford University researchers found that women reported more pain with disorders in the musculoskeletal, circulatory, respiratory, and digestive systems, as well as more acute sinusitis and neck pain.[22]

Are there evolutionary reasons for sex differences in pain?

There might be. Females may have evolved sensory mechanisms that allow for greater acuity across sense organs in general.[23] Females are more sensitive to changes in smell, temperature, visual cues, and other stimuli that may signal danger, so the fact that they are more attuned to pain makes some sense. The advantages of a woman's ability to feel and be more sensitive to a child's pain may come with the price tag of higher sensitivity when feeling her own.[24]

If females have more pain, why is most basic research done in male rodents?

Shockingly, most—in fact, 79 percent—of basic pain research in mice and rats is still done in males, even though the old rationale that menstrual cycles make females too complicated to study is no longer seen as valid.[25] In most cases, female mice tested throughout their hormone cycles display no more variability than males do, according to the National Institutes of Health (NIH).[26]

More proof of the necessity to study both male and female animals came in July 2015, when researchers led by geneticist Jeffrey S. Mogil of McGill University reported on a study of specific cells called glial cells and pain hypersensitivity. One of the hottest research areas currently is the way microglial cells, so-called glue cells that derive from the immune system but live in the nervous system, affect transmission of pain signals from nerve cells. Mogil's team found that, contrary to expectations, microglial cells were not required for mechanical pain hypersensitivity in female mice as they were for males. The team concluded that "this sexual dimorphism suggests that male mice cannot be used as proxies for females in pain research."[27]

"Sex matters," concluded the prestigious Institute of Medicine in a 2001 report: "Sex, that is, being male or female, is an important basic human variable that should be considered when designing and analyzing studies in all areas and at all levels of biomedical and health-related research."[28]

But many researchers still don't take that to heart. While the NIH requires routine inclusion of both sexes in *human* studies, much animal research "continues to eschew females," according to University of Florida pain researcher Roger Fillingim. Given that pain is mainly a female problem, this means research that excludes females is incomplete at best and invalid at worst.[29,30]

In May 2014, the NIH issued new guidelines mandating equal representation of both sexes in preclinical research except in cases where the research pertains to diseases that affect only males or only females.[31,32] It remains to be seen how well this policy will be enforced.

What is the experimental evidence that females have more pain?

It's not just clinical pain conditions that reveal the unequal burden of suffering. Sex differences have also shown up in lab experiments where people voluntarily let scientists test their responses to painful stimulation, though recent research suggests these differences may not be as significant as once thought.

One intriguing finding is that the sex of the experimenter—not just the sex of the subject—affects how men and women volunteers report pain, perhaps because of cultural expectations.[33]

In the pain lab, when the experimenter is a woman, men tend to report *less* pain. But women's reports of pain, some research shows, do not seem to be influenced as much by the gender of the experimenter.[34] In one study, a British team took two groups of male and two groups of female college students. A female experimenter tested one group of males and a male experimenter tested the other; the female students were tested similarly, one group by a man, the other by a woman. In all cases, the experimenters were dressed to emphasize their gender roles.[35]

The men tested by a woman showed higher thresholds for pain—that is, they seemed to be tougher—than those tested by a man. For the female students, ratings of pain were the same whether the experimenter was a male or female. After University of Florida researchers told men in one experiment that women had tolerated the procedure better, the men then scored the highest pain tolerance of all.[36]

On the other hand, other studies show that *both* men and women report less pain to an opposite-sex experimenter.[37] In one study, for instance, German researchers showed that both men and women tolerated pain longer when tested by an experimenter of the opposite sex, perhaps to look good to that person, but also found that both men and women rated pain intensity higher when tested by female experimenters.[38]

Other research, however, has found no effect of experimenter gender on pain reports in both men and women.[39] And still other research suggests that, depending on where a woman is in her menstrual cycle, she may be more tolerant to pain when queried by a male experimenter.[40]

Even lab rats respond to male and female researchers differently. At McGill University, researchers found that in the presence of male experimenters—or even in the presence of just a T-shirt worn by a male—rats exhibited a greater stress response, which temporarily suppressed the response to pain stimuli.[41,42]

Historically, women in lab studies have been shown to be more sensitive to experimental pain stimuli than men—with lower pain *thresholds* (i.e., they report pain at lower levels of stimulus intensity) and lower *tolerance* (they can't bear intense painful stimulation as long).

The existence of this difference is highly consistent across studies. Women are more sensitive than men across virtually all types of pain stimuli, though the magnitude of the difference varies depending on a variety of factors, including the type of pain stimulus used.[43] Researchers use different stimuli in different experiments—heat, cold, mechanical pressure, electrical stimulation, or ischemia (i.e., pain caused from tourniquets cutting off blood supply.)[44]

Pain induced by mechanical pressure, for instance, produces big sex differences in sensitivity.[45] Electrical stimulation, too, is more painful for women[46]—ditto for pain induced by heat and cold.[47]

The cumulative experience of pain, called "temporal summation" and measured by the gradual increase in a person's pain ratings as brief, potentially painful stimuli are delivered to the skin every 3 seconds, is also greater in women.[48,49,50] This is important. If women's brains accumulate pain sensations more than men's, that may be one reason why women are more susceptible to *chronic* pain—pain that adds up over time.[51]

And it's not just what men and women *say* about their pain when they're being tested in pain labs that highlights sex differences—it's also what their brain scans show. With heat as the painful stimulus, positron emission tomography (PET) scans show that women exhibit more pain sensitivity than men at the same level of thermal stimulation of the inner arm (122 degrees Fahrenheit).[52]

In a different PET scan study that used rectal distention as the painful stimulus, University of California, Los Angeles researchers looked at 23 women and 19 men with irritable bowel syndrome.[53] Women's brains showed more activation in the limbic system, which processes emotions, while men's showed more activation in cognitive, or analytic, regions. Harvard Medical School researchers have documented similar findings with migraines—women's brains react differently from men's, especially in the emotional reaction to the pain.[54] This difference fits with the idea that women often express pain in more emotional terms—and may indeed have stronger emotional responses to pain.

Why do women have more pain?

One theory is that the chemical pathways that are activated inside nerve cells may be different in males and females. In some studies with rats, the "secondary messengers" (chemicals that relay pain signals) are different in females and males. Male rats use three different secondary messengers; females use one.[55] In women, there are more nerve endings in the skin than in men.[56] Moreover, the nerve cells that convey information about intense stimulation are studded with receptors for the sex hormones testosterone and estrogen. These two hormones are believed to explain a lot, though far from all, of the sex differences in pain responsiveness.[57]

As young children, boys and girls show comparable patterns of pain until puberty. But once puberty hits, certain types of pain are strikingly more common in girls. Even when the prevalence of a pain problem is the same in both sexes, pain *severity* is often more intense in girls than boys.[58,59,60,61,62]

Overall, testosterone seems to protect against pain. If newborn male rats are castrated, for instance, they are unable to produce testosterone later, during puberty. The result? The animals become less sensitive to the pain-reducing effects of the opioid morphine.[63] If newborn female rats are *given* testosterone, they obtain *better* pain relief from morphine. As adolescence progresses, boys actually develop more pain *tolerance*, perhaps because of cultural expectations but partly also because of the flood of testosterone.[64]

But if the role of testosterone is relatively straightforward (more testosterone, less pain), the role of estrogen is anything but.

Estrogen levels, of course, vary significantly across the menstrual cycle, and so do reports of pain. In one study of temporomandibular pain (formerly called TMJ), pain levels were highest at times of lowest estrogen, but increased pain was also associated simply with rapid changes in estrogen levels.[65]

Gene researchers have found that estrogen downregulates—or reduces—the activity of a pain gene called *COMT*. The job of the *COMT* gene is to get rid of stress hormones. So, if *COMT* activity is too low, the body can't rid itself of stress hormones effectively. Since stress hormones act directly on nerves to rev up pain, the net result of estrogen acting on *COMT* is more pain.[66]

At the University of Maryland, neuroscientists have tested the pain sensitivity of female rodents, then surgically removed their ovaries (which make estrogen). When tested again, without their ovaries, these females act more like males; that is, they're less sensitive to pain.[67] If they are then given back estrogen, the females soon go back to feeling pain, just as in the bad old days before their ovary surgery.

We could think of menopause as the human version of this experiment. At menopause, women's ovaries stop pumping out estrogen, almost as if the ovaries had been surgically removed. To combat the symptoms caused by this precipitous drop in estrogen, many menopausal women begin taking exogenous estrogen (i.e., estrogen not made naturally in the body but taken as a drug). If the general theory—that estrogen increases pain—is true, we would expect that hormone replacement therapy would make pain worse. The confusing thing is, sometimes it does sometimes it doesn't, and sometimes it makes it better.

Several studies have shown that menopausal women who take hormone replacement therapy do have more chronic pain.[68,69,70,71] But other studies show no link between hormone replacement therapy and pain in older women. And still others show that when postmenopausal women *stop* taking hormone replacement therapy, their pain goes up, just the opposite of what the theory would predict.[72] Indeed, some women who used to have migraines begin getting them anew within a couple of weeks of *stopping* estrogen therapy.[73] And some pain conditions like trigeminal neuralgia that are more common in women typically don't start until after menopause.[74]

Here's more food for thought: Have you ever wondered what happens when transsexuals take hormones to enhance the sexual characteristics of their "new" sex? Italian researchers wondered exactly that. In a preliminary study, they tracked male-to-female human transsexuals, who take estrogen to enhance female sex characteristics, and found that approximately one-third develop chronic pain, especially headaches. They also looked at female-to-male transsexuals, who take testosterone to enhance male characteristics, and found that their chronic pain goes down.[75] All of this fits with the overall theory.

No one is quite sure why these hormones would be linked to these effects on chronic pain. One theory is that testosterone dulls the *excitatory* pain pathways in the brain that crank up pain, while estrogen may block the pathways for *inhibiting* responses to potentially painful stimuli, thus yielding more pain.

What makes unraveling the estrogen–pain link even more complicated is that in premenopausal women, estrogen levels go up and down over the course of each menstrual cycle, with striking fluctuations in pain responsiveness at different points in the cycle. Pain in a number of conditions, including irritable bowel syndrome, TMD, headache, and fibromyalgia, changes significantly over the cycle—but not always in the direction one might expect. Some women feel *more* sensitive to pain during times in their cycles when estrogen is low.[76] Yet, during pregnancy, when estrogen levels are high, some women have *fewer* migraines and TMD pain. After childbirth, when estrogen falls abruptly, the number of migraine attacks increase. Go figure.

Given such complexity, a growing number of researchers now suspect that it's not the absolute level of estrogen that is key for pain but rapid *changes* in hormone levels; in other words, it's the change that produces the change.

Are women in pain undertreated?

In medicine in general, there is evidence that, across a number of different conditions, including heart attacks, women may be undertreated.[77,78] There's some data suggesting the same holds true for pain too.

To be sure, a 2003 study by researchers from the Albany Medical Center did not find such a pattern. In fact, they found that, overall, comparable doses of opioids (narcotics) were given to men and women.[79] A 2011 review article also found there is no evidence of systematic bias against women, at least for musculoskeletal pain.[80]

In addition, a 1995 study from Stanford University found that women sometimes receive even more aggressive pain treatment than men. Women in the emergency room who came in with headache, neck pain, or back pain were perceived by providers as having more pain and received more powerful pain-relieving drugs.[81]

Overall, though, women do often come up short when seeking care for pain.[82] One reason may be that when women talk about their pain, they use more emotional language and thus are often perceived by health-care providers as exaggerating. Indeed, according to criteria developed by psychiatrists, women are often deemed histrionic—that is, dramatic and emotional.[83] That's a shame, given that other evidence suggests that, at the level of brain function, women may truly have more intense emotional responses to pain.

In one study, researchers from Georgetown University videotaped professional actors portraying people with chest pain. The researchers showed the videos to more than 700 primary care physicians and provided them with data about each hypothetical patient. The doctors were much less likely to believe that the women had heart disease.[84] Similarly, when European researchers looked at the records of 3,779 heart patients, 42 percent of them women, they found that women were not worked up as thoroughly.[85] It was the same story in a Mayo

Clinic study of 2,271 men and women who went to the emergency room with chest pain.[86]

Though diagnosing heart attacks can be tricky, even less complicated medical problems, like the knee pain of osteoarthritis, exhibit the same pattern. Women are three times less likely to receive the hip or knee replacement that they need, and they often don't have the surgery soon enough, according to Mary I. O'Connor, who heads the orthopedic surgery department at the Mayo Clinic in Jacksonville, Florida. When women do have the surgery, the results may not be as good because the disease is often more advanced.[87,88]

An unconscious bias may make doctors less likely to recommend surgery to a woman with moderate knee arthritis. Canadian researchers asked 38 family physicians and 33 orthopedic surgeons to evaluate one "standardized," or typical, male patient and one standardized female patient with moderate knee arthritis.[89] The odds of a surgeon recommending knee replacement were 22 times higher for the male patient than the female.

Women are undertreated for abdominal pain too. In Philadelphia, emergency room doctors kept track of 981 men and women who arrived with acute abdominal pain. The men and women had similar pain scores, but women were significantly less likely to receive any kind of pain medication and were 15 to 23 percent less likely than men to receive opioids specifically. Women also had to wait longer before they received any kind of pain medicine—65 minutes, on average, compared to 49 minutes for men.[90] Women with cancer and AIDS are also more likely than men to receive inadequate pain treatment.[91,92]

A fascinating Swedish study similarly revealed gender biases. Using a modified version of a national exam for young doctors, the Swedish researchers described hypothetical neck-pain patients. Some of the hypothetical patients were male and some were female; all were described as bus drivers who were living in tense family situations. The interns were more likely to ask female patients psychosocial questions and more likely to request lab tests in the males.[93] Female interns were just as biased as males.

If pain in men and women is so different, should medications be sex-specific?

One of the most pressing questions in pain research today is why some opioid drugs (i.e., narcotics) work better in one sex than the other. That there are such sex differences in opioid analgesia is clear. What's less clear is the direction and magnitude of these differences.[94,95,96] Even less clear is why findings on opioid responses in lab rats don't necessarily translate to people.[97]

In the nervous system, there are three major classes of opioid receptors: *mu, delta,* and *kappa*. These receptors are like magnets into which painkilling opioids fit. This lock-and-key set-up is the same whether the opioids come from inside the body (endorphins) or are taken as drugs. Wherever the opioid comes from, a filled opioid receptor is a happy receptor—it acts quickly to reduce pain.

Morphine, the most commonly used opioid, binds to *mu* receptors, the largest of the three classes of receptors. Fentanyl, a drug that is 100 times more powerful than morphine, also binds to *mu* receptors. Codeine does not bind strongly to *mu* receptors, but after the body turns codeine into morphine, it binds just fine.

Other, less frequently used drugs, such as Talwin, Nubain, and Stadol, are different. They bind primarily to *kappa* receptors. This is important because response to *kappa* opioids varies depending on sex and may even be specific to certain pain situations, such as tooth extraction.[98] (So far, there are no drugs designed to fit into *delta* receptors.) For complicated genetic reasons, women with red hair respond especially well to *kappa* opioids.[99]

All three receptors, *mu, kappa,* and *delta,* work roughly the same way. When the receptors are filled, they trigger a cascade of chemical events inside the nerve cell that ultimately blocks production of pain-boosting chemicals such as substance P. Blocking substance P results in decreased pain.[100]

At Georgia State University, neuroscientists are trying to unravel the mechanics of sex differences in response to opioids.[101] They have found that female rats require twice as much morphine as males to produce the same level of anesthesia.[102] Reasoning that the answer may lie in the *mu* receptors, they counted the *mu* receptors in a particular area of the brain and found out there were twice as many in male as in female rats. That fits with a 2003 study at Tufts University Medical School in Boston that found that, following surgery, women report more intense pain than men and need at least 30 percent more morphine.[103] But other researchers doubt that it's just a question of how many *mu* receptors a person has.[104]

Adding to the complexity is the fact that the efficacy of opioids in females can vary a lot depending on where she is in the menstrual (or, in animals, the estrus) cycle. In the Georgia State research in rats, it turns out that when estrogen is highest, morphine is the least effective, perhaps because estrogen *downregulates,* or reduces, the efficacy of *mu* receptors; when estrogen is low, morphine works better, possibly because of more *mu* receptors. But in humans, researchers from the University of Michigan have found just the opposite: when women are in the high-estrogen phases of their cycles, there is an *increase* in *mu* activity.[105]

It's actually even more complicated than that. In studies in which real patients control their own analgesia—by pushing a button to release a dose of drug intravenously—men consume more opioids.[106] But that does not necessarily mean that women feel less pain; it may be that women deliberately underdose themselves because they have worse side effects from opioids, including negative mood, nausea, and vomiting.[107]

Ultimately, the differences in the way women and men process opioids may mean, as pain geneticist Jeffrey Mogil of McGill University puts it, that someday we may need pink pills for women and blue pills for men.[108]

Does race influence pain prevalence?

Yes, and this is a major concern because the United States is an increasingly diverse nation, with non-Caucasians now comprising about one-third of the total population By 2042, minorities are expected to constitute the majority, and by 2050, minorities will comprise 54 percent of the population.[109] Racial disparities in pain epidemiology, access to quality pain care, and treatments have been documented consistently for years.

In 2009, researchers from the University of Texas, the University of Michigan Schools of Medicine and Public Health, and the Duke Institute on Care at the End of Life conducted a major review of studies on racial disparities in pain.[110] Among other things, the review team found persistent racial and ethnic disparities in acute, chronic, cancer, and palliative pain care all across the lifespan, with minorities receiving lesser quality pain care than whites.

And it's not just lesser care that is a problem. Some data suggests that blacks and Hispanics also *have* more pain than whites. One 2005 study found that blacks with cancer pain had significantly higher pain intensity, more pain-related distress, and more disruption of daily functioning than white patients.[111] A 2007 study of adults ages 51 and older found that blacks and Hispanics were at higher risk for severe pain than whites.[112] Other studies, though, have not found such clear racial disparities.

In experimental labs, are blacks more sensitive to pain than whites?

In some studies, yes. In one study, blacks were more sensitive to pain (in this case, immersion of one hand in ice water) than whites.[113] Other studies have also found evidence of racial disparities in experimental pain.[114] A 2012 review of 26 studies of experimentally induced pain showed that blacks had consistently lower pain tolerance (the maximum stimulus intensity that a person can stand) and, to a lesser extent, lower pain thresholds (the minimum stimulus intensity needed to elicit pain).[115] A 2014 study of older adults with knee osteoarthritis found that blacks had more experimental pain sensitivity than whites, as well as more clinical pain and poorer function, although the differences in clinical pain "became nonsignificant when the analyses were controlled for education and annual income. . ."[116]

Are there genetic differences that might account for higher pain sensitivity in blacks and Hispanics?

In their 2009 report, the researchers from the University of Texas, the University of Michigan, and Duke noted several differences in genes known to be involved in pain among different racial groups.

Is the pain of blacks and Hispanics undertreated?

Often, it is. It's not totally clear why minorities are undertreated for pain, but this pattern fits with already-existing inequalities in society.[117]

In a 2011 report, the Institute of Medicine found that there is substantial undertreatment of pain among racial and ethnic minorities.[118]

Prejudice clearly influences perceptions of blacks in pain. A 2012 study by University of Virginia researchers found that whites and even blacks themselves assume that pain in black people is less intense that in whites, a misperception that can lead to undertreatment of blacks' pain.[119] In this study, volunteers were shown pictures of either a black person or a white person in pain and asked to rate that person's pain. Everyone, including nurses and nursing students, rated blacks' pain as less intense than whites'.

Also troubling was a New York City area study in 2000. A random sample of 347 pharmacies in the area found that more than 50 percent did not have adequate medication in stock to treat a person in severe pain and that pharmacies in predominantly nonwhite neighborhoods were the most likely to be poorly stocked. The authors of the study, which was published in *The New England Journal of Medicine* and called "We Don't Carry That," concluded that members of racial and ethnic minorities are at substantial risk for the undertreatment of pain.[120]

In a study from Case Western Reserve University School of Medicine and Northwestern University Medical School, researchers found that physicians in the emergency room were less likely to prescribe opioids for black pain patients than for whites.[121] A different study of 16,000 people with cancer pain found that blacks—and Latinos—faced more barriers to pain treatment.[122]

Even minority children are often undertreated for pain: A 2010 study by Seattle researchers found that Hispanic children received 30 percent less opioid analgesia than white children after their tonsillectomies.[123] Blacks taking opioids are also more likely than whites to be asked to undergo urine tests.[124]

A 2009 review by researchers from the University of Texas, the University of Michigan, and Duke University found conflicting results on racial pain disparities.[125] In emergency rooms, blacks and Hispanics are at risk for undertreatment of pain according to some studies but not according to others. With postoperative pain, some studies show that white patients are more likely to receive higher doses of opioids after surgery than Asian Americans, blacks, or Hispanics, but other studies contradict this finding.

Among women having surgery for breast cancer, black and Hispanic women appear to have more postsurgical pain than white women. With chronic noncancer pain, blacks report more severe pain than whites, regardless of age or gender.

Blacks also report significantly more pain-related disability and more symptoms consistent with depression and posttraumatic stress disorder, according to the 2009 review.[126]

With arthritis, which afflicts 20 percent of the general adult US population, blacks have a similar *prevalence* as whites but have higher rates of arthritis-related severe joint pain. Blacks with arthritis are also less likely than whites to receive hip or knee replacement surgery, even when necessary.

A review of patients with hypertension found that blacks received fewer pain-relieving medications. Minority patients with chest pain also received fewer diagnostic tests, the 2009 review noted. And, although cancer pain is often undertreated in both whites and minorities, African Americans and Hispanics seen in clinics in minority areas are three times more likely to be undermedicated than patients seen in nonminority settings. The researchers found that the disparities occur even at the end of life: minorities are less likely than nonminorities to enroll in hospice care.[127]

Is pain different in older people?

Pain is common in older people, but, contrary to common belief, it is not an inevitable part of aging.[128] It is, however, a growing challenge. In 2000, Americans over 65 represented 12 percent of the population; by 2050, older people will represent more than 20 percent of the population.[129]

Pain can also be tougher to treat in older people, in part because aging bodies metabolize medications differently from younger people and older people are more likely to suffer adverse drug reactions.

Older people, for instance, have a three to four times higher risk of bleeding complications from nonsteroidal anti-inflammatory drugs (NSAIDs) than the general population.[130] Many older people in chronic pain have to turn to opioids because they cannot tolerate NSAIDs.

Older people are also especially vulnerable to some kinds of pain, including joint pain (osteoarthritis), pain after surgery, and chronic conditions like shingles.[131] On the other hand, abdominal pain, migraine headaches, and pain from temporomandibular joint disease decrease after midlife. Low back pain, too, seems to increase until age 65 or so and then decline. The prevalence of irritable bowel syndrome also seems to peak in midlife and then decline.[132]

But teasing apart the various contributions of age and pain is often difficult, according to researchers from the University of Florida and the University of Washington.[133]

Are there biological reasons for changes in the experience of pain among older people?

Yes, but these changes can cut both ways.

One phenomenon well-known to increase with age is the shortening of telomeres, those tiny pieces of DNA at the end of chromosomes (much like the protective tips on the ends of shoelaces) that keep DNA intact during cell division. Some research suggests that chronic pain can be linked to shortening of telomeres. Oxidative damage due to free radicals is linked to aging and may also be linked to the development of increased pain.[134]

In the nervous system, there is an age-related reduction in both myelinated and unmyelinated fibers. The number and size of sensory nerves in the dorsal root ganglia decreases with age too. Older people also appear to have fewer opioid receptors (into which opioid drugs fit), which could mean less responsiveness to pain-reducing medication. Aging in general is linked to increases in systemic inflammation, which can translate into increased pain sensitivity.[135]

On the other hand, the pain threshold (the minimum stimulus intensity needed to elicit pain) *increases* with age, meaning that older people may actually become *less* sensitive to pain. Pain tolerance (the maximum stimulus intensity that a person can stand), however, shows a *decrease* in pain tolerance with advancing age in some, but not all, studies.

Do age-related fears contribute to pain problems in older people?

Yes, in particular the fear of falling. Fear of falling often makes older people afraid to exercise or move, which in turn fosters a sedentary lifestyle and constriction of social activities that can make the experience of pain worse. In addition, opioid drugs, anticonvulsant medications, and antidepressants can all increase the risk of falls, thus compounding the problem.[136]

Are older people undertreated for pain?

Yes. Just as some studies show undertreatment for women and minorities, some research also shows undertreatment for older people. In one study of more than 13,000 people age 65 and older with cancer, more than one-third were in daily pain, and those age 85 and older were 1.5 times more likely to receive no analgesia, compared to those age 65 to 74.[137]

What about children? Is their pain undertreated?

In the not-so-distant past, doctors mistakenly believed that babies' nervous systems were too immature to process pain and that, therefore, babies didn't feel pain at all.[138,139] Or, some doctors reasoned, if babies did feel pain, they wouldn't remember it. There was also the worry about anesthesia—in years past, no one knew how dangerous anesthesia drugs might be in tiny babies, so doctors figured that if surgery was necessary to save a child's life, they'd better operate anyway.

Doctors and researchers now know with certainty that children—and even fetuses—can feel pain. But in many hospitals around the world, this knowledge has not changed pain management in infants and children.

Way back in 1974, a nurse at the University of Iowa walked around the wards at her Iowa hospital and looked at the medical charts of 25 children ages four to eight who had had all sorts of surgeries—cleft palate repair, repair to the urethral opening at the tip of the penis, and other procedures. Over their entire hospital stays, the 25 children—collectively—received only 24 doses of pain medicine. Of these, only half were opioids. Thirteen children received no pain medication at all, despite having had a traumatic amputation of a foot, removal of a neck mass, partial kidney removal, or other serious procedures.

The Iowa nurse contrasted this poor pain management for children with that of 25 adults who had surgeries in the same hospital at the same time. Over their hospital stays, the adults—collectively—received 372 doses of narcotics and 299 doses of nonnarcotic painkillers.[140]

After this discovery, other researchers began documenting the undertreatment of children's pain. In 1982, one team showed that children undergoing debridement of burns—an extremely painful procedure—often received no anesthesia at all.[141] In 1983, University of Virginia researchers tracked postoperative anesthesia in 50 children and 50 adults who had had cardiac surgery. No one, not even the adults, received very good pain management. But at least the adults actually received 70 percent of the opioids that had been prescribed for them. The children received only 30 percent.[142]

That same year, Australian researchers studied 170 children who had just had surgery. They found that 75 percent had inadequate anesthesia.[143] In 1986, Boston researchers compared 90 children and 90 adults undergoing identical surgical procedures—hernias, appendectomies, burns, and fractured femurs—at a variety of hospitals. They, too, found an "enormous disparity" in pain control: Adults received twice as many doses of opioids as children.[144]

But it took research into the basic neurobiology of brain development to begin to convince the medical world that babies and children did indeed feel pain and should be treated for it, a mission that British pain researchers plunged into with vigor.

They began examining how the nervous system in newborn rats—and humans—changes under the assault of severe pain. In 1985, they published the first of a series of pivotal papers in which they tracked the postnatal growth of pain pathways. They showed that not only can local analgesics reduce the risk of subsequent chronic pain but that untreated pain in infancy can have long-term adverse effects.[145,146,147,148,149,150,151,152,153]

Then came a blockbuster analysis in 1987 in *The New England Journal of Medicine*. The authors laid out irrefutable evidence that babies, and older children as well, do feel pain.[154] Citing study after study, they made the case that babies' nervous systems are indeed mature enough to process pain signals, that they react to pain with massive release of stress hormones, and that anesthetics can—and should—be given to newborns undergoing surgery.[155,156,157,158,159,160,161]

In meticulous detail, with more than 200 citations, the authors showed that newborns have at least as many nociceptive (pain) nerve endings in their skin as adults. Indeed, pain nerves are already developed in some areas of the skin as early as seven weeks of gestation, other research shows.[162]

In fact, very young babies may actually be extra sensitive to pain because the descending, top-down pain-control signals from the brain to the spinal cord haven't kicked in yet.[163] Even during the birth process itself, research shows that babies are actively trying to cope with pain.

Not surprisingly, the idea that babies feel pain has fed into the debate over circumcision. Even as far back as the early 1970s, it was clear that if a newborn was circumcised without anesthesia, his sleep was disturbed.[164] Levels of the stress hormone cortisol rose sharply.[165] By contrast, if a newborn is given local anesthetic before circumcision, he does not show behavioral signs of pain and stress.[166]

But it took decades before it became clear that uncontrolled pain during circumcision can have lasting effects. That was demonstrated in 1997, when Canadian researchers studied three groups of baby boys. One group was not circumcised. One group was circumcised after receiving a local anesthetic called EMLA. The third group was circumcised after a placebo medication. Four to six months later, the infants were videotaped while they received standard vaccinations. The circumcised babies showed stronger responses to pain—including more prolonged crying—than the uncircumcised babies. This excessive response was blocked by EMLA.[167,168] (Today, many circumcisions are done with a different kind of anesthesia, a dorsal penile nerve block.)

Older children, too, may suffer lasting effects from untreated pain. School-age kids with cancer who undergo painful procedures such as bone marrow aspiration or lumbar puncture have more pain during subsequent procedures if they do not receive good pain control the first time around.[169]

So how well, then, do we treat children's pain?

Not well enough.

Historically, infants and young children have been underdosed with opioids for fear of respiratory side effects.[170] It is true that adverse events, both major and minor, following anesthesia are about twice as common in young children as in adults. And the risk is highest, not surprisingly, in the newest, tiniest babies.[171] In newborns, the liver is so immature that it takes longer to detoxify drugs. That means that weaning babies off opioids can take longer and must be done with exquisite care so as not to trigger a new bout of pain.[172] There is also concern about the effects of opioids on a young child's developing brain, including potential death of brain cells and developmental problems.[173,174]

But now, armed with better information, it is clear that doctors can give children, even infants, effective and safe pain relief.[175,176] Children who receive good pain management during acute episodes such as surgery fare better long term than those who do not.[177,178,179]

Interestingly, by the time children are age two to six, they can clear drugs from their systems faster than adults. This becomes tricky, however, because faster clearance may mean that the child needs a new dose of medication sooner. For example, a sustained-released oral morphine drug that an adult needs to take only twice a day may require three times a day dosing in children.[180]

If given the chance, children as young as six can learn to do patient-controlled analgesia, in which the patient pushes a button to administer a preset infusion of morphine.[181] Importantly, letting kids administer their own opioids does *not* increase drug complications, and many children prefer this approach to receiving repeated intramuscular injections of painkillers. (It's actually anxious parents who mess things up. They tend to either over- or underdose their children unless they receive a vigorous education program first.)

Some research shows that the use of opioids in children does not lead to a predilection or risk of addiction, unless that child is already at risk by virtue of genetic background and social milieu.[182]

But the pendulum is now swinging back toward increasing fear of opioids, which is raising concern among pediatric pain specialists that, once again, patients in severe pain will be denied access to needed medication.[183] Black and Hispanic children are at even greater risk of undertreatment than whites, even in cases of clear-cut appendicitis in the emergency room.[184]

Many doctors and hospitals are not as proactive as they could be in using milder, nonopioid approaches to children's pain. A number of benign interventions, including breastfeeding, pacifiers, cuddling, skin-to-skin contact, swaddling, and, for older children, self-hypnosis and cognitive behavior therapy can often help with minor pain.[185,186,187]

Consider the common hospital practice of lancing a newborn's heel to draw blood for testing. It may look like nothing to an adult. But, proportionately, it's like a knife in the foot of an adult.[188]

Mary Poppins was right: a spoonful of sugar really does help—at least during heel lances and other minor procedures, A number of studies, including a major review of 44 other studies by the Cochrane Collaboration, an international group that analyzes medical research, found that sucrose significantly reduces the length of time a newborn cries during a heel stick, though it doesn't stop that initial yelp.[189] Sucrose also reduces scores on a commonly used scale called PIPP for measuring infant pain.[190,191,192]

But perhaps the best pain reliever for infants is the one that comes naturally to mothers: "kangaroo mother care," that is, basic holding and skin-to-skin contact.[193,194] Research shows that skin-to-skin contact is more effective at reducing distress—as gauged by crying, grimacing, and heart rate increase—than swaddling a baby tightly in a crib during heel lance.[195] Familiar scents, especially that of the mother, also helps calm babies, as does simply the sound of the mother's voice.

But application of these techniques is still haphazard.

In one 1992 study, researchers interviewed 150 randomly selected hospitalized children ages 4 to 14, and later their parents, to assess children's pain in the hospital. The results were depressing. More than 87 percent of the children had had pain within the previous 24 hours, and 19 percent of these said their pain was severe. Only 38 percent had received analgesic medication in the previous 24 hours.[196]

In 2000, San Francisco researchers checked the medical records of hospitalized children who had been reported by nurses to be in pain. They found that opioid use was wildly uneven.[197] In 2002, other researchers studied 237 hospitalized children and found that more than 20 percent had significant pain.[198] In 2003, a Swedish nationwide survey of nurses and doctors showed that moderate to severe pain occurred in

23 percent of children who had had surgery and in 31 percent of children who had pain from other causes.[199] That same year, when researchers from Maine and Massachusetts examined the medical charts of 180 children ages six months to 10 years who were in emergency rooms for fractures or serious burns, they discovered that a whopping 65 percent of kids under the age of two received no pain medication at all.[200]

Researchers from the Netherlands and the University of Arkansas studied 151 preemies and recorded all the potentially painful procedures they were subjected to in their first two weeks in intensive care—an average of 14 per child per day.[201] (Some of the procedures were relatively benign, like suctioning out the airway.) They found that preemptive analgesia was given to fewer than 35 percent of the babies. And 40 percent of the newborns never received any analgesia during their entire ICU stays.

Even today, serious undertreatment of children's pain persists, according to French pain researchers. In 2008, a French team did a six-week study of 430 hospitalized preemies in and around Paris. They found that each preemie received an average of 16 painful or stressful procedures every day, though some of these procedures were minor. A stunning 79.2 percent of the time, the babies received no specific analgesia at all.[202,203]

In Canada, as recently as 2008, researchers found that only 27 percent of children in a leading hospital—the Hospital for Sick Children in Toronto—had any pain assessment in the preceding 24 hours. This was despite the fact that the children or their caregivers said the children had moderate to severe pain.[204]

Indeed, many hospitals and doctors' offices still don't do the little things to reduce pain such as giving children local anesthetic creams like EMLA before injections.[205,206,207,208,209,210] And many hospitals still do not have pain guidelines for children or attempt to assess infant pain.[211]

But here's the real heartbreaker—even children with cancer still die in pain. In 2000, Boston palliative care specialists interviewed the parents of 103 children who had died of cancer between 1990 and 1997. According to the parents, 89 percent of the children suffered "a lot" or "a great deal" in their last month of life.[212] There has since been a campaign for better palliative care for kids and a follow-up study in 2007. There was some progress.

But not enough.[213,214]

3

THE OPIOID MESS IN THE UNITED STATES

What is the "opioid mess"?

It's the fact that we have two colliding epidemics: the epidemic of chronic pain, which receives almost no media coverage, and the epidemic of opioid abuse, which receives a lot.

A 2014 report from a workshop on opioids and chronic pain at the National Institutes of Health (NIH) put it this way:

> The rise in the number of Americans with chronic pain and the concurrent increase in the use of opioids to treat this pain have created a situation where large numbers of Americans are receiving suboptimal care. ... Patients who are in pain are often denied the most effective comprehensive treatments; conversely, many patients are inappropriately prescribed medications that may be ineffective and potentially harmful.[1]

The most striking thing, the NIH report found, was that there is "insufficient evidence for every clinical decision that a provider needs to make regarding the use of opioids for chronic pain."[2] That assessment is widely shared by doctors on the front lines of pain treatment.[3]

Put bluntly, doctors, who receive a median of only nine hours of pain education in four years of medical school (veterinarians have much more), are basically flying blind when trying to treat people in chronic pain. They are also guessing when trying to treat substance abuse disorders.[4]

What's the backstory here? Why are opioids so controversial?

Americans have been ambivalent about opioids for decades, with the pendulum of public opinion swinging back and forth.[5] Opioids were used fairly freely until the beginning of the twentieth century, when the government began introducing regulations to put the brakes on opioid use and physicians' opioid prescribing.[6] These restraints triggered a pendulum swing the other way, prompting doctors, especially those trying to ease the suffering of dying cancer patients, to protest. Eventually, their complaints were heard, and advocacy effectively restored opioid treatment for pain.[7]

Along the way, opioids began to be used not just for dying cancer patients but for people with intractable pain from non-cancer causes. Pain also began to be seen as the "fifth vital sign," a measure that should be assessed regularly in hospitals, along with a patient's pulse, temperature, respiration, and blood pressure. Medical ethicists, too, began to argue that pain relief should be viewed as a fundamental human right—and the lack of adequate pain relief as akin to malpractice, even torture.

All of this, of course, was music to the ears of the pharmaceutical industry, which jumped enthusiastically into the development of newer, longer-lasting opioids, most famously OxyContin. OxyContin had a built-in time-release mechanism that, the marketing hype suggested, could actually reduce the risk of addiction, a pitch that made doctors more comfortable in prescribing it. What happened, though, was that abusers found it all too easy to defeat the time-release mechanism by simply chewing or crushing the drug, thus getting all at once a dose that was supposed to last for hours.[8]

The original formulation of OxyContin has been withdrawn from the market and has been replaced by a reformulated version designed to be even more difficult to crush, break, or dissolve—it turns into a thick, sticky gel that is hard to use as an injection or to snort.[9] Of course, this trick can be subverted simply by swallowing too many pills.

Was the marketing of the original OxyContin misleading?

Yes. It was both unquestionably aggressive and misleading[10,11,12]—so much so that in 2007, three executives with the American operation of Purdue Pharma pleaded guilty in a US federal court to misleading regulators and the public about the addiction potential of OxyContin, agreeing to pay $634 million in civil and criminal fines.[13,14] The company admitted that its "fraudulent conduct caused a greater amount of OxyContin to be available for illegal use than otherwise would have been available."[15,16] Despite that corporate setback, OxyContin is still doing well financially. It garnered $4.8 million in sales in 2015, the latest year for which figures are available through IMS Health, a health-care information company that tracks markets.[17,18]

Has pharmaceutical money driven an increase in prescriptions for opioids?

It seems that way, although there are multiple reasons for increasing pain-reliever prescriptions. With all the industry marketing hype, prescriptions for opioids, both long- and short-acting formulations, soared.[19] Between 1997 and 2005, prescriptions for oxycodone rose 588 percent; for methadone, 934 percent; for fentanyl, 423 percent; for morphine, 154 percent; for hydrocodone, 197 percent; and for hydromorphone, 224 percent.[20]

More recent data from 1999 to 2012, released in February 2015, suggest that while use of "weaker-than-morphine" opioids declined in this period, use of "stronger-than-morphine" opioids increased.[21] However, the way different pain relievers were categorized in this study is open to question.[22]

Are prescriptions for opioids still increasing?

No. There are early signs that prescriptions for opioids may be slowing.

A January 2015 study published in *The New England Journal of Medicine* showed that, in the last several years, prescriptions for opioids, though they rose substantially between 2002 through 2010, *decreased* somewhat from 2011 through 2013.[23] Similarly, the study found, although there had been large increases in the rates of opioid *diversion* and *abuse* between 2002 and 2010, those rates also flattened or decreased from 2011 through 2013; the rate of opioid-related deaths rose and fell in a similar pattern.

Does pharmaceutical money support pain patient advocacy groups?

To some extent, but pain patient advocacy groups often are run by volunteers on a shoestring. Some of the money for these groups comes in the form of unrestricted grants, which means, at least in theory, they do not have to promote drug company agendas.[24] In the wake of investigative reporting from ProPublica, an online investigative news organization, the US Senate in May 2012 launched an investigation into drug industry funding of a number of pain patient advocacy groups, including the American Pain Foundation, which received 90 percent of its money from industry.[25,26] The pain foundation immediately shut down, citing irreparable economic circumstances.

How many opioid-related deaths are there every year in the United States?

According to the latest data available from the federal Centers for Disease Control and Prevention (CDC), there were 16,235 *prescription* opioid-related deaths (not heroin) in 2013.[27,28,29] That is down from a high of 16,917 in 2011 but up a bit from 16,007 in 2012.

In 2013, only about 27 percent of the 16,235 deaths involved opioids alone—that is, without any other drugs such as alcohol or benzodiazepines.[30] In other words, people who die of drug overdoses often had a combination of benzodiazepines and opioids in their bodies.[31,32,33] In fact, benzodiazepines were involved in 31 percent of opioid-related deaths in 2011, up dramatically from 13 percent in 1999.[34] Yet opioids receive most of the blame, and, when opioids are blamed, so are pain patients and their doctors.

According to CDC data, the highest fatal overdose rates were in people ages 45 to 54. Men are more likely to die from opioid overdoses than women, though that gap is closing, in part because women have more chronic pain.[35]

How do those opioid-related death figures compare with deaths from other drugs?

They are low in comparison, although deaths from opioids are usually sudden while deaths from alcohol and tobacco are typically the result of long-term use. That said, more than 481,000 Americans die a year from tobacco.[36] Roughly 88,000 die every year from alcohol.[37] Thousands, perhaps as many as 16,000, die annually from nonsteroidal anti-inflammatory drugs like ibuprofen, some research suggests, although these figures are controversial,[38] and 30,000 hospitalizations a year are due to acetaminophen (the main ingredient in Tylenol).

In fact, a 2012 report by University of Rochester researchers who analyzed data from a registry called the Toxicology Investigators Consortium (ToxIC) found that nonopioid analgesics and psychotropic agents are more likely than opioid analgesics to be associated with drug poisoning overdose, although, again, this is a controversial finding.[39] The most common types of drugs linked to poisoning cases were, in order of prevalence, sedative-hypnotics/sleeping pills, nonopioid analgesics, opioids, antidepressants, stimulants, and alcohol.

How many people with chronic pain die from suicide every year?

The exact number is not clear. But overall, the risk of sui-cide for people in chronic pain is twice as high as for other people, and the risk is highest for people with severe, chronic headaches.[40,41] National figures show 34,000 Americans die by suicide every year. By inference, it's conceivable that half of these, or 17,000, commit suicide in chronic pain, although this has not been explicitly shown. Still, as one report put it, "In examining the various risk factors for suicide, it is appar-ent that many of these factors can be associated with living in chronic pain."[42]

Is pain undertreated in the United States? Is it overtreated?

Yes to both. Doctors often fail to recommend—and insur-ers often fail to cover—nondrug treatments for pain such as acupuncture, chiropractic, massage, meditation, hypnosis, and the like. Many doctors, pressed for time and limited by a scanty knowledge of pain management, simply write pre-scriptions for opioids as the quickest way to deal with pa-tients, a practice that a 2014 NIH workshop report noted sharply.[43]

Some doctors—and dentists—prescribe opioids too freely for relatively minor procedures and offer larger supplies of opioids than are needed for short-term, acute pain relief.

Yet opioids are underprescribed as well, including for people with persistent back pain, headaches, joint pain, and cancer, according to the New York–based nonprofit Mayday Fund. Undertreatment is even worse for minorities and the poor, Mayday figures show.[44]

In one nationwide survey, 1,204 people were randomly se-lected from the general US population and questioned during a single week. Thirty-one percent said they had experienced moderate to very severe pain in the past two weeks. Only half of those who sought medical attention said they received sig-nificant pain relief.[45]

What about pain in the military? Is that overtreated or undertreated?

Pain among soldiers returning from recent wars is a staggering problem, though whether it's overtreated, undertreated, or both is not clear. According to a 2014 report, 44 percent of soldiers in one leading unit had chronic pain and 15 percent regularly used opioids.[46]

Where do prescription drug abusers get their drugs?

This is the so-called "diversion" issue.

Contrary to widespread belief, most of the drugs that wind up on the street come from initially legitimate sources, not from bad doctors writing too many prescriptions. According to the government's 2012 National Survey on Drug Use and Health, here's where Americans 12 and older obtained their pain relievers the most recent time they abused them:[47] Fifty-four percent obtained the pain relievers they most recently used from a friend or relative for free, and another 15 percent bought them from a friend or relative. In other words, almost 70 percent obtained the drugs from a friend or relative. Another 4- plus percent stole them from a friend or relative. Fewer than 1 in 20 users (3.9 percent) received pain relievers from a drug dealer or other stranger. About 18 percent obtained the drugs through a prescription from a doctor.

What are the definitions of "abuse," "addiction," "physical dependence," "tolerance," and similar terms?

One of the main problems in the pain/opioid debate is confusion over the terms "addiction," "physical dependence," "tolerance," and "abuse." Almost everyone gets these terms mixed up, patients and doctors alike.

As a group of 25 leading pain specialists put it in a 2010 report, the general public and many health-care professionals "frequently overstate" the risk of addiction or fail to differentiate addiction from physical dependence or tolerance.[48] The important point is this: physical dependence is a normal, expected response to taking opioids long term. Addiction, abuse, and misuse, on the other hand, are *not* normal, though some specialists believe that it can be difficult to separate physical dependence from addiction.

In a 2015 study of 1,422 middle-aged people who had been in chronic pain for a median of 10 years and on opioids for a median of 4 years, Australian researchers attempted to sort out the definitional problems.[49] They found that the definitions varied widely among professional groups. There was only partial agreement, for instance, between definitions used in the *Diagnostic and Statistical Manual of Mental Disorders* (5th ed. [DSM-5], published by the American Psychiatric Association in 2013) and other definitions such as those used in the *International Classification of Diseases and Related Health Problems* (10th ed. [ICD], published by the World Health Organization in 2010). The DSM-5 criteria produced much higher estimates of opioid use disorders. The DSM-5 also expanded some criteria for the definition of opioid use disorders and abolished the distinction between "dependence" and other problems.[50] The following is a rough guide to the definitions.[51]

Substance misuse is the use of any drug in a manner other than that indicated or prescribed. *Substance abuse* is the use of any substance when such use is unlawful or detrimental to the user or others. *Abuse* can also be defined as self-administration of a medication for a nonmedical purpose, such as to get "high." Both real pain patients and nonpatients can be abusers.

Addiction is a disease—a primary, chronic, neurobiological condition characterized by impaired control over drug use, compulsive use, continued use despite harm, and craving.[52] In 2011, the American Society of Addiction Medicine released a new definition emphasizing that addiction is a chronic problem involving the reward circuitry in the brain, that is, a "chronic disease of brain reward, motivation, memory and related circuitry."[53,54,55] It is characterized by inability to consistently abstain, impairment in behavioral control, craving, diminished recognition of significant problems with one's behaviors and interpersonal relationships, and a dysfunctional emotional response. Like other chronic diseases, the society states, addiction often involves cycles of relapse and remission. Without treatment or engagement in recovery activities, addiction is progressive and can result in disability or premature death.[56]

By contrast, *physical dependence* is an expected state of adaptation manifested by a withdrawal syndrome triggered by abrupt cessation, rapid dose reduction, decreasing blood levels of the drug, or administration of an antagonist, or drug blocker, such as naloxone. In other words, if opioids are stopped or blocked suddenly, withdrawal will occur, potentially including flu-like symptoms, sweating, muscle aches, joint pain, stomach cramping, increased heart rate, goosebumps, diarrhea, muscle aches, and irritability. In some cases, withdrawal can be prolonged.[57]

Tolerance is a state of adaptation in which the drug's effects diminish over time, prompting a patient to need more of the drug to control pain. Tolerance is not an inevitable consequence of chronic opioid therapy. *Aberrant drug-related behavior* is behavior suggestive of a substance abuse or addiction disorder or both such as selling prescription drugs, prescription forgery, stealing or "borrowing" drugs from others, injecting oral formulations, obtaining prescription drugs from nonmedical sources, multiple episodes of prescription "loss," repeatedly seeking prescriptions from different clinicians ("doctor shopping"), deterioration in function at work or home, or repeated resistance to getting help despite clear physical or psychological problems.

Recently, a group of physicians called PROP (Physicians for Responsible Opioid Prescribing) who take a dim view of long-term opioids has argued that the attempt to conceptually— and clinically—separate opioid dependence from opioid addiction may constitute a distinction without a difference.[58] In

2012, PROP teamed up with Public Citizen's Health Research Group, an advocacy organization, to file a Citizen's Petition with the Food and Drug Administration (FDA) asking for label changes for most opioid analgesics.[59,60]

In the petition, the two groups voiced concern about the increase in opioid prescriptions, the fact that many pain patients continue to experience pain despite chronic opioid therapy, and the threat of addiction. The next day, several members of Congress endorsed the petition.[61]

In 2013, the FDA announced labeling changes for extended-release and long-acting opioids. The agency stated that these drugs are indicated for the management of pain that requires around-the-clock, long-term opioid treatment and for which alternative treatment options are not available. But it added that these drugs should be reserved for patients for whom alternative treatments (nonopioid analgesics or immediate-relief opioids) are ineffective, not tolerated, or would not provide sufficient pain relief.[62]

What is the risk of genuine addiction?

That's been hard to pin down. Estimates vary widely, with the current consensus hovering around 10 percent.[63] National Institute on Drug Abuse (NIDA) puts the estimate in the 3 to 26 percent range, though the agency stresses that solid, long-term data are not available. Some studies cited by NIDA put the risk among pain patients at between 0.7 and 6.1 percent; other studies cited by the agency, based on reports from pain clinics, estimate 2 to 14 percent.[64]

Overall, only a minority of people who use opioids for chronic pain become addicted, according to a 2014 report from a NIH workshop on opioids and pain.[65]

In a 2015 systematic review of 38 studies, researchers from Albuquerque and Seattle found rates of "problematic" opioid use in chronic pain patients who did not have cancer to range from less than 1 percent to 81 percent.[66] They defined "misuse" as use contrary to the directed or prescribed pattern of use, regardless of the presence or absence of harm or adverse effects; "abuse" as the intentional use of the opioid for a nonmedical purpose, such as euphoria or altering one's state of consciousness; and "addiction" as a pattern of continued use with experience of or demonstrated potential for harm (e.g., "impaired control over drug use, compulsive use, continued use despite harm and craving"). Part of the variance in rates of problematic use stems from different definitions of "abuse," "misuse," and other terms.

The team found rates of misuse averaged between 21 and 29 percent and the rates of addiction between 8 and 12 percent. But, as one commentator for this study put it, it can be difficult to truly separate misuse, abuse, dependence, and addiction.[67]

A systematic review of 17 studies involving 88,235 people by Italian researchers reported a range of 0 to 24 percent (a fairly high rate) and concluded that opioid pain relievers are not associated with a major risk of addiction.[68]

Other research pegs the risk of addiction at between 3.2 and 18.9 percent.[69] A 2008 review looked at 67 studies of opioids in thousands of people with chronic pain.[70] Overall, the risk of abuse or addiction was only 3.27 percent; although this seems like a very low number, in a large population, it translates to many people. For patients with no prior or current drug abuse or addiction problem, the rate was even lower, at 0.19 percent.

A 2010 study by a group of 25 leading pain specialists also found that if a person does not have a history of substance abuse, the risk of addiction is between 3 and 5 percent.[71] And it might even be lower. In a 2010 meta-analysis for the Cochrane Collaboration, in which data on 4,893 patients from 26 studies were pooled, signs of opioid addiction were found in only 0.27 percent.[72] (This study involved patients in clinical trials who were at relatively low risk for addiction/abuse to begin with.)

In fact, far from being drug-seekers or constantly upping their doses, people in chronic pain with no history of addictive behaviors tend to *undermedicate* themselves, frequently stopping or cutting down on their opioids.[73]

That said, it's also true that addictive disorders are often underdiagnosed, partly because most physicians who prescribe pain medications have little or no training in screening for and treating addictive disorders.[74,75]

But screening *is* possible. In a 2007 study, Harvard Medical School researchers looked at 228 people in chronic pain and gave them all a series of questionnaires designed to spot psychiatric problems and the potential for misusing drugs.[76] They used the Screener and Opioid Assessment for Pain Patients, the Current Medication Misuse Measure, and the Drug Misuse Index. The questionnaires did flag people at higher risk for misusing drugs, suggesting that if these people are also pain patients, their opioid use should be monitored more closely.

But there's an important caveat to this. In another Harvard study, researchers found that people in chronic pain who are at higher risk for drug abuse may actually be experiencing more pain.[77,78] In other words, pain intensity, not psychiatric history, may be the best predictor of opioid misuse. Other studies, though, suggest that a personal history of substance abuse is the strongest predictor of future abuse.[79]

Is there a genetic component to the risk for addiction?

Yes, there is believed to be a genetic propensity for addiction in some people, with as many as 30 different genes probably underlying this risk.[80] A study by researchers from Yale University School of Medicine and the University of Connecticut looked at 393 families in which at least one member abused opioids. By studying the family members' DNA, the team found that two sites on chromosome 17 were strongly linked statistically to the risk of opioid addiction.[81]

Are there drugs to help people get off of opioids?

Yes, but it can be tricky.

The reason it is difficult to withdraw from opioids is that, in people who have been taking opioids regularly, opioid receptors in the nervous system are used to being occupied. And they don't like it when they're suddenly empty.

Understandably, many pain patients want nothing more than to get off opioids the minute they think their pain is better. If drugs are the problem, the thinking goes, why not just rid the body of all the bad stuff as fast as possible, hoping that the underlying pain is really gone, and get on with life? And it often *is* that easy. Every year, tens of millions of people are given opioids and discontinue them without problems. As the need for pain control diminishes, they just taper the dose.[82] This is especially true for people taking opioids for a few weeks or so after surgery.

For people who *do* encounter opioid withdrawal symptoms, it's reasonable to counteract those symptoms with judicious use of other drugs. Granted, it may sound crazy to think of taking *more* drugs to combat the effects of the initial drugs. But, when done properly, it can be a safe, temporary fix to allow the body to change its biochemistry back to normal.[83]

One drug that can ease the agitation of opioid withdrawal is clonidine, a blood pressure medication that reduces the jittery feelings that are triggered when the body overproduces the stress hormones epinephrine and norepinephrine during opioid withdrawal. Clonidine blocks excessive epinephrine and norepinephrine production. Another option is a sedating antidepressant medication such as trazodone, which blunts the tendency of the heart to race and blocks some of the agitation and anxiety triggered by withdrawal. If opioid withdrawal triggers intense anxiety, benzodiazepines such as Ativan can also help. (Dependence and addiction can be a problem with Ativan but to a lesser extent than with some other drugs.[84]) Antiemetics can also be used to combat nausea and vomiting, antidiarrheals to treat diarrhea, and quinine to help with skeletal muscle cramps.[85]

What if someone is both a pain patient and a person with addiction?

One option is methadone, a substitute opioid that can be used as both a pain reliever and a maintenance drug. Methadone fills up opioid receptors to reduce symptoms of withdrawal from and craving for other opioids while also providing pain control.[86] Instead of needing an opioid every three to six hours, a person can take methadone once a day and still avoid withdrawal symptoms.[87]

When used primarily for pain, as opposed to addiction, methadone is often given two or three times a day.[88] It can be taken for years if necessary. Another benefit of methadone is that it can be taken orally instead of by injection. As long as a person stays on methadone, it reduces the risk of addictive behaviors like injecting drug use, which can lead to AIDS and hepatitis from dirty needles.[89,90,91]

A possibly better, though more expensive, option for pain patients who have become addicted to opioids is buprenorphine, which is also an opioid but one that binds to opioid receptors less strongly than other opioids.[92] Buprenorphine is sold as Suboxone and Subutex. Pure buprenorphine is Subutex; if naloxone, an opioid blocker, is added, it's Suboxone.

Buprenorphine can be prescribed in a doctor's office and taken at home.[93] In fact, Subutex and Suboxone are the first narcotic drugs available under the Drug Abuse Treatment Act of 2000 for the treatment of opioid dependence that can be prescribed in a doctor's office. This change allows more patients the opportunity to access treatment.

In contrast, methadone can be dispensed only in a limited number of clinics that specialize in addiction treatment. There are not enough addiction treatment centers to help all patients seeking treatment.

How does buprenorphine work?

When an opioid hits its receptor, the receptor changes its physical shape, which triggers a cascade of chemical events inside the cell that, ultimately, leads to pain relief. But tiny changes in the shape of an opioid can make it fit more or less securely into the receptor. Morphine, for instance, binds very well to opioid receptors or, put more technically, has a high "affinity" for these receptors.

Buprenorphine keeps opioid receptors occupied but not fully.[94] In theory, buprenorphine binds just enough to keep withdrawal symptoms away and to provide some pain relief as well. Often, for someone who has both persistent pain and addiction, a doctor trained in both pain and addiction medicine will "cross taper" regular opioids and buprenorphine.[95] It's a complicated regimen but involves slowly *decreasing* the dose of the standard opioid and gradually *increasing* the dose of buprenorphine.

Buprenorphine doesn't appear to have the same overdose risk as other opioids and also appears less likely to produce respiratory depression and tolerance. (Tolerance means a person needs more and more of a drug to achieve the desired effect.)[96,97] In the buprenorphine-plus-naloxone formulation, there's also a built-in anti-abuse feature. If someone tries to crush the tablets, mix the powder with water, and inject it to get high, the naloxone will kick in and block the effects of buprenorpine, triggering withdrawal.

In 2011, researchers at McLean Hospital and Harvard Medical School conducted the first randomized large-scale clinical trial at 10 sites nationwide with 653 people who were physically dependent on prescription opioids. Almost half were people who also had chronic pain. The researchers tested the effectiveness of Suboxone for different amounts of time and with different amounts of counseling added.[98] Short-term Suboxone treatment did almost no good—only about 7 percent of patients randomized to a two-week treatment followed by a two-week tapering period were able to get off and stay off their prescription opioids. In the group that took Suboxone for 12 weeks, followed by a four-week taper, however, almost half the group (49 percent) successfully stopped using prescription pain relievers. (The group that had the longer treatment were those who had failed with the shorter treatment.) The amount of counseling made no difference in outcomes.

But here's the bad news: Once Suboxone treatment was stopped, there was a high rate of relapse.

Buprenorphine can also be used under the tongue, transdermally (through a patch on the skin), and via implants.[99] In a study led by researchers from the University of California, Los Angeles, doctors at 18 medical centers around the country studied people with opioid dependence recruited from addiction centers. They randomized the patients to receive implants of buprenorphine or implants of a placebo medication. (The study did not include people with chronic pain requiring opioid treatment.) All were followed for six months, and they provided regular urine samples during that time. The results were impressive. The buprenorphine group had significantly more "clean" urine samples, meaning they had not taken illicit drugs during the study than the placebo group. The buprenorphine group also had fewer withdrawal symptoms and less drug craving.[100,101]

Implantable buprenorphine has the additional advantage that, once it's placed under the skin, it can't be tampered with, so is less likely than an oral formulation to be abused. A study of transdermal buprenorphine in 1,160 people with chronic back pain also yielded encouraging results.[102] On the downside, buprenorphine is no walk in the park. It can cause nausea, vomiting, constipation, headaches, leg swelling, and insomnia.[103] It is also associated with abuse and deaths.[104]

Are there other drugs available to treat opioid dependence and addiction?

Yes. In 2010, the FDA approved an extended-release form of naltrexone (marketed as Vivitrol), which acts by blocking opioid receptors but is not itself an opioid.[105]

Beyond addiction, what are other side effects of opioid use?

There are many, including opioid-induced hyperalgesia, falls and fractures, cardiac problems, immune and hormonal changes, and overdose.[106]

One of the most overlooked risks, especially in older people, is falling and breaking a hip or the pelvis. In one study of 2,341 people taking opioids for noncancer pain, the risk of fracture was double that of nonopioid users.[107] Among people taking moderate to high doses (50 milligrams a day or more), there was an almost 10 percent per year chance of fracture. While fractures may sound trivial compared to overdoses or addiction, they're not. There is a 24 percent risk of death in the first year after a hip fracture for people over 50.[108]

With chronic use, opioids may also suppress the immune system and may lower testosterone levels in men.[109] In fact, the longer a man takes daily opioids, the more likely he is to have hypogonadism (impaired production of testosterone).[110] Chronic opioid therapy can also lead to menstrual irregularities in women.[111] Opioids can also exacerbate depression and cause serious constipation, including fecal impaction. They may also decrease cognitive function.[112,113,114]

Of all the risks associated with opioids, the scariest—for good reason—is overdose. Overdoses, intentional and accidental, fatal and nonfatal, can occur both with street abusers who take opioids for nonmedical purposes and with pain patients, though overdoses happen more often with the former.

In research published in 2010 by the Consortium to Study Opioid Risks and Trends (CONSORT), scientists looked at 9,940 people who received multiple opioid prescriptions for conditions such as back pain and osteoarthritis between 1997 and 2005.[115] Not surprisingly, the team found that patients receiving the highest doses of opioids were more likely to overdose than those on low doses.

But most of the overdose cases actually occurred among people taking low or moderate doses because there were so many more people taking lower doses. For people taking fewer than 20 milligrams of opioids per day, the annual risk was tiny—0.2 percent. For those taking 50 to 99 milligrams per day, it was higher, at 0.7 percent. And for those taking more than 100 milligrams per day, it was more worrisome—1.8 percent. Still, the total number of overdoses was small—51 out of the entire sample. And, thankfully, not all were fatal; only six of the 51 overdoses in this study resulted in death.

A more recent study published in *The Journal of the American Medical Association* in 2011 supports the CONSORT findings. This study found that the unintentional fatal opioid overdose rate among patients on opioid therapy was quite low (0.04 percent) but again, the risk rises with increasing dosage.[116] This study looked at 750 overdose deaths out of a sample of 154,684 pain patients on opioid therapy. Similarly, another 2011 study also found the risk of death rose with increasing dosage.[117] Obviously, people in pain on high doses of opioids need to be very careful not to exceed what their doctor prescribes and not to increase their doses on their own. But, by and large, it's people who take opioids for nonmedical reasons—abusers, not pain patients—who are more likely to fatally overdose.

In a revealing study from West Virginia, which experienced the nation's largest increase in drug overdose mortality between 1999 and 2004, researchers looked at every person—295 in all—who died of unintentional overdoses in that state in a single year.[118] Two-thirds of the deaths (63 percent) involved *diverted* drugs (mostly opioids), in other words, drugs prescribed for someone else. Most of the people who died from diverted opioids were also young—8 to 24—with the prevalence of diversion dropping steadily with older age groups. In addition to *receiving* diverted drugs, young people are often the ones *doing* the diverting. A 2011 University of Maryland study of 192 people ages 21 to 26 found that a quarter said they diverted their analgesics to others.[119]

One of the trickiest pieces of the opioid fatality problem is methadone, the synthetic opioid developed in Germany as an alternative to morphine during World War II.[120] It is difficult to prescribe correctly because it relieves pain for only four to six hours but lingers in the body for up to three days. This prompts pain patients to take subsequent doses before the first dose is out of their systems, which leads to overdosing.[121,122,123,124,125,126]

Does naloxone (Narcan) reduce the risk of death from overdoses?

Yes, and this is very important.

One emerging idea is to provide all pain patients taking opioids with naloxone to have on hand in case of an overdose.[127] Another idea is to make it available without a prescription. Naloxone (Narcan, a nasal spray) has long been a standby in emergency rooms. Drug addicts who overdose are routinely injected with naloxone to reverse potentially fatal breathing problems. In both injected and spray forms, naloxone rapidly knocks heroin and other opioids off opioid receptors, triggering an instant, horrible withdrawal but also restoring breathing and, thus, saving lives. It has virtually no abuse potential and a favorable safety profile.[128,129]

In Wilkes County, North Carolina, in a community-based effort called the Lazarus Project, free, intranasal naloxone has been central to successful efforts to combat opioid overdose deaths.[130] Preliminary data, published in 2011 in *Pain Medicine*, show that, though Wilkes County initially had one of the highest drug overdose death rates in the nation, the Lazarus Project was linked to a reduction in deaths from 46.6 per 100,000 in 2009 to 29.0 per 100,000 in 2010.[131] The Lazarus Project involved both substance abusers and pain patients. Similar projects elsewhere have also produced impressive results.[132,133]

At the national level, the CDC announced in February 2012 that community-based programs using naloxone have prevented an estimated 10,171 opioid overdose deaths since 1996. As of October 2010, there were at least 188 such programs in the United States.[134]

But there is an obvious drawback to the naloxone "rescue" idea: to prevent death in someone who has overdosed, other people must be present—friends, relatives, or emergency medical personnel—who recognize when someone is in trouble and know how to administer naloxone.

What is Zohydro?

The unique feature of extended-release Zohydro is that it contains the opioid hydrocodone and only hydrocodone. Other hydrocodone-containing drugs such as Vicodin contain both hydrocodone and acetaminophen (the active ingredient in Tylenol.) Strange as it may seem, it's the acetaminophen that is often the dose-limiting ingredient because it can cause serious liver toxicity. So, in that sense, a hydrocodone-only pill is a step forward.

But Zohydro has been controversial, to say the least. After a long review and against the vote of its own advisory board, the FDA approved Zohydro in 2013. Critics of the action protested that the FDA approval came before tamper-resistant features had been put into the drug. They also objected to having yet another opioid on the market. Proponents hailed the drug as a safer alternative to combination medications, avoiding the liver problems associated with acetaminophen.

Contrary to many media reports, Zohydro is not more potent than other similar drugs. In April 2015, Zohydro ER was acquired by a wholly owned subsidiary of Pernix Therapeutics Holdings, Inc.

What is hydrocodone? How is it classified?

Hydrocodone is an opioid that can be taken alone (as in Zohydro) or in combination pain relievers such as Vicodin and Lortab. In 2013, the FDA recommended that drugs containing hydrocodone be placed in a different category among controlled substances, in essence putting tighter controls on it to make it harder to acquire.

The change was formalized on August 22, 2014, when the Drug Enforcement Administration (DEA) published its final rule in the Federal Register.[135] The change limits the number of refills a patient can obtain before going back to his or her doctor for a new prescription. It also means that a patient must physically take each prescription to a pharmacy, instead of allowing doctors to call the prescription in. The goal is to make it harder for drug abusers to get the drug. But for patients in severe, chronic pain and those with physical limitations, these requirements pose significant difficulties.

In bureaucratic language, the change involves moving products that contain hydrocodone from classification as a Schedule III drug to classification as a more restricted Schedule II drug. When hydrocodone-containing products were in Schedule III, a pain patient could see a doctor once a year, obtain a prescription with five refills—meaning a supply of the drug for six months—and then call the doctor for another prescription good for another six months, which the doctor could call in to the pharmacy.

The change to Schedule II means that a pain patient can obtain a supply of the drug for up to three, not six, months at a time. A patient then has to have another visit with the doctor and physically take each new prescription to the pharmacy. Instead of seeing a doctor just once a year, patients must see their doctor every three months.

This change, like everything else to do with opioids, was highly controversial.

Are opioids safe and effective for long-term use?

The answer, unfortunately, is that no one really knows, in part because most studies of safety and effectiveness by pharmaceutical companies last for only a few months, not for a year or more.

A 2015 study by leading researchers published in the *Annals of Internal Medicine* compiled data from randomized and observational studies from major databases and concluded that "the evidence is insufficient to determine the effectiveness of long-term opioid therapy for improving pain and function. Evidence supports a dose-dependent risk for serious harms."[136]

In a September 2014 report from the NIH workshop on chronic pain and opioids, experts found that many long-term patients are compliant with their prescriptions, achieve adequate pain relief, and have a good quality of life.[137] This is good news for the large number of patients who use opioids responsibly. But others quit using opioids, the report found, because the opioids proved insufficiently effective or had too many side effects. The report also noted there is little evidence to support long-term use of opioids for chronic pain.

Some researchers, among them Forest Tennant, who runs a pain clinic in W. Covina, California, are convinced that opioids can be used safely and effectively for very long periods of time. In a 2010 article in *Practical Pain Management*, Tennant reviewed outcomes for 100 noncancer pain patients whom he and three other doctors had treated with opioids for 10 years or more. This was purely anecdotal evidence, however, not a clinical trial. Nonetheless, most patients appeared to be doing well and almost half had not had to increase their dosages for at least three years.[138] In addition, for "breakthrough" pain in patients on long-term opioid therapy, there is good evidence that buccal fentanyl (opioid medication absorbed through mouth) or intranasal fentanyl (medicine absorbed through the nose) work better than oral opioids, though these studies looked at extremely short-term effects.[139,140]

But other efforts to assess long-term opioid use are more discouraging.

In one such project, Pennsylvania researchers reviewed 17 studies involving 3,079 noncancer patients taking opioids for more than six months.[141] Many patients were so dissatisfied with adverse events or insufficient pain relief from opioids that they withdrew from the studies. The dropouts included one-third of patients on oral opioids who couldn't stand side effects such as nausea, constipation, and upset stomach and 12 percent on oral opioids for whom the drugs weren't helping. Opioids did reduce pain in the people who were able to keep taking them. The Pennsylvania group did another review of long-term opioids, this time analyzing 26 studies involving 4,893 patients.[142] Once again, they found huge dropout rates due to adverse side effects or insufficient pain relief.

Dropout rates were high in another analysis too—45 percent for people using oral opioids, 25 percent for people using transdermal (skin) patches, and 17 percent for people using intrathecal opioids (infusions into the space around the spinal cord).[143]

Researchers from Denmark, which has the world's highest per capita usage of prescription opioids, compared people in chronic noncancer pain who were taking opioids to similar pain patients who weren't.[144,145] The opioid users actually reported more severe pain, worse health, and lower quality of life than the nonusers.

The American Academy of Neurology also takes a dim view of long-term opioid use, arguing that while the evidence is clear that opioids help with short-term pain, it is not clear for persistent pain.[146]

Can opioids actually increase pain?

Yes.

There is a puzzling phenomenon called opioid-induced hyperalgesia, which means *increased* pain due to opioids. In certain people, opioids seem to rev up the nervous system instead of calming it down.[147] Opioids may increase pain by acting on a so-called glial cell receptor, TLR-4.[148]

It's not clear why this happens, but opioid-induced hyperalgesia makes treating pain even more difficult than it would be otherwise because if a pain patient taking opioids reports increasing pain, the seemingly obvious—but wrong—solution would be to increase the dosage of opioids.

Dropping the dose may help, as may switching to different opioids, an idea called "opioid rotation."[149] (Opioid rotation involves the use of so-called equianalgesic tables to guide lowering the dose of one opioid while raising the dose of another. Unfortunately, many doctors do not know how to use these tables and some tables themselves are flawed.)[150,151]

How effective are opioids for pain relief?

Effectiveness varies tremendously patient by patient, but, overall, opioids reduce pain by about 30 to 40 percent.[152,153] In other words, opioids usually do not *eliminate* pain but they can, especially in conjunction with nondrug therapies, help some patients function better and regain quality of life.

Do opioids work equally well for different types of pain?

That's unclear, which adds to the complexity of pain management. People with pain due to injury, rheumatoid arthritis, or cancer, for instance, may respond better than others to opioids, according to a 2014 NIH workshop report.[154] On the other hand, people with central pain syndromes such as fibromyalgia, irritable bowel syndrome, temporomandibular joint disorder, and tension headaches may not obtain as much relief from opioids as they do from centrally acting drugs such as antidepressants and anticonvulsants. For instance, while it was once thought that people with neuropathic pain did not respond as well to opioids, but more recent studies suggest that those with neuropathic and non-neuropathic pain may respond similarly.[155] However, it is often difficult for doctors to determine which opioids to use and how to dose them.

What about at the end of life? Are opioids used appropriately?

Opioids can reduce pain at the end of life, but often they are underutilized, particularly in developing nations. At the end of life, obviously, there is much less reason to worry about addiction, dependence, abuse, misuse, tolerance, or side effects.

But even in the United States, including in hospice and palliative care programs, pain is common at the end of life. Indeed, one-third of people in hospice report pain at the last hospice care visit before death, a report from the Institute of Medicine report found.[156] A recent study from the University of Texas M.D. Anderson Cancer Center found much the same thing— one-third of cancer patients and cancer survivors had untreated or undertreated pain.[157] That's better than 18 years ago, when Texas researchers found that 42 percent of cancer patients had inadequately treated pain.[158] But it's clearly not good enough.

Can doctors learn to prescribe less risky, lower doses of opioids?

Yes. In a study in Seattle, doctors in the Group Health Research Institute were successfully trained to prescribe lower doses of long-term opioid therapy.[159] The study also concluded that there is little evidence that chronic opioid therapy is more effective at higher doses.

Do opioid "contracts" or agreements help reduce risks?

Increasingly, pain specialists are making patients sign "contracts" or "agreements," which spell out the opioid doses to be taken, the risks of misusing the drugs, a list of rules and obligations and signs of side effects, and potential improvement to be recorded. But there is little data to support such contracts.[160,161,162,163] On the other hand, contracts may be helpful if a patient is being seen by someone other than his or her regular doctor.[164]

Contracts can be insulting and stigmatizing for patients. After all, no one makes people with other medical problems sign such things. The agreements may be a decent educational tool for informing patients about the risks and benefits of opioids. And there's no harm in reminding people not to refill prescriptions too early, increase doses on their own, and drink alcohol with medications. But contracts may disrupt the trust between patient and doctor, and some border on the offensive, such as those that state, "You will be on time for appointments," or "You will be respectful to me and my staff."[165]

Contracts may also miss the point. They shift the locus of concern from helping *patients* to protecting *providers* against the perceived risk from regulatory agencies. Contracts also address a social problem—the drug abuse epidemic—rather than a clinical problem, thus reinforcing the assumption that every pain patient is a potential criminal. [166]

Does urine testing reduce opioid risks?

Another controversial approach is urine testing, though its use is haphazard.[167] The CDC recommends such testing for any patient younger than 65 with noncancer pain who has been on opioids for more than six weeks.[168] Some physicians recommend starting urine testing before starting a patient on opioids. Urine tests can be useful in some cases to see whether a patient is taking illegal drugs or failing to take prescribed medicine properly.[169]

But, once again, there are questions: Does urine testing yield clinically meaningful results? Is it overly stigmatizing? Who is it really protecting? Who really benefits, besides urine testing companies? And how reliable can it be when patients can buy "clean" urine on the Internet?[170]

What is clear is that many people, whether intentionally or not, do not take their medications exactly as instructed. A national survey of 76,000 urine tests for prescription drug medications by Quest Diagnostics, a testing company, showed that

63 percent of patients take their medications in ways inconsistent with their doctors' orders—including missing doses and combining medications.[171,172,173]

Some urine tests also have built-in validity problems, in part because some drugs leave the body much more quickly than others.[174] Urine tests may only show a short snapshot in time and reveal nothing about longer term drug use or abuse.

Do prescription monitoring programs reduce abuse risks?

The evidence is slowly shifting toward a more solid "yes."[175] But some pain patients fear that such programs may deny them the drugs they need.

Prescription monitoring programs (PMPs), also called prescription drug monitoring programs (PDMPs), provide a means of keeping track of opioid-prescribing practices by doctors and the dispensing of such medications by pharmacies. The goal is to reduce "doctor shopping," "pharmacy shopping," and other ways patients may use to game the system.[176,177,178]

The practice raises potential confidentiality concerns, although law enforcement personnel typically must show that they have probable cause (good reason) to be interested in the information.[179] PMPs only get at the problem of drug *diversion* stemming from prescribing relationships, not the larger part of the problem—obtaining drugs from family, friends, and unlocked medicine cabinets.[180]

It's also hard to know how to interpret results if the data show opioid prescriptions are declining: this could mean that doctors are becoming more afraid of writing pain-reliever prescriptions for legitimate pain patients and might be turning to less effective medications.

In 2006, researchers for the federal Department of Justice reviewed the evidence on PMPs and concluded that, when PMPs share their data readily with prescribing physicians and pharmacists, there is a 10 percent drop in prescription sales and a reduction in prescription drug abuse.[181]

In a 2010 study, Boston-area researchers tracked 11 years' worth of PMP data from 1996 to 2006 in Massachusetts.[182] They found that it was only when people used four or more prescribers or bought their drugs from four or more pharmacies that there were signs of questionable activity.

One controversial assessment of PMPs came in 2011 from the CDC, which examined data from 1999 to 2005 across the United States.[183,184] It found that PMPs were *not* significantly associated with lower rates of drug overdose, opioid overdose mortality, or lower rates of consumption of opioid drugs. On the other hand, a 2012 study that looked at information from two drug abuse surveillance databases showed more encouraging results.[185]

In 2015, researchers writing in the *Journal of Opioid Management* found that PDMPs can be useful but should not be the sole factor that physicians rely on for making clinical decisions.[186]

Do measures to restrict opioid prescriptions harm pain patients?

It's unclear, but that is certainly patients' big fear.[187] In October 2014, the DEA "rescheduled" hydrocodone from Schedule III to Schedule II, meaning that the government feels the drug is more dangerous than previously believed. An estimated 130 million prescriptions for hydrocodone are written every year.

The change effectively limits patients to a smaller maximum supply between doctor visits. As previously mentioned, patients must now see a doctor or other provider for each handwritten prescription renewal. But a 2015 survey of pain patients—which collected 3,000 responses in the first 72 hours—showed that two-thirds of responders reported that they could not obtain hydrocodone-combination products even though they had been safely taking the medications for years. More than one-quarter of respondents reported suicidal thoughts due to being denied their hydrocodone prescriptions, according to industry-sponsored research presented at the 2015 meeting of the American Academy of Pain Medicine.[188] But it may be that patients with the biggest fears are the ones most likely to respond to such surveys.

Are babies affected by prescription opioid abuse?

Yes.

Even newborn babies are swept up in the opioid abuse problem because of opioid-abusing mothers. Among pregnant teenagers, 16.2 percent use illicit drugs, and 7.4 percent of pregnant women ages 18 to 25 do so, with the result that more and more babies are being born with neonatal abstinence syndrome, or drug withdrawal, according to a 2012 study in *The Journal of the American Medical Association*.[189] Indeed, between 2000 and 2009, the incidence of neonatal abstinence syndrome grew from 1.20 in every 1,000 hospital births per year to 3.39, with health-care costs soaring in tandem. In its 2013 labeling ruling, the FDA insisted that extended-release and long-acting opioids carry a boxed warning that use in pregnancy may result in neonatal opioid withdrawal syndrome.[190]

Does prescription opioid abuse lead to heroin abuse?

That's not totally clear, but it appears to. Overdose deaths from heroin have been increasing in recent years—in 2010, there were 3,036 such deaths, and in 2013, there were 8,257, according to the CDC.[191,192] Most of those deaths were in men.

The National Survey on Drug Use and Health, conducted annually from 2002 through 2011, found that four out of every five people who recently started using heroin (79.5 percent) had previously used painkillers *nonmedically*, that is, to get high, not to relieve pain.[193] According to NIDA, one in

15 people who take prescription pain medications nonmedically will try heroin within the next 10 years.[194] (There is little data on whether people who use prescription pain relievers properly [i.e., as prescribed for them for medical reasons] later turn to heroin. The number is believed to be very small.)[195]

In a 2014 report from a workshop at the NIH, researchers noted that, historically, the most common first opioid used by people who became heroin addicts was heroin itself. By 2000, this pattern had changed dramatically: The most common entry drug for heroin use was a prescription opioid.[196]

Tragically, OxyContin, in part because of its abuse-deterrent features, also seems to be spurring heroin use. Data from a 2015 study show that reformulated, that is, abuse-deterrent OxyContin is associated with a reduction in abuse of OxyContin, just as its designers had hoped. But determined abusers have simply turned away from OxyContin and switched to heroin, which is much cheaper, instead.[197] Heroin use has also morphed from being primarily an inner-city, minority-centered problem to one with a more widespread geographic distribution involving mostly white men and women in their late 20s living outside of large urban areas.[198,199]

Is there a vaccine to prevent heroin addiction?

Not yet, but researchers are working on it. In rats, a prototype "dynamic" vaccine appears to block heroin and its metabolites from entering the brain.[200,201]

Are there new biotechnology techniques to make heroin and opioid painkillers?

Not yet, but they are in the works. Researchers are already looking at ways to produce morphine from yeast, a process that may be as simple as brewing beer. The process mimics the way poppies make opiates.[202]

So is there an opioid abuse epidemic, a pain epidemic, or both?

Both.

The trick is to address the abuse problem without harming legitimate pain patients who genuinely need opioids to function. Ideally, this would mean, among other things, better education on the basics of pain for doctors and other providers, better addiction treatment, greater use of naloxone to stop overdose deaths, better "after-market" studies by drug companies to obtain a more accurate picture of abuse and misuse, better pain medications, and more use of (and reimbursement for) nonpharmacological treatments for pain.[203]

It would also mean more balanced press coverage. Stories of prescription drug abuse dominate the headlines, while stories about chronic pain patients not receiving the treatment— including opioids—they need almost never do. This is critical. The mainstream media has contributed substantially to the opioid mess by lopsided reporting, a "biased" practice criticized in September 2014 by experts at a workshop on opioids and chronic pain convened by the NIH.[204] According to that report,

> Stories that focus on opioid misuse and fatalities related to opioid overdose may increase anxiety and fear among some stable, treated patients that their medications could be tapered or discontinued to "prevent addiction." For example, one workshop presentation indicated that a typical news story about opioids was likely to exclude information about the legitimate prescription use of opioids for pain, focusing instead on overdose, addiction, and criminal activity.[205]

Historically, public misconceptions about the relative urgency of the pain/abuse epidemics were exacerbated by the genuinely disastrous situation with "pill mills," most notably in Florida. In 2011, the DEA made headlines when it swept through South Florida to shut down the pill mills—shady operations often advertised as "pain clinics" in which unscrupulous doctors handed out prescriptions for opioids to "fake" patients—drug seekers—who claimed to be in pain.[206,207] In the massive raid by 400 law enforcement officers, 20 people, including five doctors, were arrested.[208] In a subsequent action, dubbed Pill Mill Nation II, DEA officials arrested 22 people in Orlando and Tampa, including five doctors and two pharmacists.[209]

Those DEA actions were widely applauded, with good reason. But the zeal of the DEA and other federal, state, and local law enforcers has also had what some physicians feel is a chilling effect on good doctors and real pain patients, making doctors fear prescribing opioids for legitimate pain.[210]

The reality, as the 2014 NIH workshop team concluded, is that we now have a double problem—a pain epidemic and an abuse epidemic.[211]

How bad is the opioid abuse epidemic?

Bad, but possibly improving slightly.

Beginning in 2012, opioid-related deaths dropped for the first time since 1990, and essentially leveled off, according to 2015 figures from the CDC.[212] This mirrors a similar drop in opioid-prescribing rates.

But opioid-related deaths—and nonfatal opioid abuse problems—*had* been climbing steadily for years. According to 2014 government data, for every one opioid-related death, there were 10 admissions for abuse, 32 emergency department visits for misuse or abuse, 130 people who were abusers or were dependent on opioids, and 825 people who used opioids nonmedically, such as to get high.[213]

Opioid prescribing patterns vary widely by state, with providers in some states writing three times as many opioid prescriptions per person as providers in other states.[214] The highest risk of opioid overdose deaths is in people ages 45 to 54.[215]

On the other hand, opioid-related deaths are relatively rare among pain patients, unlike among abusers. In one industry-sponsored 2013 study, opioid abuse was extremely low among pain patients, less than 0.2 percent.[216]

How bad is the chronic pain epidemic?

Bad, and not clearly improving.

As the Institute of Medicine reported in 2011, 100 million American adults live in chronic pain.[217] According to the NIH, of these, approximately 25 million "experience moderate to severe chronic pain with significant pain-related activity limitations and diminished quality of life."[218]

Pain is the primary reason Americans are on disability, the NIH report added, noting that an estimated 5 million to 8 million Americans use opioids for long-term management of their chronic pain. It is not totally clear why there are growing numbers of people in pain—although the population is aging, more people are surviving cancer and its treatments, and many people are overweight and underexercising, all of which can contribute to chronic pain. The result is that

> 40 to 70 percent of people with chronic pain are not receiving proper medical treatment, with concerns for both over- and under-treatment of chronic pain ... Together, the prevalence of chronic pain and the increasing use of opioids have created a "silent epidemic" of distress, disability, and danger to a large percentage of Americans.[219]

The result is what the 2011 Institute of Medicine called the "opioid conundrum."

While access to opioids has become difficult for many pain patients because of exaggerated fears of abuse and addiction, street abusers obtain them easily and sometimes become addicted. Most pain patients never become addicts.[220,221]

What is the government doing to combat these two epidemics?

Not much for chronic pain—more for opioid abuse.

With chronic pain so prevalent, one might assume that the federal government would be spending frantically on pain research. It is not. Although spending on pain has increased ever so slightly over the past five years, since 2004 less than 1 percent of the massive budget for the NIH has been targeted for primary pain research.[222,223] In 2012, the NIH spent only about 0.63 percent of its budget on pain research, according to an independent analysis by the Pain Research Center in Salt Lake City.[224]

In the 2014 NIH budget of slightly over $30 billion, only $499 million, or about 1.6 percent, was targeted for pain research.[225,226,227] The NIH tends to classify more research projects as aimed at basic pain research than outside analysts do, so the true percentage is probably lower.[228,229]

The basic problem is that no one is really in charge of pain research at the NIH. Although there are "institutes" and "centers" within the NIH for almost every other disease, there is no such "home" for pain, even though chronic pain is now considered a disease of the nervous system in its own right.

"Because there is no single institute funding pain at NIH, there is not a coordinated allocation," according to Philip Pizzo, emeritus dean of the School of Medicine at Stanford University and chair of the Institute of Medicine committee that wrote the 2011 pain report. "Pain costs the nation more than cancer, heart disease and diabetes together. But the funding for pain research is only a fraction of that allocated to these disorders."[230]

There are two efforts in the federal government to address chronic pain. One is the Pain Consortium, set up in 1996 and rejuvenated in 2003, which tries to coordinate pain efforts. But it doesn't have much clout.[231] As one 2012 report from the Senate Committee on Appropriations noted, "It is clear that the NIH must do more. Although every Institute and Center deals in some way with pain, none of them 'owns' this critical area of research."[232]

The other government group trying to coordinate pain research is the Interagency Pain Research Coordinating Committee (IPRCC). This group has come up with a National Pain Strategy that has been turned over to the Department of Health and Human Services for vetting.[233] The goal of the strategy group was to operationalize recommendations from the 2011 Institute of Medicine report, but, so far, it doesn't have a funding mechanism and not much has happened.[234,235]

Both the NIH Pain Consortium and the IPRCC are administered out of the Office of Pain Policy, which is in the National Institute of Neurological Disorders and Stroke.[236]

That's it for pain.

By contrast, a slew of federal agencies are zealously combatting the opioid abuse problem, including the DEA, CDC, NIDA, the Substance Abuse and Mental Health Services Administration, and the White House–based Office of National Drug Control Policy, among others. It's difficult to put a dollar figure on the federal effort to combat opioid abuse because the federal drug control budget does not break out opioids from other drugs that can be abused.[237]

Has the "war on drugs" been a failure?

Many people now think so, including the Global Commission on Drug Policy, an elite group that included former heads of state as well as Kofi Annan (the former secretary-general of the United Nations), Paul Volcker (former chairman of the Federal Reserve), and George P. Shultz (former US Secretary of State).

"The global war on drugs has failed," the commission reported in June 2011.[238] Vast expenditures on criminalization and repressive measures directed at producers, traffickers, and consumers of illegal drugs have clearly failed to effectively curtail supply or consumption.[239]

According to the Global Commission,

> When the United Nations Single Convention on Narcotic Drugs came into being 50 years ago and when President Nixon launched the US government's war on drugs 40 years ago, policymakers believed that harsh law enforcement action against those involved in drug production, distribution, and use would lead to an ever-diminishing market in controlled drugs such as heroin, cocaine, and cannabis and the eventual achievement of a drug-free world.[240]

It hasn't worked, concluded the Global Commission: "In practice, the global scale of illegal drug markets—largely controlled by organized crime—has grown dramatically over this period."[241]

4

THE OPIOID MESS WORLDWIDE

On June 1, 2014, in India, the parents of an eight-year-old boy watched in horror as he writhed in pain from a severe genetic disorder. The hospital, like most other hospitals in India, had no morphine. Eventually, the parents did the only thing they could think of to stop his pain. They killed him. Then they committed suicide, leaving behind a note saying they could not stand to watch him suffer.[1]

Morphine costs almost nothing—in some countries, as little as 3 cents a dose. Yet because of man-made barriers to manufacture and distribution, it never reaches millions of people around the world, leaving them to live—and far too often die—in agony.

This is not a natural disaster like an earthquake or tsunami. It is a result of deliberate, often well-intentioned but short-sighted and unbalanced policies.

Pain itself, of course, is ubiquitous—and increasing, as the world's population explodes and ages. In one study involving tens of thousands of people in 17 countries, researchers found that about 40 percent of people live in chronic pain, most of them women.[2][3]

Yet, all too often, the opioids that might mitigate some of this suffering are not available.

M. R. Rajagopal, India's most famous palliative care physician, put it this way in an op-ed piece for the *Los Angeles Times*.

In the United States, where doctors write more than 250 million prescriptions for painkillers a year, the frequency of abuse and overdose represents a public health crisis. . . . More than 15,000 Americans died from an overdose of prescription opioids in 2013. In other parts of the world, however, the crisis is that strong painkillers such as morphine aren't available at all.[4]

He tells the story of one man he knew.

A few years ago, Gopalan, a man with an ugly scar around his neck, came to see me. When I asked about the scar, he looked away in shame. He had tried to hang himself to end the leg pain caused by a disease of his blood vessels. His teenage children discovered him and saved his life.

Gopalan had, only at this desperate stage, been sent to my palliative care center by his hospital, which had no morphine or any doctor trained in its use. I could treat his pain here only because palliative care centers, unlike hospitals, have access to morphine. He got to spend his last few weeks with his family reasonably free of pain. In the end, however, he died not from his disease, but from kidney damage caused by the high doses of over-the-counter painkillers he had taken before.[5]

With morphine so cheap, asks Rajagopal, "Why was it nearly impossible to get in most parts of India?"

In the United States, as Rajagopal notes, people are so focused on opioid abuse that it is easy to ignore the larger problem elsewhere in the world: the suffering caused by lack of availability to morphine-type drugs.

One of those on the front lines of the global pain crisis is Meg O'Brien, managing director of Global Cancer Treatment for the organization Treat the Pain, part of the American Cancer Society. In many countries, she says, the hard truth is that

> no one is getting pain treatment. People are dying of burns, cancer, HIV, and there is no pain relief. It is appalling. There are cancer hospitals with no morphine. People are dying like animals. People with cancer are dying with tumors breaking through the skin and we have nothing to give them. With burns, you can't imagine a burn unit with no opioids, but they are all over Africa.[6]

If anything, things are getting worse, in part because of the controversy in the United States over opioid abuse. "This has had a killing effect on people around the world," says O'Brien. "People are afraid of morphine—that is the only thing that doctors have absorbed—that it's dangerous. Nobody knows how to use it or that it's quite useful."[7]

Felicia Knaul, a health economist, former head of the Harvard Global Equity Initiative and chair of the Lancet Commission on Global Access to Palliative Care and Pain Control, has studied health inequalities around the world. "The most heinous of all is access to pain control," she has found. "It is incredibly feasible to close that divide and incredibly unconscionable that it exists. All over the world there are archaic restrictions on physicians for prescribing morphine."[8] It is "grossly inequitable."[9]

James Cleary, an oncologist and palliative care expert at the Pain & Policy Studies Group at the University of Wisconsin, has also spent decades studying cancer and pain control around the world. "The most essential service we could offer cancer patients is palliative care, in part because in poorer countries, cancers are so advanced at the time of diagnosis that money would be better spent on pain control than treatments like chemotherapy. Yet palliative care is often not available."

Statistics can only begin to tell the story. But they are powerful.

In 2010, researchers looked at opioid availability for cancer in one of the most developed parts of the world: Europe. They studied 21 eastern European and 20 western European countries and found significant access problems because of costs and regulatory barriers.[10] In some countries in eastern Europe such as Lithuania, Tajikistan, Albania, Georgia, and Ukraine, some essential opioid medications were virtually unavailable, creating what the researchers called "a public health catastrophe."

In less developed parts of the world, the situation is even more critical. Millions of people in Asia, Africa, the Middle East, and Latin America are dying in severe pain.[11] Fourteen countries reported *no consumption of opioids at all* between 2006 and 2008. That means that there was no relief available through legitimate channels to treat moderate to severe pain, according to Human Rights Watch (HRW), an independent, nonpolitical organization that tracks human rights abuses.[12] Eight other countries, HRW found, were in almost as bad straits. And thirteen other countries do not have enough opioids available to treat even 1 percent of their dying cancer and AIDS patients.

Even in some of the world's most populous and *not* necessarily poorest, countries—including China, India, Indonesia, Nigeria, Russia, and South Africa—opioids are so scarce that at least 100,000 people in each of these countries die every year from cancer or AIDS without access to adequate pain relief.[13]

HRW estimates that 80 percent of the world's population is without adequate access to opioids.[14] The World Health Organization (WHO) estimates that 5 billion people live in countries with no or insufficient access to treatment for moderate to severe pain.[15] The Harvard Global Equity Initiative says 5.5 million people dying of cancer and 1 million people with end-stage HIV/AIDS have inadequate pain control.[16]

Indeed, some research shows only 7 percent of the world's population does have adequate access to morphine.[17]

Even long before the end of life, routine pain control after surgery is not available in many poor countries.[18] And nearly a million people who have had accidents or been the victims of violence, people with chronic illnesses, and women in labor suffer from lack of access to strong painkillers.[19]

Moreover, the gap in access between rich and poor nations is getting worse.[20] In countries like Uganda and India, consumption of pain medications is less than 1 milligram per capita.[21] People in the United States and Canada generally have access to sufficient morphine—averaging about 100 milligrams per capita. Put differently, in the United States and Canada, the average person dying in pain of AIDS or cancer has access to 336,000 milligrams of opioids; in the poorest countries, the average person dying of AIDS or cancer receives only 160 milligrams.[22,23,24,25]

So what is the problem?

There are many underlying problems, of course, including poverty, lack of education on pain management for physicians, lack of a national history of using opioids for pain relief, and laypeople's fears that needing opioids means death is near.

But one of the thorniest problems is "opiophobia," the extreme fear of opioids, which all too often means that pain patients who need opioids are unable to obtain them because of excessive governmental efforts to control drug abuse.[26]

It becomes a bureaucratic vicious cycle. Cautious physicians prescribe opioids at low rates. That leads governments to underestimate the *need* for opioids and to submit low estimates of need to the International Narcotics Control Board (INCB), which in turn approves only small amounts of opioids for these countries. That keeps opioid consumption low, far lower than it should be given the need for pain control, especially at the end of life.[27]

The INCB, an independent, quasi-judicial monitoring body, was set up in 1968 in accordance with the Single Convention on Narcotic Drugs of 1961. (Most countries have signed on to this agreement.) Anyone who wants to import or produce opioids in any country must receive approval from the INCB.[28] For instance, a pharmaceutical company seeking to make opioid products must obtain a permit from the INCB to import the raw material from whatever country is supplying it, and the exporting country also must have an INCB permit. In theory, this allows the INCB to obtain data on consumption of narcotics in every country, though, in practice, many countries do not give the INCB regular updates.[29] The goal is for the INCB to use information on projected consumption to tell growers of opium poppies how much to grow—ideally, enough to meet legitimate pain control needs but not so much that there is excess opium floating around the world.[30]

The 1961 agreement actually *requires* that the INCB not just control drug abuse but also assure the availability of opioids for legitimate medical needs.[31] Yet most countries still have policies that severely restrict opioid prescribing, tipping the balance toward heavy regulation and away from pain control—this, despite the fact that the WHO has long recognized the necessity for strong opioids such as oral and injectable morphine and had guidelines designed specifically to promote policies that both minimize diversion of opioids for illegal use and maximize the availability of opioids for moderate to severe pain.[32,33]

Is the opioid access problem equally bad in all countries?

No: quite the opposite.

Access to health care *in general* is uneven all over the world, with large inequalities in maternal mortality, child mortality, and access to antibiotics, clean water, sanitation, and other measures. But, of all the health inequalities, the most shocking is the unequal access to pain control. To some who study the issue, it is the most unequal of all of the unequal distributions of resources, the most insidious injustice.[34,35,36,37] Rich countries, which contain only 15 percent of the world's population, consume 94 percent of the world's morphine; the rest of the world is left to live—and die—in pain:[38,39]

How solid is the evidence for the unavailability of opioids?

Overwhelming, but to some extent inferential.

The data on actual consumption of opioids comes from the INCB. Armed with that data, various groups such as Treat the Pain, HRW, the Harvard Global Equity Initiative, and academic groups such as the Pain & Policy Studies Group at the University of Wisconsin analyze the data in various ways.

The Treat the Pain project, for instance, takes the INCB consumption data and compares that to data from the United Nations (WHO) on the numbers of people dying from particular diseases, say, AIDS and cancer. The researchers then *estimate* the actual need for opioids from disease-specific death numbers. (Two countries with roughly the same population may have different needs for opioids at the end of life depending on how many of their people have cancer or AIDS.)

Are there price differences in the cost of morphine in different countries?

Yes. Although morphine and similar drugs are off-patent and inexpensive, the pain relievers can cost as much as five times more in poor countries—16 cents a dose versus 3 cents.[40]

But isn't morphine considered an "essential medicine"?

Yes.

Morphine has long been on the WHO's list of "essential medicines." According to the WHO,

> Essential medicines are those that satisfy the priority health-care needs of the population and are selected with due regard to public health relevance, evidence on

efficacy and safety, and comparative cost-effectiveness. Essential medicines are intended to be available within the context of functioning health systems *at all times in adequate amounts*, in the appropriate dosage forms, with assured quality and adequate information, and at a price the individual and the community can afford.[41]

Among the opioids listed as essential medicines by the WHO are codeine and morphine, in various forms. Also listed as essential by the International Association for Hospice and Palliative Care are oxycodone, fentanyl, and methadone.[42]

What is a drug formulary?

A drug formulary is a list of a particular country's approved medicines.

If a drug, such as an opioid, is on a country's formulary, does that mean it is available?

No. Many drugs, including essential medicines such as opioids, can be on a country's formulary but not be available because of tight legal restrictions, prescribing regulations, cost, and other factors.

Is adequate relief of pain a human right?

It depends on whom you ask. Yes, according to many organizations of health-care professionals. But it is not yet enshrined in human rights conventions.[43] That said, the WHO and the INCB both recommend that opioids be available for all patients with moderate to severe pain and that physicians be allowed to prescribe opioids according to the individual needs of each patient.[44]

Human Rights Watch puts it this way: A government's "failure to ensure that cancer hospitals offer pain treatment may violate the prohibition against torture and cruel, inhuman and degrading treatment because of the widespread nature and severity of the suffering it causes." Worldwide, the group says, governments "have an obligation to ensure that essential medicines, including morphine, are available to patients and that health care workers receive adequate training in their use."[45,46]

Let's get specific: What is the opioid access situation in India?

With its vast population (1.3 billion), India is one of the best-studied countries in the world in terms of access to pain relief. And the findings are grim. In general, with the notable exception of the state of Kerala, the only opioids available in India are codeine and morphine, with very limited access to oxycodone, methadone, and fentanyl.[47]

In 2009, HRW reported on a large study of palliative care in India.[48,49] It found that access to pain control is severely hampered by overly restrictive drug regulations, a lack of training for health-care professionals, and a health-care system that often fails to provide pain medications, even though they are inexpensive. Many Indian states, for instance, have strict narcotics regulations that make it difficult for hospitals and pharmacies to obtain morphine.

Under a 1985 law, the cultivation of poppies and the manufacture of morphine is controlled by the central government, leaving the states to control the sale and distribution of morphine, according to researchers from the Global Opioid Policy Initiative (GOPI).[50]

The hope behind that law was to control drug abuse. The effect was to cut morphine consumption by 97 percent, even as morphine consumption elsewhere in the world grew. Morphine basically disappeared from India's hospitals and pharmacies.[51]

The 1985 law (the regulations take up 1,642 pages) called for a 10-year mandatory prison sentence for violations involving narcotic drugs, prompting many pharmacies to cut their stocks to avoid potential penalties.[52] It also called for mandatory imprisonment for any error with an opioid prescription—even a minor, unintentional error that did not lead to any abuse.[53]

The tide began to change in 1998 when the federal government changed its recommendations, allowing states to simplify their opioid regulations. But many states still adhered to the old restrictions.[54]

In 2007, the Indian Association of Palliative Care convinced the Indian Supreme Court that all states must provide morphine at no cost to its residents, but even so, the progress of reform countrywide continues to be slow.[55] In 2014, the Indian Parliament amended the 1985 law, softening some of its harshest features.[56] However, to this day, it is typically not financial constraints but drug regulations that prevent wider access to morphine.[57]

Many major cancer hospitals in India still do not provide patients with morphine even though more than 70 percent of the patients in those hospitals have advanced cancer upon arrival, meaning that pain management is their only option, HRW researchers found. Most large hospitals do not have staff trained to deliver palliative care, morphine, or other strong pain medications.[58] The same situation holds true for people with HIV/AIDS, paraplegics, people with advanced renal disease, and elderly people with a variety of medical conditions.

The resultant suffering is barely imaginable. One woman from Hyderabad told the HRW researchers, "It felt as if someone was pricking me with needles. I just kept crying [throughout the night]. With that pain, you think death is the only solution."

A Nepali man with bone cancer in Hyderabad said, "My leg would burn like a chili on your tongue. The pain was so severe I felt like dying. I was very scared. I felt that it would be better to die than to have to bear this pain. [I thought] just remove the leg, then it will be all right. Just get rid of the leg so I'll be free of pain."

A woman with breast cancer said, "I would sleep maybe an hour and a half per night. I could take any number of sleeping pills [without effect]. With morphine, I can relax. This place [a palliative care unit] is heaven-sent."

By HRW's estimate, more than 1 million cancer patients in India experience severe pain in any given year. Yet, as GOPI researchers confirmed, there is only enough morphine available to treat 40,000 of these patients, or about 4 percent.[59]

One of the most wrenching ironies is that because morphine is so cheap, profit margins for pharmaceutical companies and pharmacies are small, which means they have little incentive to stock it.[60] Another irony is that although India grows opium in its three northern states, it exports most of it to be made into analgesics for people in other countries, with the result that India has lower opioid consumption than most of its neighboring countries.[61]

Training in basic pain biology and pain management is also sorely lacking in India.[62,63] Most medical students and young doctors receive no training on pain treatment and palliative care because the government does not include such instruction in relevant curricula. As a result, most doctors in India do not know how to assess or treat severe pain.

What is the opioid access situation in Africa?

Terrible.

In Sierra Leone, a woman named Zainabu Sesay lay dying of breast cancer. The tumor had burst through the skin, looking, as a *New York Times* reporter wrote, "like a putrid head of cauliflower weeping small amounts of blood at its edges."[64] A local healer had wrapped her tumor with clay and leaves, but the smell of her rotting skin, the woman said, made her feel ashamed.

"It bone! It boooonnnne lie de fi-yuh [It burns like fire]," she said. There was no morphine for her.

Opioid access for the 1.1 billion people in the 50 countries in Africa is the worst in the world, according to research by GOPI.[65] This is particularly tragic given the inevitability of severe pain from Africa's HIV/AIDS epidemic and its growing cancer problem.

The GOPI researchers obtained data on opioids for cancer pain in about half of the countries (about 66 percent of Africa's population). Many of the countries had almost no access to opioids; only 15 countries had morphine available in oral and injectable forms. Despite the fact that the population of Africa is relatively young, cancer is a growing health problem on the continent, with new cases expected to double by 2030 as the population grows and ages. Palliative care is rare. Only four African countries (Kenya, South Africa, Tanzania, and Uganda) even include palliative care as part of their health-care systems.[66] Rwanda and Swaziland have established separate national palliative care policies.[67]

In addition, in many African countries, legal restrictions make access to opioids extremely difficult. In some cases, obtaining opioids requires special authorization for outpatients, inpatients, and even hospice patients. In others, even just acquiring the proper forms on which to write opioid prescriptions is difficult. Several countries make physicians pay for those forms.

The human cost of opioid unavailability in Africa is staggering. In one HIV/AIDS clinic, 44 percent of the patients said they had moderate to severe pain. Yet 29 percent of the patients from rural areas and 55 percent of the city patients were not receiving *any* pain treatment at all.[68]

As in the rest of the world, African physicians' knowledge of pain and pain management is lacking. In Nigeria, a survey of pain knowledge among physicians even at teaching hospitals found that 90 percent had no formal education on the topic.

What is the opioid access situation in Asia?

Unlike Africa, where lack of access to opioids is widespread, Asia's situation is quite variable. Access is good for cancer patients in Japan and South Korea but very poor throughout the rest of Asia, with particular problems in Bangladesh, Myanmar, Afghanistan, Kazakhstan, and Laos.[69] Even when opioids are listed on a country's formulary, they are often unavailable.

Asia is home to a disproportionate share of the world's liver, esophageal, and stomach cancer, according to GOPI researchers. Smoking is on the rise in Asia, as are lung and breast cancers. Yet most cancer patients are not diagnosed until they are at advanced stages of disease, which means they already need significant pain relief and palliative care.

To be sure, palliative care services are robust in places like Singapore and Hong Kong, but in countries such as Afghanistan, Pakistan, Laos, and Cambodia, palliative care systems are underdeveloped. As in Africa, some countries in Asia require physicians to pay for prescription forms for opioids. And many countries limit the prescription of opioids to two weeks or less.[70]

There are financial twists too. In some Asian countries, transdermal fentanyl (a powerful opioid) is comparatively easy to obtain because this medication is profitable for manufacturers, while the cheaper oral opioids are not.

And, as elsewhere, many Asian physicians receive almost no training in palliative care and pain management.[71]

Is the situation different in Vietnam?

Yes.

The opioid situation in Vietnam is particularly complex for historical reasons, resulting in both extensive opiophobia *and* widespread heroin abuse. For years, the French financed their colonial regime in Vietnam through opium importation, refining, taxation, and sales. Today, heroin use is endemic in Vietnam, with an estimated 200,000 addicts, the highest prevalence of injection drug use in Southeast Asia.[72] Injection drug use, in turn, is fueling the HIV/AIDS epidemic, which increases the prevalence of pain.

The understandable fear of heroin abuse in Vietnam has led to particularly intense and widespread fear of morphine even for legitimate pain relief, according to researchers from the Pain & Policy Studies Group at the University of Wisconsin. As a result, Vietnam's consumption of morphine for medical use is tiny: Vietnam ranks 122 out of 155 countries studied.[73] But (see chapter 8) the country has made major strides in palliative care recently.

Is access to morphine any better in Latin America and the Caribbean?

Somewhat, though it varies by country. Morphine is moderately available in Argentina, Brazil, Chile, Colombia, Cuba, Mexico, Costa Rica, Uruguay, and some of the Caribbean but much less available in Guatemala, Honduras, and Bolivia.[74]

Strikingly, official formularies in many Latin American countries *do* list many morphine formulations—in contrast to other parts of the world. But, in practice, widespread overregulation impairs access all across the region.[75]

Complicating the situation is the fact that Latin America has the highest income gap in the world. Some countries, like Brazil, are booming, but other Latin American countries are among the poorest in the world. Cancer is becoming widespread, and mortality rates from cancer are higher than in North America, Europe, and Japan in part because many patients have advanced disease at diagnosis. (Breast cancer in particular is caught late—in Brazil, 80 percent of newly diagnosed patients have advanced disease and in Mexico, 90 percent.)[76]

On the plus side, palliative care is growing in a few Latin American countries, most notably, Chile, Mexico, and Argentina, though it is almost nonexistent elsewhere in the region. Another good sign is that in Cuba and Uruguay, medical schools are now offering palliative care training.

And the Middle East? How is opioid access there?

Mixed, but generally bad.

Access to opioids is good in Israel and is at least on the formularies in Qatar and Saudi Arabia. But in many other countries in the region, opioids are not even in formularies and, even when they are, are unobtainable in reality.

The worst opioid access problems, according to INCB standards, are in Afghanistan, Iraq, Lebanon, Libya, Palestine, and Tunisia. (The ongoing political and religious strife in the region adds to the difficulties in opioid availability.)[77] Once again, lack of good pain control is exacerbated by the fact that many people in the Middle East with cancer are not diagnosed until their disease is advanced.

There are some bright spots. The Middle East Cancer Consortium has recently invested in programs to boost palliative care education for health-care professionals.

But negative views of opioids persist. In a survey of final-year medical students in Saudi Arabia, half of respondents said that cancer pain is untreatable and 40 percent said cancer pain is a minor problem.

Worldwide, how common is it for countries to lack palliative care policies?

Very.

In a study of 40 countries by HRW, only 11 countries (Argentina, Brazil, Indonesia, France, the Philippines, Poland, South Korea, Turkey, Uganda, the UK, and Vietnam) had national palliative care policies.[78] And even in some countries that did, such as Argentina and Brazil, it is not clear whether these policies are actually implemented.[79]

How common is it for countries to lack medical education on pain and palliative care?

Again, it's extremely common. Most countries surveyed by HRW had little education in pain and palliative care for healthcare practitioners, and several countries (Cameroon, Ethiopia, Jordan, and Tanzania) had none.[80] In only five of the countries surveyed (France, Kenya, Poland, Uganda, and the UK) was there pain education for all medical students. Doctors around the world still fear opioids because they do not know how to prescribe them or understand the laws that restrict them.[81]

What is the bottom line on opioid unavailability?

Access to morphine and other opioids is still severely lacking throughout much of the world. Of 40 countries surveyed by HRW, 33 nations imposed more restrictive regulation of opioids than was actually required by international drug treaties and conventions.[82]

In many countries, "excessively zealous drug controllers or policy makers, or poorly considered laws and regulations to restrict the diversion of medicinal opioids into illicit markets, profoundly interfere with medical availability of opioids for the relief of pain," according to researchers from the GOP.[83]

The end result, according to GOPI researchers, is that patients "must cajole doctors, chase after permits, wait excessively in inconveniently located pharmacies, and return for frequent refills of prescriptions or any correction on a prescription that many not have been written with adequate attention to detail."[84]

Are people aware of the enormity of the global pain crisis?

No. Pain patients, of course, are all too aware of it, as are researchers who study the problem. But, by and large, the lack of access to pain and palliative care is not on the world's radar.

Researchers from the Harvard Global Equity Initiative put it this way: "The chronic deficit in outrage and outcry is a moral failure that requires remedy."[85]

5

MARIJUANA

What is marijuana?

"Marijuana" refers to the dried leaves, flowers, stems, and seeds from *Cannabis sativa*, a psychoactive plant with significant healing properties that has been around for millennia. It contains more than 400 different chemical compounds, including more than 100 cannabinoids, some of which can be used to treat a range of illnesses or symptoms.[1,2,3] Cannabinoids occur naturally not just in the marijuana plant but are also made in the body and can be synthesized in the lab. Whether they come from the plant, the lab, or our own bodies, cannabinoids act by locking into cannabinoid receptors in the body, producing distinct effects.

The first cannabinoid, isolated in 1964 by Raphael Mechoulam, an Israeli chemist, is the psychoactive tetrahydrocannabinol (THC).[4] Another important, nonpsychoactive cannabinoid is cannabidiol, or CBD. Other cannabinoids are also increasingly well-studied.

Usually smoked as a cigarette, marijuana is the most commonly used illegal substance in America, according to National Institute on Drug Abuse (NIDA).[5] In 2012, there were 18.9 million current users—about 7.3 percent of people age 12 or older—up from 14.4 million (5.8 percent) in 2007. In recent years, marijuana has been gaining widespread acceptance for both recreational and medicinal use in the United States.

What is medical marijuana?

The term refers to the whole, unprocessed marijuana plant or its extracts when used for medicinal purposes, though these uses are not recognized or approved as medicine by the US Food and Drug Administration (FDA).[6]

In practice, though, cannabis is one of the oldest and most potent herbal medicines in the world. Flowers from the female cannabis plant were found in the 2,700-year-old tomb of a medicine man in northern China. From China, the medicinal use of marijuana spread to India. There, a British surgeon "discovered" its healing properties and introduced it into Western medicine in the 1840s.[7,8,9] Among its many ancient uses, cannabis was used to treat migraines not just in the Chinese and Indian cultures but in Egyptian, Assyrian, Greek, and Roman cultures as well.[10,11]

Do our bodies make our own, natural marijuana?

Yes. As mentioned, all human beings are born with the ability to make cannabinoids as well as the cannabinoid receptors into which they fit.[12] The two most important endogenous (body-made) cannabinoids are anandamide and 2-arachidonyl-glycerol, or 2-AG. These are lipids that have a wide range of biological functions, including pain processing.[13] Basically, their job is to make us "relax, eat, sleep, forget and protect."[14,15]

In recent research, scientists have shown that people—and mice—who have a particular mutation in a gene called FAAH, which makes an enzyme that destroys anandamide, are less anxious. The mutation causes less of this destructive enzyme to be made, thus leaving more anandamide in the system, which has a calming effect.[16,17]

Cannabinoid receptors can be activated not only by endogenous cannabinoids but also by those from the marijuana plant itself and by synthetic cannabinoids made in the lab.

To scientists' surprise, cannabinoid receptors turn out to be among the most abundant receptors in our bodies.[18] Presumably, evolution favored us with all these cannabinoid receptors for practical reasons such as dampening pain but perhaps also to reward us with that "feel-good" experience of the "runner's high," which turns out to be triggered not just by endorphins, as is well known, but by endogenous cannabinoids as well.[19]

Are low levels of endogenous cannabinoids linked to greater pain?

It appears that way. People deficient in endogenous cannabinoids may be more susceptible to certain pain conditions, including migraine, fibromyalgia, and irritable bowel syndrome.[20,21] Certain mutations in the receptor for anandamide can also raise the risk of migraine.[22] Furthermore, *boosting* levels of endocannabinoids—by blocking substances that break them down—may also reduce pain.[23] In fact, some pain medicines that we already use, such as NSAIDs (nonsteroidal anti-inflammatory drugs), may work in part by stopping this breakdown of endocannabinoids.[24]

What are the main receptors for cannabinoids?

The two most important cannabinoid *receptors* are CB1 and CB2. The CB1 receptors reside mostly in the central nervous system and on peripheral nerves, while CB2 receptors are mostly in immune cells and, to a lesser extent, in the central nervous system.[25,26] These receptors are vital to survival. Mice genetically engineered to lack CB1 receptors show increased anxiety and susceptibility to depression.[27] They don't respond normally to reward stimuli.[28] They eat less and lose weight.[29] CB1 receptors also seem to play a role in the placebo response.[30]

How do cannabinoids produce their effects?

THC triggers a high when it lands on CB1 receptors.[31] Curiously, CBD doesn't bind strongly to *either* CB1 or CB2 receptors, but it does partially block the binding of THC to CB1, a potential benefit for those seeking marijuana's medical benefits without the "high."[32] When CB2 receptors are activated, inflammation and activity in spinal cord pain relay centers are reduced.[33,34,35]

The holy grail of marijuana pharmaceutical research is to unravel the exact roles of the two major receptors and the role of the many cannabinoids. In theory, teasing apart this biochemistry will allow the creation of fine-tuned marijuana strains that *decrease* the psychoactive effects of marijuana—the high—and *increase* pain-killing effects.

There's a catch in this theory, though. It may be that a little of the psychoactive effect is what helps pain patients dissociate emotionally from their pain. A 2013 study from Oxford University showed that cannabis does indeed make pain less unpleasant.[36] Using functional magnetic resonance imaging (fMRI) brain scanning, the researchers found that while THC did not reduce the *intensity* of pain, it did reduce the *emotional* impact. So the very mood-altering effect of THC may actually be an important part of the overall therapeutic response.[37]

What are the major medical benefits of marijuana or its synthetic cousins?

In recent years, there have been major reviews of more than 100 randomized, double-blind, placebo-controlled clinical trials of marijuana or its synthetic cousins involving thousands of patients with a variety of medical conditions.[38,39,40]

Studies of cannabis or its synthetic cousins suggest that cannabis compounds may be effective at combating nausea, vomiting, appetite loss, glaucoma, irritable bowel disease, muscle spasticity in multiple sclerosis, muscle spasms, Tourette's syndrome, epilepsy, and symptoms of amyotrophic lateral sclerosis (Lou Gehrig's disease).[41,42,43,44,45]

There may be another benefit as well. In 1974, researchers at the National Cancer Institute found a hint that cannabis might have an anti-cancer effect.[46,47] In 2003, Spanish researchers reviewed evidence showing that marijuana can block the growth of tumors.[48] Specifically, cannabinoids seem to fight tumors by blocking inflammation and cell proliferation, other research shows.[49,50] It may also be possible to block cancers that start in immune cells by targeting cannabinoid receptors on those cells.[51] In 2013, California researchers found that CBD was able to block a gene that controls the spread of aggressive breast cancer cells from mice.[52]

As for its potential for treating pain specifically, put bluntly, marijuana works—not dazzlingly, but about as well as opioids. That is, it can reduce chronic pain by about 30 percent,[53,54] and with fewer serious side effects. It may be too soon to declare marijuana and synthetic cannabinoids a first-line treatment for pain.[55] But then again, that may be too cautious a view.

Marijuana and its prescription cousins show a significant analgesic effect compared to placebo in people with all sorts of chronic, noncancer pain, according to a 2011 review of 15 high-quality studies.[56] One of the huge advantages is that marijuana may allow people in severe pain to take *lower* doses of opioids. While doctors often shy away from prescribing opioids if they know a patient also uses marijuana, this may be backwards: there's evidence that marijuana can make opioids *more* effective, thus allowing people to take lower doses.[57,58,59] Marijuana seems to work best, ironically, for people with the most intractable pain. It is less effective for acute pain, such as pain after surgery.[60,61] It has only mixed efficacy against acute pain intentionally induced in research labs.[62]

Some conditions in particular seem amenable to the pain-reducing effects of cannabis—neuropathic pain, fibromyalgia, and pain from multiple sclerosis. With neuropathic pain, which affects 1 to 2 percent of the population, cannabis is a promising treatment, according to California researchers.[63] Canadian researchers have come to the same conclusion.[64] Interestingly, considerable pain reduction can come from the first marijuana cigarette.[65]

In recent years, a steady drumbeat of studies has confirmed the effectiveness of cannabis for neuropathic pain relief. In a 2008 University of California, Davis study, 38 patients rated their neuropathic pain after inhaling cannabis or placebo: Smoking cannabis clearly reduced their daily pain.[66] In 2009, other researchers followed 28 patients who puffed away— under direct observation in a hospital. Again, cannabis yielded significant pain relief, as well as improvements in mood and daily functioning.[67] In 2010, a different study set researchers buzzing at the annual meeting of the International Association for the Study of Pain.

The study was done McGill University researchers who looked at 21 neuropathic pain patients and found that one puff through a pipe three times a day for five days yielded significant pain relief, as well as better sleep. Patients smoking marijuana with the highest concentrations of THC received the most benefit.[68,69]

People with fibromyalgia also seem to be helped by marijuana or the synthetics. A 2008 randomized, double-blind, placebo-controlled Canadian study of Cesamet (nabilone) in 40 fibromyalgia patients found that the patients receiving Cesamet experienced pain relief, though they complained of side effects such as drowsiness, dry mouth, vertigo, confusion, and dissociation.[70] A 2011 Spanish study compared 28 fibromyalgia patients who inhaled cannabis or consumed it orally to 28 nonusers. The cannabis users had less pain and stiffness, were more relaxed, and had increased feelings of well-being. They also scored higher on a questionnaire for mental health.[71]

For multiple sclerosis pain, the prescription medication Sativex (nabiximols) may help reduce pain and sleep problems more than placebo.[72] As for migraines, marijuana should work for migraines because it can activate CB1 receptors, but more data are needed.[73,74,75]

What are the overall medical risks of marijuana?

When researchers look at medical use, they don't find much harm. In a review of 23 randomized controlled trials and eight observational studies of medicinal use, McGill University researchers found that the overall risk of adverse events for short-term (two-week) use of cannabinoids and cannabis extracts was minor.[76] The most common problem was dizziness. Overall, the rates of serious adverse events did not differ between people taking medicinal cannabis and controls.[77]

What are the risks of dependence and addiction with marijuana?

Dependence is a physiological adaptation that can occur with regular drug use and results in withdrawal symptoms when drug use is abruptly discontinued. In that sense, according to NIDA, in some people, marijuana can cause dependence because they can develop tolerance to its effects and experience withdrawal when they stop using it.[78] (Tolerance is a condition in which higher doses of a drug are needed to produce the same effect as initially.)

Addiction is different—it's a primary, chronic, neurobiological condition characterized by impaired control over drug use, compulsive use, continued use despite harm, and craving. Put differently, it is a "chronic disease of brain reward, motivation, memory, and related circuitry. Dysfunction in these circuits leads to characteristic biological, psychological, social, and spiritual manifestations," according to the American Society of Addiction Medicine.[79]

But many people, including doctors, researchers, and staff at federal agencies, confuse the two terms. With marijuana, there are reports of withdrawal symptoms in both adults and adolescents, especially among heavy users.[80] But even when mild physiological withdrawal does occur in heavy users, the symptoms are not as impairing as those caused by alcohol.[81]

NIDA says that marijuana users run the risk of both dependence and addiction.[82,83,84] And that's somewhat true. But the research shows that cannabis has a *lower* rate of dependence/ addiction than alcohol, cocaine, heroin, or tobacco, although the risk increases with dose.[85] Among users of tobacco, for instance, 32 percent become addicted, according to NIDA. For heroin, it's 23 percent; for cocaine, 17 percent; for alcohol, 15 percent; and for marijuana, 9 percent.[86,87]

On its website, NIDA asks, "Is marijuana addictive?" and answers "Yes." Over time, it says, "Overstimulation of the endo-cannabinoid system by marijuana can cause changes in the brain that lead to addiction, a condition in which a person cannot stop using a drug even though it interferes with many aspects of his or her life." But in the next sentence, the agency uses the word "dependent" instead of "addiction," saying, "It is estimated that 9 percent of people who use marijuana will become dependent on it," adding that this number goes up to 17 percent for those who start in their teens.[88]

What is the risk of cancer from marijuana use?

Historically, one of the big fears about smoking marijuana was that it might raise the risk of cancer. This does not appear to be the case. A 2009 study by researchers at the University of Leicester in England did find that cannabis smoke can damage DNA, raising the theoretical possibility that the damaged DNA could produce cancer.[89]

But the bulk of the evidence points the other way. In human studies, once the effect of smoking *tobacco* is accounted for, there's no extra risk from smoking marijuana, as a landmark 2006 California study showed. In this research, scientists from France, the University of Michigan, the Albert Einstein College of Medicine, the University of California, Los Angeles, and other medical centers pooled their efforts to study 1,212 people with lung and oral cancers and 1,040 people without.[90]

The team asked all the participants about marijuana habits using a standardized questionnaire. When the researchers controlled for tobacco smoking, there was no positive association of the cancers and marijuana. The researchers had hypothesized that long-term heavy use of marijuana would increase the risk of lung and head and neck cancers. But after controlling for cigarette smoking, they found no evidence of that.[91] (NIDA takes a more cautious view, saying that it is not yet known whether smoking marijuana raises the risk of lung cancer.[92])

In 2009, many of the same researchers looked more specifically at head and neck cancers. They pooled data from other studies involving more than 4,000 people with these cancers and more than 5,000 people without and asked them about marijuana use.[93] Once again, there was no elevated risk of the cancers from marijuana.

The National Cancer Institute notes that while cellular and molecular studies would suggest that inhaled marijuana is carcinogenic, the epidemiologic evidence of such a link is still inconclusive.[94] One possible exception to this is a 2012 study that found somewhat increased risk of testicular cancer in men who smoke marijuana.[95]

What are the risks of schizophrenia and other psychoses?

There has been serious concern about whether marijuana raises the risk of psychosis, especially schizophrenia. This is not a big concern for older people who use marijuana medically, but it may be for adolescent and young adult recreational users whose brains are still developing and who are at the age when schizophrenia is most likely to develop.

In 2002, British researchers analyzed data on more than 50,000 people (97 percent of all males age 18 to 20) who had been drafted in 1969–1970 into the Swedish army.[96] The study, published in the *British Medical Journal*, found that cannabis use was linked to a higher risk of schizophrenia, and the more the men smoked, the higher the risk. The link could not be explained by the use of other drugs or personality traits. In that same issue of the journal, other British researchers studying 759 New Zealanders also found that early adolescent use of cannabis was a risk factor for schizophrenia, with use at age 15 carrying more risk than use after age 18.[97]

That same year (2002), yet another team, this time a group of Dutch, British, and French researchers, came to similar conclusions.[98] These researchers looked at more than 4,000 psychosis-free people and 59 others who been diagnosed with a psychotic disorder. They tracked all the subjects' marijuana use for three years. They found that smoking marijuana increased the risk of both becoming newly psychotic and faring poorly if the person already had a diagnosis of psychosis. In 2004, a different Dutch team reviewed five other studies and found that cannabis use seemed to raise the risk of schizophrenia, especially in vulnerable people.[99] In 2007, a meta-analysis of data pooled from 35 other studies further strengthened the link. If a person smokes cannabis during his or her youth, this analysis found, there's a significantly increased risk of psychosis later in life.[100]

Other studies hammer this home. In 2010, Australian researchers found that teenagers who started using cannabis early, around age 15, and kept smoking for six years until they were 20 had more than twice the normal risk of psychosis.[101] In 2011, Australian researchers who analyzed pooled data from 83 studies concluded that cannabis users who develop psychosis do so at an earlier age (by about two years) than nonusers.[102] (Some researchers theorize that pre-schizophrenic teenagers self-medicate with cannabis because they find it improves their thought disorders, but it's difficult to tease apart cause and effect.[103])

But if marijuana use really does increase the risk of schizophrenia, this should show up in large populations as marijuana use has increased over the years. It doesn't.

In 2009, United Kingdom researchers from Keele University looked at the medical records of almost 600,000 people, more than 2 percent of the entire UK population age 16 to 44. They studied the years from 1996 to 2005, when there was a substantial rise in cannabis use. They found no evidence of increasing schizophrenia or psychoses in this time period.[104]

The latest thinking is that if there is a link between marijuana use and schizophrenia, it may be because of genetic susceptibility to psychosis that is exacerbated by marijuana use.[105] Marijuana users who have a specific variant of a gene called *AKT1*, for example, are at increased risk of psychosis. This gene controls an enzyme that affects the neurotransmitter dopamine. (Altered dopamine signals are involved in schizophrenia.) People who use marijuana every day and who have a particular variant of the *AKT1* gene are at seven times the normal risk of psychosis than people who use marijuana infrequently or not at all.[106]

Similarly, a specific variation in a gene called *COMT* also raises the risk of psychosis in people who use marijuana.[107] The *COMT* gene governs an enzyme that breaks down dopamine. People who used marijuana as teenagers and who also have one or two copies of the so-called Val form of the *COMT* gene are at higher risk of schizophrenia-type disorders as adults.

The genetic susceptibility idea was echoed in a carefully designed 2014 study by Harvard Medical School researchers. They found that having a family history of schizophrenia may be the underlying basis for schizophrenia in marijuana users, not smoking pot per se.[108]

The bottom line is that more research is needed on potential links between marijuana use and serious mental illness.[109,110] Meanwhile, the prudent take-home lesson is that adolescent, recreational users should be cautious, particularly if there is a family history of schizophrenia. But older people using marijuana medically probably need not worry.[111]

What are the risks of other psychiatric problems?

Research on potential links between cannabis and anxiety or depression is inconclusive. In 2002, Australian researchers reported that teenage girls who inhaled marijuana at least once a week were twice as likely as less frequent users to have depression or anxiety over the next seven years.[112] But other research shows that, while anxiety, paranoia, and disorientation do occur in new cannabis users, these problems are uncommon in regular users. Indeed, a systematic review of the data does not find a strong association between chronic cannabis use in young people and psychosocial harm.[113] In other words, the putative links between marijuana use and depression, anxiety, suicidal thoughts, and personality disorders in teenagers constitute unsettled science.[114]

What are the risks of cognitive problems?

Cognitive problems attributed to marijuana have also been a concern, but again, the jury is still out.

In 2002, researchers from Harvard's McLean Hospital studied 122 long-term heavy cannabis users and 87 people who had minimal cannabis exposure and subjected them all to a number of cognitive tests. As hypothesized, the people who started using cannabis earlier in adolescence did do more poorly on cognitive tests. But it's not clear how to interpret this. The heavy cannabis users may have been on a bad track to begin with. As the authors put it delicately in this and a subsequent study, these people may already have "eschewed academics and diverged from the mainstream culture."[115,116] In 2008, Australian researchers used MRIs to scan the brains of 15 men in their late 30s who had inhaled more than five joints a day for an average of almost 20 years. The men had not used other drugs or had any neurological problems. They were compared to 16 similar men who had not used cannabis. The brains of the marijuana group showed reduced volume in two areas key to emotional and cognitive functioning, the amygdala and the hippocampus, suggesting possible damage.[117]

In 2009, a different group of Australian and Irish researchers used fMRI scans and also documented changes. They found that several brain regions, particularly the anterior cingulate cortex and right insula, were underactive in chronic cannabis users.[118] This is troubling, as was a 2013 study from McLean Hospital that found that age of initial heavy use of marijuana was crucial, especially in terms of white matter development in the brain and greater impulsivity.[119]

In 2012, researchers from Duke University's Center for Child and Family Policy analyzed data on 1,037 people from birth to age 38 and found that those who were diagnosed with marijuana dependency as teenagers and who continued to use it had cognitive declines.[120]

NIDA says on its website that marijuana's effects include difficulty with thinking and problem-solving as well as disrupted learning and memory. When heavily used by young people, NIDA states, these effects on thinking and memory may be permanent, even if a person quits as an adult.[121]

This is pretty worrisome, to be sure. But other data suggest that once a person stops using marijuana, some cognitive changes like memory bounce back to normal.[122,123] When San Diego researchers pooled data from a dozen studies on 704 cannabis users and 484 nonusers, they found that while chronic marijuana users sometimes showed a decreased ability to remember new information, other cognitive functions weren't affected at all.[124] An Oxford University pharmacologist who reviewed the data concluded there is "little evidence" that long-term cannabis use causes permanent cognitive impairment and that, overall, when compared to other drugs used recreationally, cannabis is a relatively safe drug.[125]

What are the cardiac risks of marijuana?

Overall, the cardiac risk from marijuana appears small.

Marijuana can increase heart rate and blood pressure and can increase the risk of heart attack in the first hour after smoking, which suggests that people with uncontrolled hypertension or active heart disease should be cautious about marijuana use. Marijuana also lowers the resistance in blood vessel walls, meaning that if a person stands up suddenly, there can be a sudden drop in blood pressure. There have also been a few reports of minor strokes (transient ischemic attacks) right after marijuana use. But overall there appears to be no link between marijuana use and hospitalization or death from cardiovascular disease.[126,127,128]

What are the risks of respiratory problems?

Since the main way marijuana is taken in to the body is by inhalation, one of the persistent concerns has been whether smoked cannabis causes respiratory damage.

Obviously, smoking is not an ideal drug delivery system because of potential respiratory risk. (The good side of inhalation of *any* drug—whether marijuana or inhaled analgesia—is that if the goal is to get the drug to the brain quickly, inhalation does the trick.)

The challenge for researchers has been to tease apart potential respiratory damage from smoking marijuana from that due to smoking tobacco, because the same people often do both. New Zealand researchers studied 339 people from four different groups—those who smoked only cannabis, those who smoked only tobacco, those who smoked both, and those who smoked neither.[129] In 2007, they reported that smoking one marijuana joint had similar adverse effects (in terms of airflow obstruction) as 2.5 to 5 cigarettes, although inhaled marijuana was not linked to chronic obstructive pulmonary disease, as cigarettes are.[130]

In a 2012 American study of more than 5,000 men and women in four cities, researchers found that occasional and low cumulative marijuana use was not associated with adverse effects on pulmonary function.[131] In a higher tech study, Canadian researchers used smoking machines to compare the ingredients in smoke from tobacco and smoke from marijuana.[132] They found that ammonia was 20 times more prevalent in marijuana smoke, as were other substances, but different potentially harmful ingredients were less prevalent. In yet another study, a different Canadian team scoured 79 research papers on adverse effects of cannabis published from 1966 through 2004. Long-term, heavy cannabis smokers did contract more bronchitis. And inhaled marijuana did contain many of the same constituents as tobacco smoke, as well as higher concentrations of polyaromatic hydrocarbons, which are known carcinogens.[133]

But—and here's the surprise—the researchers couldn't find any lung damage in long-term users, nor any link between smoking pot and the cancers typically linked to tobacco smoking.

Is vaporizing better than smoking marijuana straight?

Yes.

Whatever the respiratory risks of smoking marijuana, they probably can be at least partially offset by vaporizing (inhaling marijuana smoke through a gadget that delivers just the vapor). This allows the active ingredient of marijuana, THC, to get into the bloodstream without toxic carbon monoxide, a constituent of both marijuana and tobacco smoke.

Vaporizing heats the cannabis to between 180 and 200 degrees Centigrade. This releases the cannabinoids on the surface of cannabis flowers and leaves but avoids the combustion (which happens at 230 degrees Centigrade or higher) that yields smoke toxins. In a pivotal 2007 study, California researchers asked 18 healthy subjects to inhale standardized marijuana for six days and measured the carbon monoxide in their expirations. When the subjects used vaporizers, they found little if any increase in carbon monoxide.[134] Researchers from the State University of New York at Albany confirmed the benefits of vaporizing in a 2010 study.[135]

Is marijuana lethal?

No.

Overall, marijuana has a good safety profile. In fact, there are no deaths attributable directly to marijuana, according to the federal Centers for Disease Control and Prevention.[136] In stark contrast, government figures show that nearly 500,000 Americans die prematurely every year from cigarette smoking and 88,000 die annually from excessive alcohol use.[137,138] Even NSAIDs (like ibuprofen) are more lethal than marijuana—killing thousands of Americans every year.[139]

The main reason marijuana is so nonlethal is that, unlike opioids, it does not cause respiratory depression. With marijuana, overdosing is extremely rare and is usually accompanied by the use of other drugs, such as alcohol, as McGill University researchers noted in a 2005 review.[140] In fact, a lethal dose of THC has never been reported. Two other large studies support this, showing no increase in deaths attributable to cannabis.[141]

This safety profile has held true for decades, as even an administrative law judge for the federal Drug Enforcement Administration (DEA) noted in 1988 in an official finding of fact: "There is no record in the extensive medical literature describing a proven, documented cannabis-induced fatality." (By contrast, the judge noted, aspirin causes hundreds of deaths a year.)[142]

Although marijuana does not kill directly, it can contribute to risky behavior, such as driving while stoned and drunk.[143]

Is marijuana a "gateway drug"?

Not really.

One of the most often-alleged risks of marijuana is that it is a "gateway" to other illegal drug use. This is only partly true. Because it is the most widely used illicit drug, marijuana is predictably the first illicit drug most people encounter, acknowledged a 1999 review by the Institute of Medicine, an arm of the National Academy of Sciences.[144] "Not surprisingly," the report said, "most users of other illicit drugs have used marijuana first."

But here's the catch. Most drug users *begin* their drug use with the legal drugs alcohol and nicotine. Because underage smoking and alcohol use typically precede marijuana use, the report said, marijuana is not the most common, and is rarely the first, "gateway" to illicit drug use.

Some studies on the gateway hypothesis yield mixed results, among them a 2006 study by New Zealand researchers.[145] They found that regular or heavy cannabis use was associated with an increased risk of using other illicit drugs, but this risk declined with age, and the causal mechanisms underlying the gateway hypothesis remain unclear.

In other words, for most people, marijuana is not a gateway drug; the main driver of drug problems is more likely to be the mental state of the user.[146] Put differently, it is not marijuana per se that leads to more serious drug use but a propensity to use drugs, period, that is the major factor.[147]

In addition, the fact that marijuana is still illegal in many states may underlie a progression to more serious drugs by "forcing" would-be marijuana buyers to buy from drug dealers, who also peddle "harder" drugs.[148]

In a major study using 24 years' worth of data from more than 1 million American teenagers in 48 states, researchers found *no evidence* that legalizing marijuana for medical purposes increased use among adolescents.[149]

The researchers, from Columbia University, used data from the Monitoring the Future survey of adolescent behavior funded by NIDA. They found that marijuana use by teenagers does not increase after a state legalizes medical marijuana; in states that have passed medical marijuana laws, adolescent marijuana use was already higher than in other states.

How many states have approved the medical use of marijuana?

The latest White House figures show that 23 states have now approved the medical use of marijuana.[150] By other tallies, 34 states and the District of Columbia permit some form of marijuana consumption for medical purposes.[151] Altogether, about 74 percent of the US population now lives in states where, one way or another, marijuana laws have been relaxed.[152] (Currently, four states plus Washington, DC, had approved the *recreational* use of marijuana as of February 2014.[153])

What is the status of marijuana in terms of federal law?

It's a work in progress.

President Obama was open-minded on the issue. In a 2014 interview with *The New Yorker,* Obama recalled his own use of marijuana "as a kid" and "up through a big chunk of my adult life . . . I don't think it is more dangerous than alcohol." Asked if he thought it was *less* dangerous, Obama said he thought it was "in terms of its impact on the individual consumer. It's not something I encourage, and I've told my daughters I think it's a bad idea, a waste of time, not very healthy." What really troubles him, he said, is the disproportionate arrests and incarcerations among minorities.[154]

In February 2015, Surgeon General Vivek Murthy also signaled a shift in federal thinking, acknowledging that there is "some preliminary data showing that for certain medical conditions and symptoms marijuana can be helpful. . . . We have to use that data to drive policymaking, and I'm very interested to see where that data takes us."[155]

Congress has also been increasingly positive toward marijuana. In December 2014, Congress quietly ended the federal government's ban on medical marijuana.[156] This means that federal agents are now prohibited from raiding retail marijuana sales operations in states where medical marijuana is legal.

But the DEA still sees things differently. The DEA continues to classify marijuana as a Schedule I drug under the Controlled Substances Act, which means it is considered to have no currently accepted medical use and a high potential for abuse. Other drugs in this, the "worst" category, are heroin, LSD, ecstasy, and peyote.[157]

The federal government's long-term anti-marijuana stance has seriously hampered marijuana research in this country. Without that research, the government claims it cannot reschedule marijuana.[158,159]

Actually, even the government may not be so sure marijuana is medically useless. In October 2003, the Department of Health and Human Services took out a patent on cannabinoids for potential use as antioxidants and neuroprotectants.[160]

Most telling, in April 2015, in a little-publicized move, the same department posted a notice announcing the availability of funding for the "therapeutic potential of cannabinoids and endocannabinoid system across a variety of pain conditions."[161]

Should marijuana be reclassified?

That's more a political than a medical question.

In 1995 and 2002, the Coalition for Rescheduling Cannabis filed petitions to have marijuana taken out of Schedule I, arguing that there *is* enough evidence of its medical usefulness that the government should not claim it has none.[162,163] It suggested that marijuana be regulated as a Schedule III, IV, or V (over-the-counter) substance or simply like alcohol or tobacco.

The petition cited 87 health-care or state government entities supporting medical marijuana use, including the American Academy of Family Physicians, the American Public Health Association, the National Association of [state] Attorneys General, the National Institute of Medicine, and many others. On July 8, 2011, nine years after the second petition, the DEA finally did rule—it denied the petition.[164,165]

In June 2011, the Global Commission on Drug Policy, an august, nonpartisan group, also recommended the rescheduling of certain drugs—cannabis, coca leaf, and MDMA (ecstasy)—because the current scheduling has "obvious anomalies."[166]

But other groups disagree, among them Smart Approaches to Marijuana, which argues that rescheduling marijuana is "neither necessary nor desirable."[167]

What is "synthetic marijuana"?

In popular culture, so-called synthetic marijuana products (which are *not* the same as pharmaceutical marijuana substitutes) are being sold illegally with names such as Spice, K2, fake weed, Yucatan Fire, Skunk, Moon Rocks, and the like. These products are illegal and very dangerous.[168,169,170,171,172]

What are the major pharmaceutical forms of marijuana?

In the early 1970s, there was a perfect balance of THC and CBD in natural cannabis plants from Afghanistan. This balance produced a modulatory effect. The CBD blocked the intoxication, rapid heartbeat, and sedation of THC alone but also boosted the good effects—pain control and reduced inflammation.[173]

Drug companies have been trying to come up with manufactured equivalents. Several have tested CB2-only drugs, but, so far, the results have been disappointing.[174,175,176,177] As for the two synthetic cannabis medications on the US market, the jury is out. Both drugs act on both CB1 and CB2 receptors, and Marinol (dronabinol), which contains THC, can produce a high if the dose is sufficient. So far, both Marinol and Cesamet (nabilone) are approved only for anorexia and nausea, though they can be used "off-label" for pain, as well as for improving sleep.[178] Marinol has shown to have efficacy as an add-on to opioid therapy in some people with chronic pain.[179]

Other marijuana-related substitutes being studied include dexanabinol, CT-3 (ajulemic acid), cannabinor, HU-308, HU-331, rimonabant (Acomplia), and taranabant (MK-0364), but none have been FDA-approved.[180]

In truth, nothing manufactured appears to be as effective—or as quick—for pain relief as inhaling the cannabis plant itself.[181,182] Cesamet is perceived to produce more undesirable side effects, to take a long time to work, and to be more expensive than smoked cannabis.[183] It can be hard for people to find the right dose because of individual variations in how digestive systems absorb the drug.[184]

Another marijuana substitute is Sativex, made by a British company (now handled by a Japanese company) and legally available in a number of countries, but not yet the United States, though it has been "fast-tracked" for cancer pain relief by the FDA.[185] The company, GW Pharmaceuticals, announced in January 2015 that in the first of three trials, the drug did not reduce pain in cancer patients better than placebo.[186] Sativex is scientifically interesting because it is not a synthetic but an oral spray that contains extracts of the marijuana plant itself.[187]

Can marijuana cut deaths from opioids?

It appears so, and this is important.

The idea that marijuana might help prevent opioid overdoses first took hold in California when researchers began testing marijuana in chronic pain patients in a federally funded study. Patients inhaled vaporized marijuana three times a day for five days while taking their regular opioid pain relievers. In 2011, the researchers reported that pain was significantly reduced—by 27 percent—when inhaled marijuana was added to the opioid regimen. This suggests that marijuana may have a synergistic effect, potentially allowing pain patients to obtain significant pain relief with lower doses of opioids, but this needs to be replicated in other studies.[188]

In another potentially significant finding, in July 2014, Pennsylvania researchers analyzed opioid overdose deaths from 50 states between 1999 and 2010 and tracked the implementation of medical marijuana laws in the 10 states that had such laws during this period.[189] The team found that states that had legalized medical marijuana had a 24.8 percent lower average annual opioid overdose death rate compared to states that had not. In 2010, that translated to about 1,729 fewer deaths than expected.

Should marijuana be legalized?

In a word, yes.

Even some conservative thinkers now believe it should. In March 2012, Pat Robertson told *The New York Times*, "I really believe we should treat marijuana the way we treat beverage alcohol. I've never used marijuana and I don't intend to, but it's just one of those things that I think: this war on drugs just hasn't succeeded."[190]

More recently, Republicans Jeb Bush, former Florida governor, and Ted Cruz, a senator from Texas, admitted to using marijuana in their younger days, and Kentucky senator. Rand Paul has not been specific but noted he was no "choir boy" in college.[191]

More and more Americans want legalization.[192,193] A Gallup survey in October 2011 showed that 50 percent of Americans think the use of marijuana should be made legal, up from 46 percent the year before.[194] By 2014, that number was up to 51 percent.[195] This attitude has been growing steadily since Gallup first asked the question in 1969, when only 12 percent of Americans favored legalization.

In July 2014, the *New York Times*, in an editorial titled, "Repeal Prohibition, Again," the newspaper said flatly, "The federal government should repeal the ban on marijuana."[196] It went on to say

We reached that conclusion after a great deal of discussion among members of the *Times*'s editorial board, inspired by a rapidly growing movement among the states to reform marijuana laws. There are no perfect answers to people's legitimate concerns about marijuana use. But neither are there such answers about tobacco and alcohol and we believe that on every level—health effects, the impact on society and law-and-order issues—the balance lies squarely on the side of national legalization.

The editorial also noted that the social costs of current federal marijuana policy are vast: there were 658,000 arrests for marijuana possession in 2012, according to FBI figures, compared with 256,000 for cocaine, heroin, and their derivatives. This cost is borne disproportionately by young black men. The *Times* added that "the evidence is overwhelming that addiction and dependence are relatively minor problems, especially compared with alcohol and tobacco" and that moderate marijuana use "does not appear to pose a risk for otherwise healthy adults." The paper did advocate prohibition of sales for people under 21.

On the other side, some groups, including the American Society of Addiction Medicine, strongly oppose legalization, arguing that "addiction associated with cannabinoids is a significant public health threat and marijuana is not a safe product to use."[197]

In a position paper issued in January 2015, the American Academy of Pediatrics reaffirmed its position against legalization of marijuana and its opposition to medical marijuana "outside the FDA regulatory process" but also recommended that marijuana be decriminalized and that exceptions be made for some children who may benefit from cannabinoids and cannot wait for a meticulous and lengthy research process.[198,199]

Would legalizing marijuana violate international conventions?

In 1961, many of the world's countries signed an agreement called the Single Convention on Narcotic Drugs, and, by 1972, 184 nations had agreed to be parties to the treaty.[200] If the

United States, or any other signatory to the treaty, legalized marijuana possession and production for nonmedical purposes, this would be a violation of the treaty. However, each country can make its own decisions about what any punishment would be.

Are there potential economic advantages to legalization?

Yes.

In 2005, a Harvard University economist calculated that legalizing marijuana could save $7.7 billion per year in enforcement of marijuana prohibition, most of which would accrue to budget-strapped states but some to the federal government as well. Also, taxing legal marijuana would yield $2.4 billion if it were taxed like all other goods—that figure would be a whopping $6.2 billion if it were taxed comparably to alcohol and tobacco.[201]

Those estimates have been updated.[202] In 2010, the calculation suggested that legalizing drugs would save roughly $48.7 billion per year in enforcement costs. Approximately $13.7 billion of the savings would result from legalizing marijuana, $22.3 billion from legalization of cocaine and heroin, and $4.0 billion from legalizing other drugs.

There's a downside to this, though. In states that have embraced legal marijuana, some marijuana shops say they have to pay very high federal income taxes because of an old law originally designed to stop drug dealers from claiming smuggling costs and couriers as business expenses.[203]

So is marijuana a law-and-order issue or a health and human rights issue?

That depends on one's point of view.

But consider the evolution of thinking by Gustin L. Reichbach, a pancreatic cancer patient and justice of the State Supreme Court in Brooklyn. In May 2012, Reichbach wrote an op-ed piece in the *New York Times*. He noted that he did not "foresee that, after having dedicated myself for 40 years to a life of the law, including more than two decades as a New York State judge, my quest for ameliorative and palliative care would lead me to marijuana." Despite ongoing mainstream treatment, he continued,

> nausea and pain are constant companions. Every drug prescribed to treat one problem leads to one or more drugs to offset its side effects. Pain medication leads to loss of appetite and constipation. Anti-nausea medication raises glucose levels, a serious problem for me with my pancreas so compromised. Sleep, which might bring respite from the miseries of the day, becomes increasingly elusive.

To his surprise, Reichbach found that

> inhaled marijuana is the only medicine that gives me some relief from nausea, stimulates my appetite and makes it easier to fall asleep. The oral synthetic substitute, Marinol, prescribed by my doctors, was useless. . . . I find a few puffs of marijuana before dinner gives me ammunition in the battle to eat. A few puffs more at bedtime permits desperately needed sleep.

"This is not a law and order issue; it is a medical and a human rights issue," the judge went on. "Because criminalizing an effective medical technique affects the fair administration of justice, I feel obliged to speak out as both a judge and a cancer patient suffering with a fatal disease."

He concluded his piece poignantly: "Medical science has not yet found a cure, but it is barbaric to deny us access to one substance that has proved to ameliorate our suffering."[204]

Judge Reichbach died two months later.[205]

6

WESTERN MEDICINE TREATMENTS FOR CHRONIC PAIN

Overall, how effective is Western medicine at treating chronic pain?

Not very, which is especially discouraging for people with low back pain, headaches, joint pain, and neck pain—the biggest causes of chronic noncancer pain in America.[1] Indeed, more than 28 percent of all people with chronic pain have pain in their lower back and another 15 percent have it in their neck.[2] (This includes both *axial* pain, which doesn't radiate down an arm or leg, and *radicular* pain, which does.)[3]

In recent years, chronic pain has resulted in dozens of highly promoted interventions, thousands of studies, millions of lost work days, and billions of dollars spent, according to *The Spine Journal*.[4] But more often than not, these treatments do not eliminate pain and functional limitations, according to researchers from the Oregon Health and Science University, the University of Washington, Stanford University, Harvard Medical School, and other institutions.[5]

Unfortunately, "Few nonsurgical interventional therapies for low back pain have been shown to be effective in randomized, placebo-controlled trials," concluded a separate team of researchers.[6]

Something must help, at least somewhat. What about electrical stimulation?

Electrical stimulation is actually just a fancy way of rubbing. It activates nonpain nerves that respond to temperature, pressure, or vibration, and this, in effect, swamps the nervous system, inhibiting the transmission of pain signals.[7]

Animals, including people, have instinctively used rubbing, or electrical stimulation, to ease pain for millennia. Dogs lick or rub a hurt paw to make it feel better. Mothers rub children's stubbed toes and bumped knees. Rubbing a sore area fits with the famous *gate control theory* proposed in 1965 by Ronald Melzack and Patrick Wall.[8]

How does electrical stimulation work?

Nerves carrying painful signals from the periphery and those carrying sensations of touch and vibration all converge in a structure in the spinal cord called the dorsal horn. When nonpain nerves are stimulated, this can overwhelm incoming signals from pain nerves, in essence, jamming the signals. The new signals change the message heading toward the brain from "here comes pain" to "here comes a gentle vibration."[9] In other words, electrical stimulation induces white noise so that the brain doesn't recognize the incoming signal as pain.[10]

What is "scrambler" therapy?

This therapy involves neurocutaneous stimulation with a device that delivers signals with surface electrodes placed on the skin. In one small trial involving patients with postherpetic neuralgia (pain following shingles), pain scores diminished fairly quickly.[11] In another study of 147 patients with various kinds of chronic pain, more than one-third benefitted from this type of therapy.[12,13]

What is TENS? Is that electrical stimulation too?

Yes.

TENS stands for transcutaneous electrical nerve stimulation. A small device is used to send mild electric currents noninvasively through the skin. It is inexpensive and very low risk.[14]

Does it work?

Probably not. A 2007 meta-analysis of pooled data from 38 studies showed that TENS was effective for musculoskeletal pain.[15] But a slew of other studies found no clinically significant benefit.[16,17,18,19,20] In March 2012, Medicare announced it would withdraw most coverage of TENS treatments.[21]

What about PNFS? That's another type of electrical stimulation, right?

Yes.

PNFS, or peripheral nerve field stimulation, is a slightly more invasive approach than TENS. It involves stimulating peripheral nerves by putting electrodes through a needle under the skin. After implanting the electrode, surgeons withdraw the needle; the electrode is hooked up to a power pack implanted under the skin. A drawback of this procedure is that the electrodes can migrate away from where they were inserted. On the other hand, it can help some people. In a 2014 paper, Austrian researchers used PNFS devices on 105 people with chronic low back pain and found statistically significant improvements in reported pain and reductions in medication use.[22]

What about PNS?

A still more invasive technique is peripheral nerve stimulation (PNS). PNS is sometimes done through a needle but more often is done through an open surgical incision through which an electrode is placed directly on a nerve. (As with PNFS, the electrode is hooked up to a battery pack implanted under the skin.) Typically, a temporary electrode is implanted for a week to see whether it reduces the patient's pain; if it does, a permanent one is then implanted.[23]

The procedure can provide short-term relief, but it's not clear how good the long-term results are.[24] These electrodes can migrate, too, especially if they are inserted in areas—like limbs—that move a lot. So, once again, the results are mixed.

And SCS?

The big gun in this whole approach is spinal cord stimulation (SCS). An electrode is implanted either through a needle or an open operation into the epidural space around the spinal cord. This is a permanent implant, and the procedure carries the risk of complications such as infection, bleeding, and electrode migration; surgeons usually insert a temporary implant first to see whether the patient will truly benefit.

Sadly, the main reason people undergo spinal cord stimulation is because they have "failed back syndrome"; that is, they have already had back surgery for pain and ended up worse than where they started. Sometimes this occurs because back surgery was the wrong approach in the first place. Other times, back surgery was appropriate but didn't work. There is growing concern that surgeons are doing too many back surgeries.[25,26,27]

On the plus side, several studies have shown positive results for SCS.[28,29,30] Most recently, it has been shown to significantly reduce the pain of diabetic neuropathy.[31] If chronic pain is severe, SCS may be worth a try. Both SCS and PNS appear to be more useful for neuropathic pain than other kinds of pain.[32]

And, finally, what about deep brain stimulation?

There's one last type of electrical stimulation for pain control, and it's the most invasive: deep brain stimulation (DBS), in which an electrode is surgically implanted deep in the brain. This procedure has been used for 50 years for various purposes, but it's still not clear how well it works for chronic pain relief. The research is encouraging, with the best results occurring when electrodes are placed in brain regions called the periventricular/periaqueductal gray and the sensory thalamus/internal capsule.[33] Stimulating the motor cortex, as opposed to deeper layers in the brain, may also help.[34] But this is brain surgery, and not to be undertaken lightly.

How is transcranial magnetic stimulation for pain different?

Transcranial magnetic stimulation is a *noninvasive* procedure in which plastic-covered coils of wire are placed on the skull to induce electrical currents that activate specific brain regions.[35] It can be used both to diagnose certain chronic pain conditions and, increasingly, to treat them.

With TMS, the physician passes a strong electrical current through a coil of wire. This creates a magnetic field that goes through the skin, scalp, and skull.

In the brain, the electrical stimulation from TMS can decrease the excitability of specific regions involved with pain. And because the skin and skull bone don't respond to the magnetic field, strong currents can be applied without causing pain. This is in stark contrast to electroconvulsive shock therapy (ECT), which uses direct electrical currents—not magnetic fields—to treat severe depression. Unlike TMS, ECT does cause intense pain, which is why ECT is administered under general anesthesia.

TMS has considerable potential for pain relief, in part because it can target brain regions very specifically, unlike drugs, which travel all over the body. So far, most research on TMS has focused on depression. But researchers are now studying its potential for pain relief, including handheld devices that a patient can place on his or her head at critical times, such as at the onset of a migraine to abort the headache's progress.

One early French study suggested that TMS can provide short-term pain relief in some patients.[36] A 2004 study similarly showed that TMS can temporarily reduce chronic pain, as did a 2009 study.[37,38] A 2009 meta-analysis of five other studies showed that TMS works better for pain originating in the central nervous system than for pain from the peripheral nervous system.[39]

More recently, a 2010 study of people with migraines showed TMS reduced pain two hours after treatment.[40] A 2010 randomized study in Barcelona involving 39 people with neuropathic pain following spinal cord injury showed that TMS, combined with "walking visual illusion," significantly reduces pain.[41] (In the illusion group, patients watched a movie of legs walking. It was projected under their own head and trunk and reflected in a mirror so that they could imagine that they were walking.) And a small French–Brazilian study in 2011 showed that repeated TMS treatments significantly reduced pain intensity in people with fibromyalgia.[42]

But it remains to be seen how long these pain-relieving effects last.[43,44,45] Some research has been discouraging, including a 2010 Cochrane Collaboration review that found that, at least at low frequencies, TMS was *not* effective for chronic pain.[46]

Repetitive TMS (rTMS), in which a series of pulses is delivered in rapid succession in a single session, may be more promising.[47] A technique in which TMS is combined with peripheral nerve stimulation may also prove more promising than TMS alone.[48]

But a potential drawback of TMS is that, so far at least, it can only reach brain regions close to the skull.

What is transcranial direct-current stimulation? Does it work for pain?

This relatively new technology involves sending a low electrical current to the brain to treat a number of conditions, including pain.[49] So far, studies have been small and meta-analyses have been inconclusive. The technique (called tDCS) is not yet approved by the US Food and Drug Administration, but doctors at a few hospitals in New York and Boston have been trying it. At Beth Israel Deaconess Medical Center in Boston, researchers have shown that the technique can reduce pain in people with spinal cord injuries and fibromyalgia.[50,51] Other researchers are finding encouraging results for pain in multiple sclerosis, trigeminal neuralgia, poststroke pain, back pain, and fibromyalgia.[52,53]

What about injections for pain relief? What works and what doesn't?

Overall, research suggests that injections carry small benefits and can be expensive.[54,55,56,57] But there are several different kinds of injections.

Do steroid injections reduce pain?

Epidural steroid injections, that is, injections into the space around the spinal cord, have been used for more than 50 years for low back pain—and often for neck pain as well. In fact, for low back pain, epidural steroid injections are the most common intervention in pain clinics worldwide.

However, of around 35 controlled studies evaluating such injections, only a bit more than half show any benefit, according to a 2011 editorial in the *British Medical Journal*.[58] Even in the trials that did show a benefit, the benefit was short-lived— 8 to 12 weeks.

The occasion of this editorial was a study by Norwegian researchers, who divided 461 chronic low back pain patients into three groups.[59] One group received "sham" (fake) injections under the skin in the back. The second group received real injections into the epidural space but, instead of medicine, the injections contained only saline (salt water). The third group received genuine steroid injections. The result? There were no differences among the groups in disability, pain, or quality-of-life scores.

Unfortunately, that fit with previous studies. In the 1990s, studies in the *New England Journal of Medicine* had already questioned the value of steroid injections.[60,61] Some data had suggested that steroids might work if combined with local anesthetics.[62] But in 2007, a review of 30 studies of low back pain concluded that steroid injections did not help, a finding repeated by other studies in 2008 and 2010.[63,64,65,66]

In a more recent blow to epidural steroids, a Johns Hopkins University team studied 84 people with low back pain and sciatica in 2012 and found that steroids may provide some pain relief. But this relief is modest and short term and may involve nothing more than normal healing.[67] In a 2013 study, other researchers also found that epidural steroids didn't help.[68]

Worse, it's not just *epidural* steroids that can't be counted on to relieve spinal pain. Steroid injections into *facet joints* don't work so well either.[69] (Facet joints are the bony protrusions that stick out from vertebrae and help stabilize the spine.)

Steroid injections can also carry risks, as a 2012 outbreak of fungal meningitis showed. More than 100 people with low back pain came down with meningitis after being injected with contaminated steroid injections, prompting criticism, once again, that such injections are among the most overused procedures in the United States.[70]

Do "nerve block" injections reduce pain?

Doctors often inject ordinary local anesthetics such as lidocaine and bupivacaine, the same medications that dentists use before drilling teeth, into painful areas. Called "nerve blocks," these injected anesthetics can be used both diagnostically, to stop pain temporarily in a particular area so that doctors can determine exactly which nerves are causing the pain, and therapeutically, to temporarily control pain.[71] Typically, local anesthetics are tested first, and, if they work, the doctor may inject alcohol or phenol (carbolic acid) as a longer-lasting block. Increasingly, doctors now use continuous peripheral nerve blocks, in which a particular nerve is blocked for longer periods with the anesthetic supplied by a portable pump.[72]

Nerve blocks can reduce pain, perhaps for as long as 6 to 12 months. But there are risks, including paralysis and damage to the arteries that supply blood to the spinal cord and accidental injection of alcohol or phenol into an artery.[73] Overall, the evidence for effectiveness is scant.[74]

Do Botox injections reduce pain?

Some people with chronic pain, including pain from muscle spasms, are helped by injections of Botox, or botulinum toxin. Botox is also used—and, since 2010, has been FDA-approved—to treat chronic migraine.[75] But a 2012 study in the *Journal of the American Medical Association* found that Botox had only small benefits for chronic migraine.[76] And Botox is *not* FDA-approved for treating temporomandibular joint disorder (TMJ).[77] On the other hand, small preliminary studies suggest Botox may help with arthritis pain.[78]

Until recently, researchers have not understood why Botox might reduce pain from migraines. A 2014 study by Harvard Medical School researchers suggests that the toxin selectively calms sensory neurons that detect pain caused by mechanical pressure.[79] In other words, Botox seems to block the ability of nerves to become activated by mechanical pain, that is, pressure.[80]

What are "trigger point" injections? Do they work?

Saline (salt water), local anesthetics, or other substances are often injected into "trigger points," which are hyper-irritable spots in taut bands of muscle. There's little evidence that these trigger point injections work for low back pain.[81] The jury is still out on whether they work for myofascial pain, a type of chronic pain in the tissue surrounding muscle.[82]

What is "prolotherapy"? Does it work?

Prolotherapy involves injections of irritating substances into ligaments to trigger a controlled, acute inflammation that supposedly can lead to stronger ligaments and reduced pain, after an initial period of increased pain. But a Cochrane Collaboration review of five studies on prolotherapy came out negative,[83] as did another review in 2008 and another in 2009.[84,85] A 2011 review by Ohio State University researchers found prolotherapy "promising" but noted that much more research is needed.[86]

What about pain in knees and other joints? Do injections help?

Maybe. In 2012, Cleveland Clinic researchers looked at published studies on knee injections and concluded that steroid injections for rheumatoid arthritis and osteoarthritis were linked to significant improvements in pain and function, with the benefit sometimes lasting as long as a year.[87] Injections of a lubricating substance called hyaluronic acid may have even longer-lasting effects.

But Swiss researchers reporting in 2012 pooled data from 89 other studies involving 12,667 adults with knee osteoarthritis and found the studies were too poorly done to draw conclusions.[88] Injections of hyaluronic acid did reduce knee pain moderately, but it made it worse in some people. A 2013 study showed that steroid injections did not help with tennis elbow.[89]

On the other hand, injections with platelet-rich plasma may help. This technique involves taking a patient's own blood, spinning it down, separating out and concentrating the platelets, then reinjecting them into the painful joint. In one 2013 Indian study in people with osteoarthritis of the knee, the technique proved helpful, although the benefit diminished after six months.[90] In another 2013 study, researchers also found a decrease in pain, although other outcome measures were mixed.[91]

Can injections or infusions with stem cells help with pain relief?

Stem cells are increasingly being studied for pain relief. (Stem cells are undifferentiated cells that can give rise to many other kinds of cells that arise by differentiation.) In one trial, people with knee arthritis who had had surgery to remove part of the meniscus experienced some improvements in pain after such injections.[92]

Stem cell injections may also help replace lost cartilage in osteoarthritic joints. While doctors have tried to replace lost cartilage by simply harvesting cartilage cells from a patient's own joints, growing up the cells in culture, then reinjecting them, that method appears to work primarily if the area of lost cartilage is small.[93] But a recent study by MIT researchers published in the *Proceedings of the National Academy of Sciences* suggests that stem cells can be used to nudge bone marrow cells to behave like cartilage, a promising approach to cartilage repair.[94]

Researchers at Duke University have shown that a certain type of stem cell called bone marrow stromal cells relieves neuropathic pain (pain caused by nerve injury) in mice.[95] Unlike pain relief achieved through standard drugs, the pain relief from this technique lasts for four to five weeks. The stem cells appeared to work by raising levels of a natural, body-made chemical called TGF-B, an anti-inflammatory chemical that people in pain typically do not make enough of.[96] Other researchers have shown that stem cells can reduce the pain of degenerative disc disease.[97]

Why not just kill pain nerves to get rid of pain?

It's a tempting idea, but nerve-killing, technically called *denervation*, is not very helpful for chronic pain. To be sure, there's no shortage of ways to kill nerves—for example, injections of alcohol or phenol, scalpels, lasers, and radio-frequency waves.[98] But while wiping out nerves can sometimes relieve chronic pain, it also can make things a lot worse. If a doctor cuts a peripheral nerve, the result can be a neuroma, an overgrowth of nerve tissue that itself can become a source of pain. (There is an important exception to this though: cutting branches of the trigeminal nerve in the face can reduce the pain of *tic douloureux*, a painful, stabbing pain—at least until the nerve regrows).[99]

But the biggest problem with nerve killing is that peripheral nerves are multifunctional. If doctors cut a nerve, this can deprive the patient of all sorts of necessary incoming sensory stimulation, not just pain.

Moreover, cutting doesn't work for all types of pain. If the pain is neuropathic—that is, caused by damage to the nerve itself—cutting nerves can make things worse. When nerves grow back, they are sometimes more damaged than before.[100]

On the other hand, cutting nerves *may* help with nonneuropathic pain, such as pain from arthritis. When arthritis causes pain in the facet joints along the spine, the tiny peripheral nerves feeding the facet joints can be cut safely. In fact, cutting these tiny nerves has become standard for treating some types of facet joint pain.[101]

It's also possible to cut nerves in the spinal cord. This technique, called *cordotomy*, has been used—with some success—for nearly 100 years, especially in advanced cancer patients who don't have long to live. Traditionally, cordotomies have been done under direct vision with a small scalpel, so the surgeon can see what he or she is doing. When it works, the operation reduces pain from the spot where the spinal nerve was destroyed to about three levels (vertebrae) down the spinal cord.[102] But it's far from risk free: cutting spinal nerves can lead to paralysis and phantom limb pain.[103,104]

Is radio-frequency ablation a better way to kill nerves?

It may be, and, increasingly, cordotomies are being done with radio-frequency energy. In this method, a needle containing an electrode is inserted through the skin (under X-ray guidance) toward the spot where the nerve is believed to be, and then the radio-frequency current is turned on, killing the nerve. Radio-frequency energy produces a kind of controlled burn—the heat is generated from the friction of electrons vibrating rapidly. Radio-frequency ablation is a more accurate way to kill nerves than simply dousing them with alcohol or other chemicals, which can ooze all over, hitting neighboring nerves as well as target nerves.

But the trouble is, doctors can't see what they're doing. They can use X-rays to find the patient's bony structures, and they can use their general knowledge of anatomy to make an educated guess as to where the target nerves *probably* are in relation to the bones. But the nerves themselves do not show up on X-rays.

To get around this, doctors first inject a nerve block. If the numbing medication yields pain relief, doctors know they are in the right place and can go on to kill nerves with radio-frequency waves. In some cases, it may not be necessary to do this preliminary step—and skipping it could save money, as a 2010 study suggested.[105] But this study also revealed a depressing reality: More than half of the patients did not get lasting pain relief from radio-frequency ablation.

In some situations, like pain in the sacroiliac joint in the lower back, radio-frequency ablation may provide a reasonable option, according to a 2010 review of 10 studies.[106] But another review concluded that radio-frequency ablation doesn't help.[107] Once again, better research is needed.[108]

What about surgery for back pain? Does that help?

Sometimes, but sometimes, as already noted, it can make things worse, creating the condition called failed back syndrome.

Back surgery is a veritable gold mine for doctors. The average cost of such surgery is about $70,000 per patient.[109] In recent years, billions of dollars have been spent worldwide on surgery for back pain.[110]

For spinal fusion surgery, for instance, in which two adjacent vertebrae are grafted together to reduce pain and increase stability, rates of surgery soared dramatically in the 1980s and even more so in the 1990s, according to Dartmouth Medical School researchers. In fact, between 1992 and 2003, Medicare spending for lumbar surgery more than doubled, even though this explosion of surgical procedures far outpaced any evidence that it worked.[111]

Couldn't doctors do a better job at figuring out who needs surgery?

Ideally, yes, but it's not that easy. There's surprisingly little correlation between what X-rays and MRI scans show and the back pain a person feels. Some people with horrible MRIs feel little or no pain, while others with severe pain have fine scans.[112]

Is surgery contraindicated for some types of neck and back pain?

It depends. With neck pain that stems from irritated nerve roots (radiculopathies), surgery may help somewhat if the goal of the surgery is to decompress the area around the nerve root, though studies show little benefit to surgery compared to nonsurgery after two years.[113] The best treatment is often conservative—acupuncture, physical therapy, chiropractic, and time—in other words, treatments that can make a person feel better while the body heals itself.

When is surgery the right treatment? How well does it work?

These are thorny questions, and the data are mixed. In a clinical trial conducted between March 2000 and November 2004, Dartmouth researchers randomized 501 back pain patients from 13 spine clinics in 11 states to surgery or nonoperative care.[114] All had been deemed good candidates for surgery on the basis of persistent pain and scans that showed herniated spinal discs. (Discs are the soft, cushioning material that act as shock absorbers between vertebrae. If there is a tear in the outer ring of a disc, the soft, central part of the disc bulges out, releasing inflammatory chemicals that can cause severe pain. A bulging disc can also press directly on small nerves or the spinal cord itself, which also causes pain.)

The goal of the study, published in 2006, was to see which worked better—surgery or nonsurgical care—up to two years later. The first surprise was that things didn't work out as planned. Half of the patients who had been randomly assigned to have surgery opted out for one reason or another. And almost a third of those who were *not* supposed to have surgery did. Even more surprising was that over the course of two years, there was substantial improvement in pain and disability symptoms in *both* groups. The people who had surgery did a little bit better, but the differences were small and not statistically significant, although the surgery patients did feel better faster.

In a 2009 review of a 161 randomized trials, researchers from the Oregon Health and Science University concluded that outcomes are so iffy that doctors should tell potential surgery patients the truth: that there is only a small to moderate average benefit from surgery.[115] The majority of people who undergo surgery do not wind up with minimal or no pain.

To be sure, the Oregon team was talking specifically about fusion surgery, not other types of back surgery such as discectomy (the removal of a herniated disc).[116] The evidence is better for discectomy and decompression for spinal stenosis than for fusion in people with nonspecific, nonradicular low back pain. Surgery can also be a good solution for other problems, including trauma and deformity, in which the biggest need is to restore stability to the back.[117,118,119]

But overall, fusion in the lower back appears to offer limited benefits, and artificial discs rate the same tepid assessment.[120] Basically, spinal fusion should be a last, not first, resort for back pain stemming from degenerated discs.[121]

What is the relationship between pain and depression?

Complicated, real, and bidirectional. The lifetime prevalence of depression in people with chronic pain is much higher than in people without, and people who are depressed are at higher risk of developing chronic pain after an injury or other pain problem. People who are depressed also tend to feel more pain at lower thresholds (lower intensity of pain stimulus) than nondepressed people.[122] (For alternative medicine treatments for pain with depression, see chapter 7.)

Overall, epidemiological evidence suggests that in the general population, at least 20 percent of people in chronic pain have a serious mood problem. The good news is the flip side— 80 percent don't. In other words, mood problems are not inevitable. Among pain patients in primary care clinics, the number of mood problems is higher: about 40 percent. And of those who go to pain clinics, it's even higher—60 to 75 percent.[123] This still means that one-quarter of people in miserable pain do not become seriously depressed or anxious.

For years, psychiatrists and psychologists—wedded to the theory of "somatization"—that is, the tendency to express emotional distress in terms of bodily symptoms—leaned heavily toward the view that depression comes first and is expressed as chronic pain later.

In one fascinating experiment, researchers from Oxford University and Harvard Medical School gathered 20 healthy volunteers.[124] The volunteers rated their mood on standard scales, then underwent "mood induction," which meant reading depressing statements such as "I feel worthless" while listening to depressing music (Prokofiev's "Russia Under the Mongolian Yoke," which was played at half speed.) In the alternate condition, they read neutral statements such as "Cherries are fruits" and listened to cheerier music, the largo movement from Dvorak's "Symphony from the New World." During all this, the volunteers lay in fMRI scanners and were given painful (heat) stimulation.

During the down moods, the volunteers had more negative thoughts and rated their pain as significantly more unpleasant. The volunteers' brain scans reflected this—marked by increased activity in the prefrontal cortex, anterior cingulate cortex, and hippocampus. In other words, being depressed made the pain experience worse.

But the emerging view today is that in most cases where people have both pain and depression, it's the chronic pain that comes first and mood problems later.[125]

Many studies have looked at this chicken-and-egg question, but one of the most important involved people with disabling occupational spinal injuries. The researchers found that psychiatric disorders were much more likely to develop *after* the onset of the work injury, which shows that the injuries are probably the initiators, not the consequences, of mood problems.[126] Another example is a 2012 Boston study showing that women with migraine headaches are 40 percent more likely than women without to develop depression.[127] In other words, most of the time, depression *follows* the onset of chronic pain and is not preceded by it.[128]

Even when this isn't true, there is little clinical benefit to be gained by debating which came first. When people have bad chronic pain and cannot be active, do their jobs, sleep, or even hang out with friends, that's just plain depressing—and a vicious cycle.[129] And when a person is caught up in that cycle, neuroimaging studies show, his or her natural pain relievers (endorphins) become less effective, as do exogenous opioids (drugs prescribed for pain).[130,131]

So if someone has both pain and depression, should both be treated?

Yes. If one treats just the depression, pain may get a bit better but not as much better as the depression. And just treating the pain if there is still depression is not optimal, either. Depression should be treated too.[132,133,134]

Does that mean taking antidepressant drugs?

Not necessarily. There are many good, nondrug treatments such as cognitive behavior therapy for the double-whammy of pain and depression. (See chapter 7.)

As for the *pharmacological* approaches, the rule of thumb for treating both pain and depression is to use antidepressant medications that have independent analgesic (pain-killing) effects as well as effects on mood.[135,136,137]

There are different classes of antidepressants. The class known as selective serotonin reuptake inhibitors (SSRIs) and serotonin and norepinephrine reuptake inhibitors (SNRIs) work against depression by boosting levels of these neurotransmitters in the brain.

These drugs, especially the SNRIs, can also somewhat damp down pain signals traveling up to the brain from the peripheral nerves and spinal cord. SNRIs that work against the "double hurt" of pain and depression include duloxetine (Cymbalta), venlafaxine (Effexor), and milnacipran (Savella). (Cymbalta is approved not just for neuropathic pain but also for musculo-skeletal pain, including back and joint pain.)[138,139,140]

Older-style antidepressants called tricyclics can also help with both pain and depression. These include nortriptyline (Pamelor and Aventyl), amitriptyline (Elavil, Endep, and Vanatrip), and desipramine (Norpramin and Pertofrane).[141,142,143] In some cases, the pain-relieving features of tricyclics may kick in at lower doses than that needed for the antidepressant effects. An additional benefit of tricyclics is that they can also enhance sleep, which is often disrupted in people with chronic pain.[144]

Beyond antidepressants, other classes of drugs may also help with both pain, particularly neuropathic pain, and depression. One example is the class of drugs called anticonvulsants (antiepileptics), such as Neurontin, though this is more powerful at pain relief than mood improvement. Similarly, antipsychotic drugs such as olanzapine (Zyprexa) might help with both pain and mood problems, though this is controversial.[145] For severe muscle spasms, carisoprodol (Soma), cyclobenza- prine (Flexeril), and diazepam (Valium) may help.[146,147,148,149]

Sorting out exactly how well the different drugs work has not proved easy. In one review, Australian researchers pooled data from six studies and separately examined data from two other studies. They concluded that antidepressants were not effective at relieving low back pain.[150] But a team from the United Kingdom also did a review and asked spe- cifically whether the antidepressant duloxetine (Cymbalta) relieved the pain of diabetic neuropathy or other chronic pain.[151] They came to a more encouraging conclusion. At 60 milligrams a day (but not at lower doses), Cymbalta was ef- fective against both diabetic neuropathy and fibromyalgia, although side effects forced 16 percent of patients to stop taking it.

Another review looked at 61 randomized controlled trials of 20 different antidepressants in 3,293 people with neuropathic pain.[152] It concluded that tricyclic antidepressants such as Elavil were somewhat effective against pain, as is venlafaxine (Effexor), but that there was only limited evidence of efficacy for SSRIs such as Prozac.[153]

The best approach is to combine antidepressants with "self- management" skills such as coping with negative emotions, increasing physical activity, and muscle relaxation.[154]

What can be done for pain triggered by cancer chemotherapy?

Sometimes cancer-related pain comes not from the spreading cancer itself but from the treatments, specifically chemother- apy, used to treat it.

In most cancer patients, chemotherapy does not lead to pe- ripheral neuropathy (damage to pain nerves). But in some it does, and, of these, some people wind up with numbness and pain, which can be severe. Painful peripheral neuropathy is the most common reason for stopping chemotherapy.[155]

Many different chemotherapy drugs can trigger neuropathy.[156] They are believed to cause pain by poisoning mitochondria—tiny powerhouses that produce energy in every cell—in the axons of nerve cells. (Axons are long projections from nerve cell bodies that carry pain signals from one nerve cell to the next.)

If chemotherapy actually *killed* all sensory nerve fibers, patients would feel no pain in response to a stimulus. The reason chemotherapy patients do feel pain is that nerve cells still function to some extent but with a severe energy deficit because of the injured mitochondria. Instead of dying outright, the axons degenerate, which causes them to fire spontaneously, causing pain. There are two drugs that may protect mitochondria against this damage —at least in animals. One is a dietary supplement called acetyl l-carnitine (ALCAR), which has to be taken with chemotherapy, not afterward.[157] The other is olesoxime, which is currently under study for various neurological problems.[158] Cannabidiol, a component of marijuana, may also guard against chemotherapy-induced pain.[159]

Are there new pain relievers in the pipeline?

Yes, though not nearly enough.

At Harvard Medical School and Duke University Medical Center, researchers are working on chemicals called resolvins, protectins, and maresins that have the potential to shut down runaway inflammation, a major cause of pain. These lipid mediators are derived from omega-3 polyunsaturated fatty acids, the kind found in fish oils.[160,161,162,163,164,165] Interestingly, low-dose aspirin (81 mg) has been shown to boost the production of resolvins, the chemicals that dampen down the inflammatory response.[166]

Around the world, other scientists are working on ways to block cytokines and chemokines, substances made in the body that promote potentially painful inflammation.[167]

Adenosine, already on the market as Adenocard, Adenoscan, and Pentostatin, is another promising strategy, though the current formulations have drawbacks for pain control. Adenosine is made naturally in the body from the energy molecules adenosine triphosphate and adenosine monophosphate. Recently, researchers have shown that acupuncture reduces pain in part by triggering release of adenosine.[168]

At the University of North Carolina, researchers are looking for other ways to boost adenosine, including an enzyme called PAP (a so-called ectonucleotidase).[169,170,171,172,173] Some research suggests that adenosine may turn out to be more powerful than opioids.[174,175,176]

Another potential drug target is an enzyme called AC1, a chemical messenger made inside nerve cells that enhances transmission of pain signals. Blocking this enzyme is a potential way to block pain.[177,178,179]

Monoclonal antibodies, specialized molecules designed to attach to tiny markers (proteins) on cells, may also help control pain by blocking nerve growth factor, a chemical made in the body that stimulates nerves to grow.[180,181,182] The drug company Pfizer has spent years testing its monoclonal, called tanezumab, for knee and hip pain from osteoarthritis.[183,184] In two studies, tanezumab showed promise in reducing the pain of this type of arthritis.[185]

Another encouraging study was published in 2010 in the *New England Journal of Medicine*.[186] In this study, researchers looked at 450 people with knee arthritis who took tanezumab and found it reduced pain a remarkable 45 to 62 percent, far more than the 30 percent achievable with opioids. But a number of patients wound up requiring joint replacement surgery, perhaps because the drug reduced pain *too* much, allowing patients to overdo physical activity and damage their knees and hips to the point where they needed surgery.[187,188] It's also possible that the problem was caused by taking tanezumab along with nonsteroidal anti-inflammatory drugs (NSAIDs).[189]

At the request of the US Food and Drug Administration, Pfizer suspended its studies of tanezumab for arthritis, back pain, and diabetic neuropathy in the summer of 2010.[190] In the fall of 2012, Pfizer was allowed to resume its studies.[191] The latest news on this has been good. In 2013, a new study found that tanezumab was better than placebo at reducing hip pain.[192]

A totally different monoclonal antibody aimed at a sodium channel called Nav1.7 (which triggers pain signals) appears to block pain signals at both peripheral nerve and spinal cord sites.[193]

Can drugs not specifically designed to treat pain help reduce it?

Yes. A number of drugs initially designed for other problems can also reduce pain and can legally be used for this purpose. In some cases, pain relief has been added as an official FDA-approved "indication" for these drugs; in others, the drugs are not specifically approved for pain but can be used off-label to treat pain.

Anti-epileptics are a prime example. Gabapentin (sold as Neurontin, Fanatrex, Gabarone, Gralise, and Horizant), can help with pain, as can its close cousin, pregabalin (Lyrica), which is often prescribed for people with fibromyalgia. (Both gabapentin and pregabalin are FDA-approved for pain.)[194,195,196]

What about over-the-counter pain relievers: What's the story?

There is a huge irony here. While many people are highly fearful of opioids, they are often not fearful enough of over-the-counter drugs, most notably NSAIDs and acetaminophen (Tylenol). These drugs can be effective for moderate pain and are an appropriate first step for many types of pain. Acetaminophen, however, appears to be relatively ineffective for low back pain.[197]

But, while opioids, for all their much-publicized risks, do *not* cause specific organ toxicity such as damage to the liver, kidneys, brain, or other organs, acetaminophen and NSAIDs can.[198,199]

What are the risks of acetaminophen?

Acetaminophen is the active ingredient in Tylenol. But it is not just in Tylenol, and that's part of the problem. Acetaminophen is everywhere —mixed in with cold and cough medications as well as with opioid-combination drugs such as Vicodin, Lortab, Percocet, Tylox, and Darvocet.

In 2008, 25 billion doses of acetaminophen were sold in the United States, according to the FDA. While acetaminophen is reasonably safe used by itself, because it is in so many other medicines and because it has such a narrow therapeutic index (the dose at which it helps is very close to the dose at which it harms), it is potentially dangerous.

In fact, acetaminophen is a leading cause of acute liver failure. There are roughly 30,000 hospitalizations a year linked to acetaminophen overdose, according to government figures.[200] It's especially dangerous in combination with alcohol, which is why the FDA says flatly, "Do not drink alcohol when taking medicines that contain acetaminophen."

In January 2011, the FDA issued a safety announcement asking drug manufacturers to limit the amount of acetaminophen in combined products to 325 milligrams per dose. It also demanded that labels carry a "boxed warning" to highlight acetaminophen's potential for severe liver damage.[201]

But the FDA only specified that this limitation apply to *prescription* acetaminophen, not over-the-counter formulations, a serious problem, according to an investigative report from ProPublica, the online news organization.[202]

Counterintuitive as it sounds, many chronic pain patients have to limit their usage of products like Vicodin, not because of the opioid (hydrocodone) it contains but because of the acetaminophen.

A significant public controversy arose in 2013 when the FDA, after a long review and against the vote of its own advisory committee, approved a new painkiller, Zohydro, whose chief attribute is that it contains only hydrocodone, with no acetaminophen added. Anti-opioid activists were outraged, while many pain specialists applauded the action, arguing that the hydrocodone-only drug was a step forward.[203] (The fierce controversy led to poor drug sales, prompting the maker of Zohydro, Zogenix, to sell the drug to another company in March 2015.[204])

How safe are NSAIDs?

NSAIDs, the most famous of which is ibuprofen, the main ingredient in Motrin and Advil, are hardly risk-free either. NSAIDs can cause severe and potentially fatal bleeding in the stomach and intestines, among other problems.[205] Since April 2005, the FDA has required boxed warnings on NSAID labels. In its 2009 guidelines, the American College of Gastroenterology noted that gastrointestinal bleeding and perforation send 100,000 people to the hospital every year and cause 7,000 to 10,000 deaths, particularly in people at high risk.[206]

Unfortunately, as the American Geriatric Society noted in its 2009 guidelines, increasing age puts people at high risk.[207] The risk of a serious NSAID-associated gastrointestinal bleed for people age 16 to 44 is 5 in 10,000, with the risk of death being 1 in 10,000; for people 75 and over, the risk of a serious bleed is 91 in 10,000, and the risk of death from the bleed, 15 in 10,000.[208] The implication is sobering: some older people in pain cannot take these drugs and must turn to opioids for lack of better options. But advocating for opioids in older people poses a potential conflict of interest: Since 2009, the American Geriatrics Society has received $344,000 in funding from opioid manufacturers, according to the *Milwaukee Journal Sentinel* in a May 2012 report.[209]

NSAIDs have also been linked to a small but potentially important increased risk of atrial fibrillation (an abnormal heart rhythm that can increase the risk of stroke) in a huge Danish study in 2011 involving more than 32,000 patients.[210] Other studies have also raised concern about cardiac risks with NSAIDs. In 2010, a different Danish study showed that NSAIDs can raise the risk of cardiovascular problems, with rofecoxib (Vioxx) and diclofenac (Voltaren, Cambia) among the more dangerous and naproxen (Aleve) among the least.[211]

In 2011, Swiss researchers analyzed pooled data from 31 trials involving 116,429 patients who had taken different NSAIDs.[212] Once again, Vioxx was associated with the highest risk of heart attack; ibuprofen was linked to the highest risk of stroke, and naproxen appeared to be the least harmful.

Canadian researchers also recently reviewed NSAID use in 2.7 million people—the largest study to date—and came to similar conclusions, namely that naproxen (Aleve) and low-dose ibuprofen were the least likely to raise cardiovascular risk whereas diclofenac (Voltaren, Cambia) carried more risk.[213] British researchers, too, have studied the issue, finding in a meta-analysis of 639 randomized studies involving more than 300,000 patients that NSAIDs raise by about one-third the risk of major vascular events such as nonfatal heart attacks, strokes, and death.[214] In July 2015, the FDA strengthened its heart attack warnings for NSAIDs.[215]

What about topical pain relievers applied to the skin?

Topical treatments have an obvious advantage over pills. With swallowed pills, the chemical ingredients pass through the stomach, enter the bloodstream, and then pass through the liver, where they are processed in such a way that the concentration of active medication is reduced by as much as half.

This means that half the drug is wasted before it can begin to fight pain.[216]

When medications are absorbed through the skin, lower doses can be used. The simplest topicals are ice, to reduce inflammation, and heat, to relieve muscle soreness. Over-the-counter topicals include "counter-irritants" containing menthol or camphor such as Icy Hot and Biofreeze. [217]

Capsaicin, the substance used in pepper sprays for crowd control, is also useful.[218,219,220,221,222] It reduces pain by destroying a particular type of pain nerve fiber called unmyelinated C-fibers.[223]

There are also creams and patches containing the anesthetic lidocaine.[224] These, too, can be effective for minor pain. On the other hand, salicylate skin creams such as Aspercreme or Bengay Arthritis do not seem to help with osteoarthritis pain.[225]

Can gene therapy reduce pain?

Potentially, yes. Gene therapy is an experimental technique that uses genes to treat or prevent diseases. Researchers are exploring techniques such as replacing a gene that causes disease with a healthy copy of the gene, inactivating a gene that is malfunctioning, or even introducing a new gene into the body.

At Massachusetts General Hospital, researchers are using a virus called adeno-associated virus (AAV) to treat schwannomas, benign tumors that grow in nerves, causing severe pain. The AAV carries a gene that makes an enzyme that chews up the tumors.[226] Other researchers are testing a form of the herpes virus to carry pain-dampening genes to nerves.[227]

In a different twist on gene therapy, Stanford University scientists are exploring a sophisticated technique called optogenetics to turn off pain signals using light. The researchers take the AAV virus and insert into it a gene that makes a light-sensitive protein called an opsin. Using a needle as thin as a human hair, the researchers then inject the opsin-carrying virus into the sciatic nerve of mice. The mice undergo minor surgery to lightly compress the sciatic nerve, a standard technique for inducing neuropathic pain.

A couple of weeks later, the mice are put in a cage with a Plexiglas bottom so that light shone from below can reach the animals' paws. When the researchers use one opsin and shine *blue* light through the glass, the animal's pain nerves fire more, thus increasing pain. When the researchers use a different opsin and shine *yellow* through the glass, pain is inhibited.[228]

What is the bottom line?

Western medicine has a long way to go to come up with safer, more effective pain control approaches. It will take considerable federal and private investment to make serious progress.

7

COMPLEMENTARY AND ALTERNATIVE MEDICINE TREATMENTS FOR CHRONIC PAIN

What is "complementary," "alternative," or "integrative" medicine?

The names are confusing, but people now use the terms "complementary" and "integrative" to refer to acupuncture, massage, herbs, guided imagery, hypnosis, meditation, yoga—the list goes on and on—to convey the idea that these techniques are used along with, not instead of ("alternative"), mainstream medicine.[1]

How popular is complementary medicine?

Very, regardless of quite uneven evidence of efficacy. Almost 40 percent of adults now use complementary medicine, and chronic pain is the main reason they do so.[2,3,4,5,6,7]

The most recent data show that Americans are increasingly ingesting fish oil, probiotics, and melatonin and shying away from products with more questionable efficacy, such as glucosamine/chondroitin and echinacea. Yoga is soaring, now practiced by 21 million adults; meditation attracts 18 million; and chiropractic remains extremely popular, with 20 million aficionados among adults.[8]

Overall, how effective is complementary medicine?

It varies tremendously, but overall, the evidence of efficacy is limited.[9]

When *Consumer Reports* surveyed 45,601 subscribers online and asked how well complementary medicine worked for them, the readers reported that complementary medicine was "far less helpful than prescription medicine" for most of the conditions studied.[10]

Despite the caveats, the evidence for complementary medicine appears strong enough that in September 2014, the National Institutes of Health and the Department of Veterans Affairs launched a five-year, $21.7 million project involving 13 research projects to assess the effectiveness of chiropractic, self-hypnosis, meditation, and other techniques as alternatives to opioids for returning troops. (Roughly half of troops returning from Iraq and Afghanistan suffer from chronic pain, a higher rate than the civilian population.)[11,12] The US Navy and Army already use acupuncture for people with chronic pain.[13,14,15]

A sampling of the promising treatments are as follows: For fibromyalgia, gentle exercise such as t'ai chi, yoga, massage, and acupuncture can help.[16] For headache, some dietary supplements (see later discussion) can help, as may relaxation training, biofeedback, acupuncture, and spinal manipulation.[17] For low back pain, cognitive behavioral therapy (CBT), exercise, spinal manipulation, and interdisciplinary rehabilitation can be beneficial, as can acupuncture, massage, and yoga.[18] For osteoarthritis, exercise—particularly t'ai chi—and strength training can be somewhat effective, and, in some cases, acupuncture may help too.[19] For rheumatoid arthritis, omega-3 fatty acids seem to help.[20]

What is acupuncture?

Acupuncture is the ancient Chinese practice of inserting thin needles into one or more of 360 specific points in the skin that lie along 12 putative "meridians" through which a postulated kind of energy called qi (pronounced "chee") flows.

In Chinese theory, the beneficial effects of acupuncture come from releasing blocked qi.[21,22] Despite multiple attempts, no one has ever been able to find the acupuncture meridians along which qi is supposed to flow.

Does acupuncture work?

Yes. There is growing evidence that it helps with some conditions and is more than a placebo, though some skeptics disagree.[23,24]

For pain relief specifically, can acupuncture help?

The answer is a qualified yes.[25]

In terms of published studies, it's hard to sort things out, in part because there is a publication bias at work.[26,27,28,29] Over the years, a gullible mainstream press has hyped stories on acupuncture, taking its cues from the scientific and medical journals, which are also more likely to publish positive studies. Thus negative or inconclusive results may never see the light of day. When researchers, such as those from the Cochrane Collaboration, an international, nonprofit group that analyzes research results, take the time to look systematically at multiple studies at once, the data on acupuncture's effectiveness become less clear.

One of the biggest problems in trying to assess acupuncture is deciding what kind of control groups to use: Do we just compare acupuncture to no acupuncture? That could miss a lot of subtleties, including whatever benefits might accrue from the calming ritual of acupuncture procedures. A better way is to compare real acupuncture—sticking needles into known acupuncture points—to "sham" or fake acupuncture. Sham acupuncture can be done in various ways—sticking a toothpick on the skin in real acupuncture points but not penetrating the skin, sticking needles into the skin but on points other than acupuncture points, and even using fake, nonpenetrating needles on real points. (With fake needles, the needle slides up inside the shaft so it looks like it's inserted.)

Some researchers also use lasers for sham acupuncture. Unlike fake acupuncture with a toothpick, which slightly stimulates the skin and hence the nervous system, cool laser acupuncture creates no apparent sensation, thus making it a potentially better control.[30] In still another twist, some researchers compare real electro-acupuncture—in which small electric currents are passed through the needles—with a sham procedure in which researchers insert the needles and turn on an electrical stimulating machine, with all the bells and whistles but without actually connecting the wires.

By rights, if Chinese theory is correct, real acupuncture should work better than sham acupuncture. And sometimes it does. With postsurgical pain, a systematic review of 15 randomized, clinical trials found that real acupuncture resulted in less need for supplementary opioids than sham procedures and that patients receiving real acupuncture reported significantly less pain.[31] For osteoarthritis of the knee, too, real acupuncture, but not sham, may improve pain and function.[32,33] That's true for low back pain and myofascial pain in the jaw as well.[34,35,36]

But in other cases, strange things happen when researchers compare real to sham acupuncture. The most perplexing is that while acupuncture often *is* superior to usual care for pain relief, sham acupuncture is nearly as effective.[37,38] In one intriguing Seattle study, researchers gathered 638 adults with chronic low back pain and randomly assigned them to customized acupuncture, standard acupuncture, sham acupuncture, or no acupuncture (usual care).[39] The acupuncture groups were treated twice weekly for three weeks, then once weekly for four weeks. Eight weeks later, everyone felt much better—*except* the folks receiving no acupuncture. A year later, all the acupuncture groups were still doing better, at least in terms of improved back function, though some of the initial improvement in pain symptoms was gone.

What does it mean if fake acupuncture is as good as the real thing? That any old kind of skin stimulation helps? That it's the placebo effect doing the magic? That some unknown mechanism is at work? And, if the benefit is real, who cares?[40]

Scientists do.

In a series of now-classic experiments, Chinese researchers linked the circulatory systems of two animals but performed acupuncture on only one. Both animals showed evidence of less pain, leading to the hypothesis that this might be due to increased endorphins circulating from one animal to the other.[41] (Endorphins are endogenous opioids that the body makes in response to pain.)

Scientists reasoned that if acupuncture *did* stimulate endorphins, a drug that blocks the effects of opioids would also block the pain-relieving effects of acupuncture. That drug, naloxone, did exactly that, as shown in a number of experiments.[42,43,44,45]

More recently, University of Michigan researchers using brain scanning technology have found that real acupuncture, but not sham, increases so-called mu-receptors (receptors into which opioids fit) in parts of the brain governing pain, another sign that the endogenous opioid system may be at work.[46]

Acupuncture may relieve pain by releasing other chemicals as well. In mice, acupuncture stimulates adenosine, a powerful, endogenous pain reliever.[47] In one human study, too, researchers found that acupuncture stimulates release of adenosine, though only if the needle is placed in the so-called zusanli point (located about four finger-widths below the knee near the shin bone) and only if the needle is rotated.[48] Curiously, caffeine consumption may inhibit adenosine.[49]

Of all the research on acupuncture, perhaps the most encouraging are the studies involving brain scans—functional magnetic resonance imaging (fMRI), positron emission technology, and other methods. These techniques can show in real time what happens during acupuncture, especially in brain regions involved in pain processing.

Researchers from Massachusetts General Hospital in Boston have found that in people with wrist pain, acupuncture can reduce pain and numbness and change patients' brain scans back to a more normal pattern.[50,51,52,53,54,55,56] Other Boston researchers have shown that people receiving real acupuncture, but not sham, showed changes in nerve pathways descending from the brain.[57]

So can we conclude that acupuncture really works for pain?

Some reviewers still think the scientific evidence for pain relief via acupuncture is only "fair" or of no benefit.[58,59] But other data, including two Cochrane Collaboration reviews, came to more positive conclusions. One review found acupuncture somewhat effective for neck pain.[60] A separate review of 35 randomized studies found that real acupuncture (but not sham) yielded short-term relief for low back pain.[61] Yet another review of 15 randomized controlled studies concluded that real acupuncture was more effective than sham and reduced the need for pain-relieving drugs in postoperative patients.[62]

Most recently, researchers from the Sloan-Kettering Cancer Center reviewed data on nearly 18,000 patients from previously published randomized studies and found that for chronic back and neck pain, osteoarthritis, chronic headache, and shoulder pain, real acupuncture was superior to both sham acupuncture and no acupuncture, a clear indication that acupuncture is more than a placebo.[63,64]

Is acupuncture safe?

Yes, overwhelmingly so. But, like anything else, it is not totally without risks. Serious adverse effects are rare, but there have been isolated cases of pneumothorax, or collapsed lungs.[65,66] Since 2000, by one researcher's count, there have been five acupuncture-related deaths in published reports.[67] But that's out of millions and millions of treatments. Less dramatic and also rare side effects include a temporary worsening of symptoms, fatigue, soreness, bruising, muscle twitching, lightheadedness, and emotional release.[68]

Does massage help with chronic back and neck pain?

Yes.

Like acupuncture, massage therapy is booming. It is a multi-billion-dollar-a-year industry, backed by fair to strong evidence that it is reasonably effective for low back pain.[69,70,71,72,73,74,75,76] For chronic pain, massage therapy has the support of the American College of Physicians and the American Pain Society.[77]

For *acute* pain, unfortunately, there's no good evidence that massage helps very much.[78,79]

Is any one kind of massage better than any other?

That's not so clear.

In one study, researchers from Seattle compared Swedish massage, which uses long strokes, kneading, and deep circular movements, to "structural" massage, which is intended to correct soft-tissue abnormalities. (Structural massage requires more training and is more often reimbursed by health insurers.)

Both massage groups had one session a week for 10 weeks. A control group of patients received usual care. By the end of the 10-week study, both massage groups showed significant improvements in disability and the "bothersomeness" of pain. They functioned better, spent fewer days in bed, and used less anti-inflammatory medication.[80] But there was no difference *between* the two massage groups.

Other researchers have found evidence that Swedish massage may do something special—perhaps by triggering the release of beneficial hormones. In a Los Angeles study, researchers assigned 53 healthy adults to one session of Swedish massage for 45 minutes or a 45-minute session of light touch with the back of a hand.[81] (Light touch was virtually a placebo.) Blood samples were taken before and after the sessions to determine levels of certain hormones and white blood cells.

Curiously, there was no difference between the groups in levels of the stress hormone cortisol, as one might expect with general stress reduction. But those who received the Swedish massage did show significant decreases in a blood pressure regulating hormone (arginine-vasopressin) and significant decreases in certain proinflammatory chemicals called cytokines.

In another study, researchers at 15 US hospices studied 380 patients with advanced cancer and randomly assigned them to massage or light touch therapy for six 30-minute sessions over a two-week period.[82] Both groups experienced immediate improvements in pain and mood, although the benefits were greater for the massage group.

Massage for neck pain seems to provide more benefit with longer and more frequent sessions. Recently, researchers found that two to three 60-minute sessions per week yielded more pain relief than fewer or shorter sessions.[83] Sixty-minute sessions, even just once a week, also yielded significant improvement in the pain from osteoarthritis of the knee.[84]

The bottom line is this: consumers clearly love massage therapy—they rate it (along with yoga and Pilates) as equal to prescription medication for low back pain.[85]

Do energy healing techniques help with pain?

Probably not.

To be sure, the idea that there is some kind of "vital energy" in and around us is thousands of years old and is prevalent in many cultures. The Indians call it "prana," the Chinese "qi" or "chi," and the Japanese "qi." Practitioners of johrei, a Japanese healing ritual, call it "divine light" energy.[86] In the West, we may simply call it "spiritual energy."

There are extravagant claims for these therapies—and hardly any data. But there are some hints that they may help with pain. A Cochrane Collaboration review of 24 studies of various touch therapies found that, though the data were skimpy, touch therapies might help with pain reduction.[87] California researchers reviewed 13 studies of various energy therapies and found evidence for reducing pain intensity, though they acknowledged the positive effects may be indistinguishable from a general relaxation effect.[88]

British skeptics Simon Singh and Edzard Ernst, authors of the provocative 2008 book *Trick or Treatment*, take a dim view of spiritual healing in general, calling energy healing "utterly implausible."[89]

And then there's therapeutic touch, which involves the practitioner placing a hand on or near the patient to stimulate the patient's "energy field" to enhance healing. In a now-famous experiment designed by a nine-year-old girl, Emily Rosa, and published in the *Journal of the American Medical Association*, 21 practitioners of therapeutic touch placed their hands on a table. A towel was hung strategically in front of them so they couldn't see what was going on. An investigator on the other side of the towel then held a hand over one of the practitioner's hands. The idea was to see if therapeutic touch practitioners could detect energy changes and figure out which of their own hands the investigator's hand hovered over. The "therapeutic touch" practitioners flunked badly, guessing right only 44 percent of the time.[90]

Does spinal manipulation (chiropractic) help with back pain?

It may, though the research is mixed.

Spinal manipulation—performed by chiropractors, osteopathic physicians, and physical therapists—is a method of applying controlled force to a joint in an effort to restore health.[91,92,93] It is the most popular form of complementary medicine for back pain. It's inexpensive (roughly

$60 a visit), and, in some cases, is covered by insurance.[94,95,96,97] Some medical guidelines include it as one option for low back pain.[98,99,100]

Some research suggests that spinal manipulation along with strengthening exercise may work as well for low back pain as prescription nonsteroidal anti-inflammatory drugs (NSAIDs) plus exercise, though other data comparing manipulation to exercise don't show much difference.[101,102,103]

An Australian study showed that spinal manipulation worked better for back and neck pain than acupuncture or medications such as NSAIDs or acetaminophen.[104] One review of six randomized controlled trials of osteopathic manipulation showed the treatment significantly reduced low back pain.[105]

Other research shows different results. In a University of California, Los Angeles study, researchers randomized 601 people with low back pain to spinal manipulation or standard medical care. People receiving chiropractic (or physical therapy) were more likely to *perceive* improvement in symptoms, but there were no *clinically meaningful* differences.[106] A meta-analysis of results from 26 randomized controlled trials came to similar conclusions.[107]

One British randomized trial compared exercise, spinal manipulation alone, manipulation followed by exercise, and regular care in 1,334 people with back pain. After three months, the researchers did find that manipulation was the best treatment—*if* it was combined with exercise.[108] In a Brazilian and Australian study, researchers randomly assigned 240 people with low back pain to general exercise, special exercises to strengthen the trunk, or spinal manipulation. It did not settle the debate. By 6 and 12 months later, the groups were equivalent.[109]

Neck pain, as opposed to low back pain, is a bit more complicated. An Australian study of 183 people with neck pain found manipulation was more effective than exercise therapy or standard care, and other studies came to similar positive conclusions.[110,111,112] But, as often happens in complementary and alternative medicine, some studies were of such poor methodological quality that it's hard to trust the results.[113]

There is also a small but lingering safety question about chiropractic for neck pain. There have been 26 reported deaths after chiropractic treatment for neck pain. Presumably, the deaths occurred because abrupt twisting of the neck can dissect (tear) the vertebral artery, potentially triggering a stroke.[114] (If an arterial dissection is already silently in progress, any sudden jerk of the head can lead to problems, not just chiropractic treatments.)

Other researchers have also tried to calculate the risk from neck chiropractic, generally finding it's tiny but not zero. One research team found that the risk of an arterial dissection following chiropractic was *one per 5.85 million* cervical manipulations.[115,116,117,118,119,120] But the debate continues. In a pair of opinion pieces in the *British Medical Journal*, one camp argued that neck chiropractic is "unnecessary and inadvisable" and the other that "manipulation benefits people with neck pain."[121,122]

Can pain be reduced through diet?

Somewhat.

A preliminary, 12-month, gluten-free diet, for instance, has recently been shown to reduce the pain of endometriosis in women.[123] In theory, a ketogenic (high-fat, low-carbohydrate) diet may also have potential benefits for reducing pain.[124,125]

Eating a healthy diet, of course, is a cornerstone of good health in general, and there are a few specific dietary habits that may be extra important if one has chronic pain. The most obvious, especially for inflammatory pain such as arthritis, is to follow what health guru Andrew Weil calls the "anti-inflammatory diet."[126,127]

An anti-inflammatory diet involves eating all the usual fruits and vegetables but also ingesting the right ratio of polyunsaturated fatty acids. These are the omega-3s, which come from fatty, cold-water fish, walnuts, canola, soy and flax seed oil, and the omega-6s, which come chiefly from corn and safflower oils.

Why are omega-3 fatty acids important?

Earlier in human history, we ate pretty close to a 50/50 ratio of omega-6 to omega-3 fatty acids. Now we consume way too many omega-6s and too few omega-3s.[128] Most fast food is loaded with the former and lacking in the latter. The goal is to fix this balance by increasing omega-3s. That's because omega-6s increase inflammation and omega-3s decrease it. In the body, omega-6 fatty acids are converted to chemical substances that rev up the immune system and inflammatory process. This is great for fighting infections but bad for problems like arthritis. Omega-6s also boost blood clotting, which is terrific if a person is bleeding to death but not so good in terms of creating blood clots that can lead to heart attacks or strokes.

Some data suggest that fish oils—from real fish or supplements—may help combat the inflammation of rheumatoid arthritis. One observational survey looked at rheumatoid arthritis patients taking at least 1200 milligrams a day of fish oil. The oil contained eicosapentaenoic acid and docosahexaenoic acid. Almost 60 percent of the patients reported decreases in pain and were able to discontinue use of NSAIDs.[129] (Fish oil supplements vary significantly, so buyer beware.)[130] Also, while the omega-3s in fish oil can reduce arthritis symptoms, they do not appear to slow progression of the disease process itself.[131]

The science is still emerging, but omega-3 fatty acids also appear to be precursors to resolvins, chemicals that shut down the inflammatory process, a potential benefit for reducing inflammatory pain.[132,133,134]

Does vitamin D help reduce pain?

Maybe.

Vitamin D is the famous "sunshine" vitamin, so named because our bodies synthesize it in response to sunlight. Vitamin D, which is actually a hormone, has long been proposed as a pain reliever, as well as a way to protect bones against osteoporosis and fractures that can cause pain. Vitamin D may also protect against a condition called osteomalacia, a softening of the bones that can lead to widespread bone pain.[135]

But making science-based recommendations for vitamin D has proven to be complicated.[136]

In 2010, after reviewing more than 1,000 published studies, the Institute of Medicine (IOM) issued new recommendations for daily vitamin D intake, at levels some endocrinologists (the specialists who treat osteoporosis, osteomalacia, and vitamin D deficiency) found puzzling.[137] The IOM recommendations called for 600 International Units (IUs) a day for adults, or 800 a day for adults 71 and over. (The IOM says that the highest safe dose of vitamin D is 4,000 IUs a day.) But whether 600 to 800 IUs a day is really enough, especially for people who live in less sunny, northern latitudes, is a subject for debate. After the IOM released its guidelines, the Endocrine Society questioned whether those were adequate because so many Americans are deficient in vitamin D.

In 2011, the Endocrine Society came out with its own guidelines.[138] These called for babies to take 400 to 1,000 IUs a day; for children age 1 to 18 to take 600 to 1,000 IUs; and for adults over 18 to take 1,500 to 2,000 IUs a day.

What about vitamin D for pain relief, not just for meeting daily requirements?

The problem is that there is limited data on vitamin D and pain.[139] One 2010 European study—based on questionnaires sent through the mail—did suggest that men whose vitamin D levels were low were more likely to report chronic pain, specifically musculoskeletal pain.[140]

Randomized, controlled clinical trials of vitamin D are hard to come by. There was a German review of four studies, but those studies weren't methodologically good enough to allow firm conclusions.[141] More encouraging is a study by researchers at Washington University in St. Louis. They found that giving extra vitamin D relieved joint and muscle pain in a specific situation—women with breast cancer who were taking drugs called aromatase inhibitors.[142] Studies in India and Turkey also suggest that high doses of vitamin D may relieve chronic pain in arthritis patients.[143,144] A systematic review and meta-analysis involving a total of 215,757 people by South Korean researchers showed higher levels of vitamin D were associated with lower risk of developing rheumatoid arthritis and lower severity of disease, but these were observational, not interventional, data.[145]

A randomized, controlled Italian trial showed that high-dose vitamin D may relieve menstrual cramps.[146] In addition, a small study from Emory University showed that giving vitamin D to veterans with chronic pain improved pain scores, sleep, general health, and social functioning, though this study had no control group.[147] A California study of nearly 500 people with multiple sclerosis showed that higher vitamin D levels were associated with lower risk of new symptoms and disability, though, again, this was not an interventional study.[148]

And what of the idea that vitamin D can prevent painful fractures? A large 2012 analysis of 11 studies involving more than 31,000 people showed vitamin D supplementation was effective, but only somewhat, at preventing fractures.[149,150]

More recently, a presentation by British researchers at a 2014 rheumatology conference suggested that low levels of vitamin D were associated with the development of widespread pain, but these results were inconclusive because it was impossible to separate the potential effect of vitamin D from confounding factors such as depression, obesity, and physical inactivity.[151]

Is any one type of vitamin D better than any other?

That's still an open question. A few years ago, researchers thought the D3 form (cholecalciferol) was better than the D2 form (ergocalciferol). But now, it seems to be a draw. In 2011, a Cochrane Collaboration review of 50 studies involving 94,148 patients did find that D3, but not D2, was linked to a lower risk of overall mortality. But these researchers didn't look at chronic pain specifically.[152] Other studies say it makes virtually no difference which form a person takes, or even whether the vitamin is consumed as a supplement or in vitamin D–fortified orange juice.[153,154]

How good are the tests for vitamin D deficiency?

There is still some debate about the accuracy of blood tests for vitamin D (the 25-hydroxy vitamin D test). Newer assays, although they are approved by the US Food and Drug Administration, can be inaccurate and may lead to an overestimate of vitamin D deficiency.[155]

Is there a bottom line on vitamin D?

Sort of.

Despite the paucity of research data, some pain specialists are convinced by their own clinical experience that high doses of vitamin D can help select pain patients.

But there are also reports of adverse side effects with high doses. A study of older women showed that those taking a very high dose of vitamin D—500,000 IUs once a year—actually broke *more* bones than those taking a placebo. It's unclear why, though it's possible that women in the high-dose group felt better and were thus more mobile, which led to their falling, and breaking bones, more often.[156,157]

The bottom line is that it's worth giving vitamin D a try, but don't exceed the 4,000 IU daily limit unless a doctor supports it.

Do other supplements help reduce pain?

The best-known dietary supplement advertised to help pain, particularly arthritis pain, is the combination known as glucosamine-chondroitin.

Too bad it doesn't work.

In 2006, a team led by researchers from the University of Utah reported in the *New England Journal of Medicine* on a carefully designed project called the GAIT study. The researchers randomly assigned 1,583 people with symptomatic knee osteoarthritis to receive daily doses of either 1,500 milligrams of glucosamine, 1,200 milligrams of chondroitin sulfate, both together, 200 milligrams of celecoxib (Celebrex), or placebo for 24 weeks. All participants were allowed to take up to 4,000 milligrams daily of acetaminophen in addition if they needed it.[158]

Overall, glucosamine and chondroitin failed to meet the predetermined threshold of reducing pain by at least 20 percent, though a subgroup of patients with moderate to severe knee pain did benefit somewhat. In 2008, the researchers reported further that the same doses of glucosamine and chondroitin failed to stop the loss of cartilage in people with knee osteoarthritis.[159] In 2010, a two-year follow-up confirmed these earlier results.[160] A 2009 report from the Agency for Healthcare Research and Quality came to similarly disappointing conclusions.[161]

Do any other dietary interventions help with pain?

Ginger comes from a plant called *Zingiber officinale* and is widely used in Asian, Indian, and Arabic traditional medicine for pain and other problems. In one study, ginger extract did appear to reduce the pain of knee osteoarthritis.[162] A British review of eight studies came to the tentative conclusion that ginger can act as an anti-inflammatory and can help relieve various types of pain.[163] Iranian researchers have found that ginger can potentiate the pain-relieving potency of morphine.[164] Researchers from Georgia found that consuming either raw or heat-treated ginger can modestly reduce muscle pain.[165] But overall, it is unclear whether ginger helps with pain.[166]

Other dietary supplements, including riboflavin (a B vitamin), coenzyme Q10, and the herbs butterbur and feverfew, may help with migraine headaches, but again, the data are shaky.

Three studies in rodents suggest that soy protein may help with inflammatory pain. A study in people with osteoarthritis pain was also encouraging, but more research is needed.[167,168,169,170,171]

Turmeric, a staple in Ayurvedic (traditional Indian) medicine and a prime ingredient in curry, is also a potential inflammatory pain reducer. In studies at the University of Arizona, endocrinologists have shown that turmeric can slow joint inflammation in animals, suggesting it may be useful for arthritis.[172,173]

Peppermint, long-known as a folk remedy for gastrointestinal problems, may help by activating a specific anti-pain channel called TRPM8 in the bowel.[174]

A few other herbal pain remedies are popular, though hard evidence, again, is lacking. Among those are feverfew (from evening primrose), gamma linolenic acid from evening primrose, avocado-soybean unsaponifiables, devil's claw, and *Boswellia* (frankincense). A Canadian review found that other herbals—Harpagophytum procumbens, Salix alba, and Capsicum frutenscens—may reduce low back pain more than placebo.[175]

There is some preliminary evidence that injections of vitamin B12 may help reduce pain, but the jury is still out.[176,177]

All of this leaves pain patients in an unsatisfying place. There are, alas, few miracles to be had from the health food store.

Do magnets help with pain?

No.[178]

Static magnets (also known as permanent magnets, the kind people put on refrigerators) have been used for centuries in hopes of relieving pain and for other health purposes. In the United States, static magnets are a booming, multimillion-dollar industry, with magnets strapped on as belts, wraps, bracelets, or necklaces or even put in mattress pads.[179] But the evidence is so weak that in 1999 Operation Cure All, a law enforcement and consumer education campaign sponsored by the Federal Trade Commission, blasted sellers of magnet therapies for making unsubstantiated claims.[180]

More recently, in a study of people with osteoarthritis, magnetic bracelets did not reduce pain compared to control devices.[181]

In addition to static magnets, there is a technique called pulsed electromagnetic field therapy (PEMF), which is also aggressively marketed. In PEMF, a magnetic field is generated on or near the body. Because this magnetic field is pulsating (i.e., not stable or constant), there is the possibility that electrical fields are induced in the body. It's also possible that the magnetic field itself may have some biological effects.[182]

In one area of medicine—healing broken bones—there is fairly clear evidence that PEMF may help. Scientists think that the cells that promote bone healing may grow and organize themselves better when exposed to a magnetic field. Since the late 1950s, researchers have steadily documented that electrical currents can stimulate bone growth.[183,184,185,186,187,188,189,190]

But here's the problem: when researchers look at PEMF for chronic pain, it doesn't appear to help.[191] And a word of warning: magnets may be dangerous for people with pacemakers or insulin pumps.[192]

Does exercise help reduce chronic pain?

Yes, yes, yes. In fact, exercise is probably the closest thing there is to a magic bullet for many kinds of pain, including low back pain, arthritis, and fibromyalgia. And it works for both prevention and treatment.

In terms of prevention, European researchers long ago proved exercise's strong preventive effects. Danish researchers tracked 640 schoolchildren over 25 years and found that those who were physically active for at least three hours a week had a lower lifetime risk of back pain.[193] Finnish researchers studied 498 adults and found that the fittest people had the lowest risk of back problems.[194] British researchers studied 2,715 adults without back pain and found that physical activity did not increase the risk of low back pain later on, but poor health and being overweight did.[195] Norwegian researchers studying 46,533 adults found that among young and middle-age people, the prevalence of chronic pain was 10 to 12 percent lower for exercisers. The difference was even bigger—21 to 38 percent—among women age 65 or older and, with slightly less dramatic numbers, among older men too.[196]

What about exercise for treatment, especially for back pain?

Exercise can help significantly.

For decades, one of the leaders in the research on exercise for back pain has been Dr. James Rainville, a spine and rehabilitation specialist at New England Baptist Hospital in Boston. First, he notes, there is no evidence that pain-inducing activity must be avoided.[197,198] Even "aggressive" exercise (Rainville's word) does not raise the risk of more back problems in the future: People with chronic low back pain should get out and "exercise, run, ski [and] play sports as they desire."[199,200]

Not long ago, the prevailing belief was that rest—weeks and weeks in bed, if necessary—was the safest and most effective treatment for back pain. Now, the opposite view ("Rest is rust") holds sway. In fact, bed rest for low back pain may actually increase disability.[201] Randomized, controlled studies of people with low back pain show that those told to rest in bed have *more* pain than those told to stay active.[202]

Years ago, Swedish researchers randomized 103 low back pain sufferers to an exercise program or usual care. All were blue-collar workers on sick leave for disability. The people who participated in exercise training returned to work much faster than those who did not.[203] Finnish scientists came to similar conclusions,[204] as did a Dutch review of data from 14 randomized controlled trials, a Swiss study, a 2010 review of nine studies involving 1,520 people, and a 2010 Dutch review of 61 studies involving 6,390 people.[205,206,207,208] A 2011 Italian study of 261 people with chronic low back pain similarly showed that those who stuck with a 12-month physical activity program wound up with significantly improved overall health, as well as significant pain improvement, compared to 310 similar patients who did not.[209]

To be sure, many people with chronic pain fear moving (a problem called kinesiophobia) in the mistaken belief that exercise will cause tissue damage and more pain. But quitting exercise can make things worse.[210] Not only does exercise usually not cause harm, but it can improve pain, function, and mobility, even if one is older.[211,212,213,214,215,216,217,218,219,220,221]

When one research team analyzed the behavior of people with back pain, they found that the more fear people had about moving, the more pain they reported *during* activity.[222] But if people can be nudged to get over this fear—with some gentle coaching—they get better. A Dutch trial of 1,572 people with low back pain found that the people most likely to still be in pain six months later were the ones clinging most tightly to their fear of movement. Other studies agree.[223,224,225,226] It's not easy, of course, to change such beliefs. But it can be done. Australian researchers spent $10 million on a three-year effort—on prime-time TV—to convince people with back pain not to fear physical activity. It worked. People with back pain, and doctors as well, changed their long-held beliefs.[227]

Once people discover the pain relief they gain from exercise, they become true believers. Several years ago, the magazine *Consumer Reports* surveyed more than 14,000 subscribers who had had back pain the previous year and asked what had helped the most. Exercise was the top-rated measure to help relieve back pain, the magazine found, with 58 percent of respondents adding that they wished they had done even more exercises.[228]

What kind of exercise is best for low back pain?

One popular approach is strength training, also called resistance training or weight lifting. An Irish review of 16 randomized controlled trials involving 1,730 people with chronic low back pain found that strength training was a particularly effective way to reduce pain.[229] On the other hand, other data suggest that, while lumbar strengthening exercise is more effective than no treatment, it may not be better than other exercise programs.[230,231]

How hard should people with chronic back pain exercise?

Pretty hard. Canadian researchers have found that intensive exercise with stretching and strengthening improves both pain and function.[232,233]

Does that mean people should do aerobic exercise like running or biking?

That's less clear. In a 2011 study of Kosovo power-plant workers, researchers found that people randomly assigned to high-intensity, aerobic exercise (treadmill walking, stationary cycling, or stair climbing) wound up with significantly less pain, disability, and anxiety three months later than those assigned to some type of passive treatment such as ultrasound, heat, or electrical stimulation.[234] Aerobic exercise also has the added benefit of increased overall fitness.[235]

On the other hand, Hong Kong researchers found that adding aerobic exercise to physiotherapy did not increase improvement of pain or disability in people with low back pain.[236]

Are group classes better than individual workouts?

Maybe. Some data, including a study of 74 women with chronic low back pain, all age 57, suggest that group exercise classes help people stick with the program. These people also take less sick leave and make less use of health services.[237] But other studies have come to more wishy-washy conclusions.[238,239]

Does exercising in a pool (water therapy) help reduce pain?

Yes. This is a good solution if exercising in a gym seems too tough or not enough fun.[240]

What about yoga? Does that help reduce back pain?

Yes, though caution is needed: gentle as it seems, yoga can lead to injuries.

Yoga is the 4,000-year-old Indian practice that combines meditation and breathing with specific poses (asanas) and movements. It is wildly popular—the number of Americans doing yoga has exploded from 4 million in 2001 to as many as 21 million in 2015.[241] Yoga is now one of the 10 most popular complementary and alternative approaches to health.[242] Many studies show a clear benefit of yoga for back pain.[243,244,245,246,247]

But there are subtleties.

In 2011, British researchers compared yoga to usual care in 313 adults with chronic low back pain. The group doing 12 classes of yoga over three months had better back *function* 3, 6, and 12 months later, but the two groups had similar scores on back *pain*.[248]

In a 2011 American study, researchers from the Group Health Research Institute in Seattle randomized 228 adults with chronic low back pain to 12 once-a-week yoga classes, conventional stretching exercise, or a self-care book.[249] The yoga group did better in terms of function and the "bothersomeness" of pain. But 15 percent of the yoga group, like 17 percent of the stretching group, suffered mild to moderate adverse effects, including, in one yoga case, a herniated disk. Only 2 percent of the self-care book group reported problems.

New York Times science writer William J. Broad has documented some of the injuries associated with yoga. In January

2012, Broad quoted a prominent yoga teacher who said he had seen so many yoga injuries that he now thinks the vast majority of people should give up yoga because it's too likely to cause harm.[250] Citing studies from major medical journals, Broad noted that certain poses in particular—including those that overstretch the neck—can be dangerous.

Is Pilates helpful for back pain?

Yes. Pilates, like yoga, focuses on controlled movements, breathing, and core strengthening, and, like yoga, it can help reduce low back pain.[251]

So should people exercise the minute they get acute back pain?

Not so fast. For *acute* back pain—when you've just "done something" and your back is suddenly killing you—the value of exercise is not clear. Dutch scientists have found that exercise does not help people in acute back pain.[252] A review of 23 randomized controlled studies involving 3,676 workers also found that if a person has acute low back pain, exercise may not speed the return to work.[253]

On the other hand, Norwegian researchers found that even with acute low back pain, people who exercise have fewer recurrences than those who don't.[254] And Australian researchers have found that with a first episode of acute low back pain, people who exercise are less likely than those who don't to have a recurrence a year later.[255]

That said, there's no harm in waiting until the acute phase is over before exercising.

Does exercise help reduce arthritis pain?

It can certainly help.

Arthritis, a grab bag of more than 100 diseases, afflicts more than 50 million Americans today and by 2030 is expected to impact 67 million.[256] It comes in two major forms.

Osteoarthritis, or wear-and-tear arthritis, is the most common and is characterized by the breakdown of cartilage in the joints, which causes bones to rub against each other painfully. Rheumatoid arthritis is a systemic, inflammatory problem that can affect multiple organs but attacks the joints as well.[257]

Not surprisingly, both forms of arthritis are so painful that exercise is often the last thing people want to do—especially if they have gained weight, as many do, because of inactivity. And for years doctors didn't push it, assuming that exercise, especially high-intensity workouts like running or jogging, could be harmful.[258,259] But that thinking has changed dramatically, thanks to a groundswell of studies showing that exercise—including exercise done in water—can be good medicine for arthritis.

Does exercise help with rheumatoid arthritis?

One of the leaders in this field is Zuzana de Jong, a rheumatologist at Leiden University Medical Center in the Netherlands. Her research shows that, except in severe cases, long-term, high-intensity, weight-bearing exercise is both safe and effective for many people with rheumatoid arthritis.[260] One study by de Jong involving 309 patients showed that those randomly assigned to an intensive exercise program called RAPIT (Rheumatoid Arthritis Patients in Training) experienced significant improvements. The exercisers sweated their way through 75-minute strength and endurance training twice a week and kept at it for an impressive two years. By and large, they did not suffer increased damage to joints, as gauged by X-rays, except for those who had a lot of damage in the large joints to begin with.[261,262] The exercisers also improved in cardiovascular fitness, an important finding because people with arthritis who remain inactive lose fitness.[263]

Equally important, another study by the de Jong team showed that people with rheumatoid arthritis not only can stick with an exercise program—they come to love it. The team looked at 146 people in the RAPIT program. By the end of the program, 81 percent were still attending classes and 78 percent said they would strongly recommend it to other rheumatoid arthritis patients.[264] Even more impressive, a follow-up 18 months later showed that the majority of patients in the original exercise group were *still* hard at it, exercising intensely, albeit a bit less frequently.[265]

The Dutch team also found that patients participating in an intensive exercise program were able to slow down their rate of bone loss.[266] Significantly, they also found that two years of intensive, weight-bearing exercise did not cause progression of joint damage in the small joints of the hands and feet and might even protect the joints in the feet, a finding confirmed by other researchers.[267,268] Other research teams have also found aerobic training safe and effective for people with rheumatoid arthritis.[269,270]

And osteoarthritis? Does exercise help with that?

Yes. Exercise, both water-based and dry-land training, can help people with osteoarthritis, many studies show.[271,272,273,274,275] But one has to stick with it to maintain improvements from exercise. A 2010 Dutch study of people with knee or hip osteoarthritis found that, after five years of follow-up, the people who kept exercising had less pain and better functioning than people who did not.[276]

What about fibromyalgia? Does exercise help reduce pain?

Yes, two kinds of exercise in particular: aerobic and t'ai chi.

Fibromyalgia, once dismissed as psychogenic, is increasingly recognized as a complex medical disorder with biological and psychological components. It is characterized by chronic, widespread musculoskeletal pain, allodynia (increased pain with simple touch or pressure), and "tender points" on at least 11 out of 18 defined spots on the body, according to the

International Association for the Study of Pain.[277,278] It is believed to be caused in part by changes in pain sensitivity in the central nervous system.

Like low back pain and arthritis, fibromyalgia is common, with more than 5 million sufferers in the United States alone and 200 million worldwide.[279,280] For unclear reasons, it affects vastly more women than men.[281] Also for unclear reasons, people with fibromyalgia often have insomnia, fatigue, anxiety, depression, gastrointestinal symptoms, headaches, and, sometimes, anatomical changes in the brain.[282,283]

Of all the remedies available (antidepressants, drugs such as Neurontin [gabapentin] and Lyrica [pregabalin]), exercise is particularly crucial.[284,285,286,287,288]

In a randomized, 16-week study from Brazil, both patients who were assigned to a walking program and those assigned to muscle-strengthening exercises fared much better than the folks in the control group, who did nothing. By the end of the study, 80 percent of the control group was still taking pain medication, compared to 47 percent in the walking group and 41 percent in the strengthening group.[289] Even for people who are couch potatoes to begin with, doing some form of physical activity at least 30 minutes a day for five to seven days a week yields significant results: fewer deficits in function and less pain.[290] And exercise minutes can be accumulated; they don't have to be done all at once.

Of the various types of exercise that can help, aerobic exercise is one of the most effective. In one review of 46 studies involving 3,035 fibromyalgia patients, Oregon researchers found that the strongest evidence was for aerobic exercise.[291] It doesn't have to be at killer levels of intensity, they discovered— the pain and fatigue of fibromyalgia were reduced with even low to moderate intensity exercise.

Researchers from the University of Saskatchewan reviewed 34 studies on exercise and fibromyalgia.[292,293] They, too, found solid evidence for aerobic exercise, ideally done two to three times a week.[294,295] The evidence for aerobic exercise in people with fibromyalgia is so convincing that guidelines of both the American Pain Society and the Association of the Scientific Medical Societies in Germany now give it their strongest recommendation.[296]

Aerobic exercise can also be done in the pool. Spanish researchers have found that exercise in warm, waist-high water relieves pain and improves health-related quality of life in women with fibromyalgia.[297] Swedish and German research teams have come to the same conclusion.[298,299]

T'ai chi is the ancient Chinese mind–body practice that began as a martial art. It combines slow, gentle, graceful movements with deep breathing and relaxation.[300,301] Like yoga, t'ai chi has been growing in popularity and is a promising approach to pain relief.[302,303]

A small pilot study from Savannah, Georgia, showed that people with fibromyalgia who participated in twice-weekly t'ai chi classes for six weeks improved their scores significantly on a widely used test, the Fibromyalgia Impact Questionnaire.[304]

But the show-stopper was a randomized, 12-week Boston study published in 2010 in the *New England Journal of Medicine*.[305] The researchers randomly assigned 66 people with fibromyalgia to either twice-weekly group t'ai chi lessons or a control group, which received twice-weekly wellness education and stretching. The t'ai chi group, whose classes were taught by a t'ai chi master with 20 years of experience, showed clinically significant improvements not just in pain but also in mood, quality of life, and sleep. The effects were still present six months later.[306]

Is there a mind–body effect in chronic pain?

Yes, and it's huge. There is no way, in terms of brain biology, to be in serious pain and not have an emotional reaction to it. At the most basic level of brain anatomy, an emotional response is intrinsic to pain. It's how we are hardwired. The parts of the brain that process emotions (the limbic system) are literally connected to the parts (the somatosensory cortex) that detect bodily sensations.

This does not mean, as chronic pain patients are often told, that pain is psychogenic, or "all in your head." What it *does* mean is that people can use techniques such as CBT, meditation, hypnosis, distraction, and the like to help manage the pain.

Is the placebo response part of the mind–body effect?

Yes. Positive expectations clearly yield benefits, even when the "treatment" is a sugar pill or sham procedure. When harnessed effectively by patients and doctors, the placebo effect can be powerful medicine.

At Oxford University in England, pain researchers applied heat to the legs of 22 volunteers, who were also hooked up to IV drip machines so that a powerful painkiller, remifentanil, could be secretly administered—or not.

The volunteers were placed in fMRI brain scanning machines.[307,308] At baseline, the volunteers rated their pain a 66 on average. Without their knowledge, they were given a dose of the painkiller, after which their pain ratings dropped, to 55. They were then *told* that they were getting a powerful painkiller, and their scores dropped even more dramatically— to 39. Finally, they were told the painkiller had been withdrawn, though in reality it had not. Their scores soared—to 64, nearly up to baseline. The changing pain scores were reflected in changing brain scans too.

Interestingly, the dogma used to be that the placebo effect works only if the person is deceived into thinking that a pill or procedure is the real stuff. But in a well-designed, paradigm-shattering study published in *PLoS ONE* in 2010,[309] Harvard researchers showed that the placebo effect works *even if patients are told the pills they are taking are fake*. The study involved 80 people with irritable bowel syndrome. Half were randomly assigned to take fake pills, and they were told the pills were fake;

the other half received no treatment but the same amount of time interacting with supportive providers.

Guess who got better? The placebo folks. The study makes clear that healing involves not just drugs but expectations, including those fostered by health-care providers.[310,311,312]

How does the placebo effect work?

It probably works by creating changes in the brain that reduce the experience of pain.[313] In some studies, positive expectations have been linked to *decreasing* activity in pain-sensitive areas of the brain, including the thalamus, insula, and anterior cingulate cortex.[314,315] The placebo effect may also work by *increasing* activity in the prefrontal cortex—where cognition and judgment occur.

Brain scanning studies suggest that positive expectations trigger the release of endogenous opioids (endorphins), which can mute pain signals traveling up to the brain from the body.[316] The endorphin theory is buttressed by a study showing that naloxone, a drug that blocks opioids, *blocks* the placebo effect.[317] Swedish researchers have found that pain relief with placebos involves the same areas of the brain that are involved in analgesia achieved via opioid drugs.[318] American researchers have shown that areas of the brain containing a type of opioid receptor (called mu) "light up" with the placebo effect.[319]

Fascinatingly, placebos can have different effects in different parts of the body. In one study, Italian researchers induced pain in volunteers (by injecting capsaicin, which causes burning pain) in four parts of the body: left hand, right hand, left foot, and right foot.[320] They also induced specific expectations of pain relief. They rubbed a cream on one area, say, the left foot, and told the volunteers it was a powerful pain reliever. The cream was actually fake—a placebo. Amazingly enough, the volunteers said that while the other three body parts hurt, their left feet, which had the cream, didn't hurt. When the experiment was repeated so the volunteers received injections of naloxone (the opioid blocker), the placebo response disappeared completely.

In addition to working via endorphins, placebos may also work through body-made marijuana-like substances called endocannabinoids.[321]

The take-home message is that emotional expectations can boost the effectiveness of pain treatments and that doctors and nurses who nurture such expectations are an important part of treatment.

What is "catastrophizing"? Does it make pain worse?

Catastrophizing is a maladaptive cognitive and emotional habit that leads to focusing obsessively on pain, imagining all sorts of worst-case scenarios and generally believing that the pain will be endless, life-wrecking, horrible, and unfixable. Catastrophizing makes pain worse, and women tend to do it more than men.[322,323,324]

There are several ways to tell how much one may be catastrophizing, including the 13-item Pain Catastrophizing Scale.[325] The scale is designed to measure the intensity of a person's tendency to ruminate, to magnify things, and to feel helpless. It's easy: just assign each item a number from zero (not at all) to 4 (all the time), then add up the score. Here are the statements:

1. I worry all the time about whether it will end.
2. I feel I can't go on.
3. It's terrible and I think it's never going to get any better.
4. It's awful and I feel that it overwhelms me.
5. I feel I can't stand it anymore.
6. I become afraid that the pain will get worse.
7. I keep thinking of other painful events.
8. I anxiously want the pain to go away.
9. I can't seem to get it out of my mind.
10. I keep thinking about how much it hurts.

11. I keep thinking about how badly I want the pain to stop.
12. There's nothing I can do to reduce the intensity of the pain.
13. I wonder whether something serious may happen.

Healthy, pain-free adults usually have catastrophizing scores in the single digits. A score is in the mid-teens indicates moderate catastrophizing. If the score creeps toward 52, the highest score possible, the person is a serious catastrophizer. People with fibromyalgia often score in the mid- to high 20s. Not surprisingly, people with chronic low back pain and arthritis also tend to have relatively high scores. Being a high catastrophizer is not just miserable; it's a bad prognostic sign. Catastrophizing can interfere with one's ability to cope, amplify the way the nervous system processes pain, and actually get in the way of benefitting from treatment.[326,327,328]

One way to reduce catastrophizing is with CBT.

What is cognitive behavior therapy? How does it help reduce pain?

Of all the coping skills shown to help people with certain chronic pain conditions, CBT is among the most effective.[329,330,331] Instead of focusing on deep, underlying emotional issues stemming from childhood (which also can be useful), CBT is very here and now–oriented. It may not make the pain go away, but it can ease one's emotional *distress* about pain, which in turn can reduce suffering.[332]

For instance, if you're thinking, "I'm a total loser," chances are you'll feel terrible. If you notice this thought, hold it in your mind for a moment and replace it by a more accurate one; you might think, "I mess up sometimes, but often I'm pretty good at things." The result is that you will probably feel better. Similarly, if you're thinking, "The pain will always be this intense forever," you might look at your diary and, hopefully, see that in fact your pain fluctuates somewhat during the day, so it won't be at its max all the time.

In a study of people with temporomandibular joint disorder (TMD), those who had four sessions of CBT training had impressively less pain than similar patients who received only education about TMD. The results also appeared to be long term, lasting at least one year.[333] CBT has been shown to reduce the pain of fibromyalgia, chronic fatigue syndrome, irritable bowel syndrome, back pain, and headache.[334]

In a massive review of 16 rigorous meta-analyses—each meta-analysis itself was a compilation of data from other studies—CBT was found very effective for psychiatric problems and somewhat effective for pain.[335]

An earlier meta-analysis of 25 previous studies by British researchers found that CBT was effective at reducing the overall experience of pain, though the improvement was modest.[336] The British team also found that between one in three and one in seven patients using CBT achieve clinically significant gains in terms of the overall pain experience and emotional distress.[337,338,339] CBT works for kids too.[340]

CBT can even work when people learn it online. Harvard Medical School researchers pooled results from 11 studies of CBT in which people with chronic pain learned the technique online: CBT helped reduce pain, though the improvements were small.[341]

CBT seems to be especially effective in people who catastrophize, even those whose pain has lasted for years.[342,343]

What other mental "tricks" help reduce pain?

One is distraction, that is, diverting one's attention away from the pain. In a meta-analysis involving pooled data from 51 studies with nearly 4,000 pain patients, music was shown to reduce pain and the need for opioid drugs. The effects were small but good enough to take the edge off.[344]

Distraction is now going high tech as a way to pry attention away from excruciating medical procedures such as burn debridement—the changing of burn dressings and cleaning of wounds to prevent infection. Psychologists at the University of Seattle studied distraction using virtual reality (complete with goggles).[345] One of their early patients, a 40-year-old man with deep burns on his legs, neck, back, and buttocks needed opioids just to get through the day. When his wounds were being cared for, the drugs barely touched the extreme pain. But virtual reality helped significantly. Granted, it does look a bit weird.

The burn patient sits hooked up to a goggle apparatus as a nurse cuts away the bandage on one hand, while the patient grips a computer joy stick with his other bandaged hand. He wears a headset and maneuvers his way through a make-believe place called SnowWorld. We can't see his face, but his body language suggests he's totally into the game. This kind of immersive experience appears to trick the brain into believing the person is somewhere else.[346,347,348]

In Germany, researchers have shown that distraction can reduce the transmission of pain signals from the spinal cord to the brain. Using a group of 20 male volunteers, the researchers used two different forms of a memory task to distract the volunteers during pain tests using a heat stimulus on the arm. During the tests, the volunteers were placed in fMRI machines that tracked neural activity in their spinal cords. An easy memory test proved too unchallenging—it wasn't enough of a distraction to block ascending pain signals. A harder test did block pain signals significantly—at the level of the spinal cord.[349] As an extra measure, the scientists then injected either a placebo or an opioid blocker (naloxone) to see if distraction blocked pain signals generated by endorphins. When given naloxone, distracted subjects were not able to block pain signals as well.

What is biofeedback? Does it help reduce pain?

Biofeedback is a technique that provides yet more proof of the intricate mind–body connection. It is defined as "a process that enables an individual to learn how to change physiological activity for the purposes of improving health and performance."[350] Pain reduction is now one of the main uses of biofeedback.[351,352]

There are several ways to do biofeedback. One is with so-called surface electromyography (sEMG). In this technique, surface electrodes are placed over certain muscles to detect signals called action potentials that trigger muscle contractions. This type of biofeedback is used for a number of pain problems, including headaches, chronic pain, neck spasms, and TMD.[353] A more elaborate technique uses electrodes placed on the scalp to detect electrical activation in the brain. Scientists are just beginning to explore how well this technique, using electroencephalograph (EEG), may help reduce pain.[354]

Perhaps the most exciting type of biofeedback for pain comes from the lab of neuroscientist Sean Mackey, director of the Stanford Systems Neuroscience and Pain Lab. It's technically called rtfMRI, neurofeedback with real-time functional magnetic resonance imaging.

Unlike traditional biofeedback, which monitors "downstream" processes like heart rate, blood pressure, and temperature as way to sense and reduce the arousal of the autonomic nervous system, rtfMRI neurofeedback focuses "upstream," on brain areas that act earlier in the experiential process. In one pivotal experiment, Mackey's team had volunteers lie in fMRI scanners and as they watched and controlled their own brains in real time.[355]

Mackey was interested in one section of the brain in particular, the anterior cingulate cortex (ACC), a key pain-processing area. The idea was to see if people could learn how to control the ACC, and, if so, whether this would lead to better pain control.[356] The answer to both was yes.

The experiment involved healthy people who were taught various cognitive strategies that would lead to increased or decreased brain activity in the ACC (such as telling themselves the pain was not so bad). As the volunteers practiced this, they watched a computer screen that was receiving signals from the ACC in their brains. The computer displayed the incoming information visually in several ways, such as having a flame look hotter or cooler, depending on the messages from their ACCs. During this, the volunteers were subjected to heat stimulation on their arms ranging from mild to fairly painful. Strikingly, they were able to amplify or damp down their own perceptions of pain at will by using the techniques they had been taught.

How about meditation? Does that reduce pain?

Just as exercise is the magic bullet among physical techniques for managing pain, meditation is probably the best mental "trick" that can be used to reduce pain. It's simple (though not necessarily easy), it's free, it's available 24/7, and it works.[357,358,359,360,361]

There are different meditation techniques, many based on thousands of years of Buddhist tradition. The idea is to sit quietly and focus one's mind on the present, becoming aware of thoughts and feelings without judging them. Many people count breaths. Some stare at a burning candle. In terms of chronic pain, meditation is a way to stop fighting with the pain and learn to work with it.[362]

The groundbreaking research showing how meditation changes activity in the front of the brain was done by meditation guru Jon Kabat-Zinn, who created the widely used eight-week Mindfulness-Based Stress Reduction program at the University of Massachusetts Medical School, and neuroscientist Richard Davidson, director of the Laboratory for Affective Neuroscience at the University of Wisconsin.[363]

In people who are stressed, the right cortex (the more emotional side) of the brain is overactive and the left cortex (the more analytical side) is underactive. Stressed-out people also show heightened activity in the amygdala, a center for processing fear. By contrast, people who are habitually calm and happy typically show greater activity in the left frontal cortex relative to the right and tend to pump out less of the stress hormone cortisol.

Davidson and Kabat-Zinn recruited stressed-out volunteers from a high-tech firm in Madison, Wisconsin. At the outset, all volunteers were tested with EEGs in which electrodes were placed on the scalp to collect brain-wave information. The volunteers were then randomized into two groups—25 in the meditation group, who took Kabat-Zinn's eight-week course, and 16 in the control group.

At the end of eight weeks, all the volunteers underwent another round of EEG tests and a flu shot. They also had blood tests to check for antibody response to the shot. Four months later, all underwent EEG tests again. By the end of the study, the meditators' brains showed exactly what the researchers had hypothesized—a demonstrable shift toward the left frontal lobe—while the nonmeditators' brains did not. The meditators also had more robust immune responses to the flu shots.

Using more modern technology and magnetic resonance scans instead of EEGs, neuroscientists Sara Lazar and Bruce Fischl at Massachusetts General Hospital in Boston studied 20 volunteers who were experienced meditators.[364] The volunteers had been meditating for years for an average of 40 minutes a day. The scientists compared their brain scans to those of 15 nonmeditators. The results? Meditation was linked to long-term changes in the brain, including increased cortical thickness all over the brain and especially in parts of the brain associated with attention, interoception (paying attention to internal, bodily stimuli such as noticing that one's stomach is "in knots"), and sensory processing.

Similarly, researchers from the University of Montreal studied 17 long-term meditators and 18 controls with magnetic resonance brain scans and found lower pain sensitivity in the meditators and greater thickness in pain-related brain regions, including the anterior cingulate cortex, the parahippocampal gyrus, and the anterior insula.[365] The researchers suspect that one way by which meditation helps is by "decoupling" the sensory component of pain from the cognitive-evaluative component.[366]

Other encouraging studies have poured out of labs all over the world.[367,368,369,370,371,372,373,374,375] In one study from Massachusetts General Hospital in Boston, meditators, but not nonmeditators, were able to reduce "pain unpleasantness" in experimental pain labs by 22 percent and anticipatory anxiety by 29 percent when they were in a "mindful" state.[376] The fMRI scans of the volunteers also hinted at that "decoupling" effect. In other words, meditation helps us notice sensations without trying to change them, in essence separating the emotional distress of pain from the sheer sensory aspect of it.[377]

Does hypnosis help?

Yes, it can. Hypnosis and self-hypnosis are similar to other techniques we've talked about in that they involve deep relaxation and focused attention. The big difference is that hypnosis also involves "suggestions" for a person to experience something different (e.g., something pleasurable rather than painful) or to do something different when "cued" (such as reach for a stick of gum instead of a cigarette). Experts define hypnosis as a social interaction in which one person responds to suggestions offered by another person, the hypnotist.[378] In self-hypnosis, the patient learns to do this for himself or herself.

There are numerous types of "suggestions" that hypnotherapists can use to help offset pain.[379] Sometimes it works to suggest that the pain is changing, perhaps diminishing or turning to numbness, or to imagine a growing sense of comfort. Sometimes the therapist can suggest that a stabbing pain be imagined as vibrations; other times, the suggestion might be that the pain is ever so subtly moving from, say, the abdomen to a leg. A person in pain can also try to imagine being dissociated from the body—moving into another, more pleasant place.

In 2011, University of Washington psychologists reported on a study of 33 adults with chronic pain, finding that those using a combination of self-hypnosis and cognitive restructuring were better at reducing pain than those using either technique alone.[380] The team also showed that self-hypnosis decreased daily pain in people with spinal cord injuries.[381] Hypnosis has also been shown to reduce pain in children undergoing painful procedures such as lumbar puncture and bone marrow aspiration.[382]

Neuroimaging studies suggest that hypnosis can block pain signals from reaching the somatosensory cortex in the brain and can also modulate emotional response to pain in the limbic (emotional processing) system.[383] In other words, if we focus our attention on something other than the pain, the brain's response to pain calms down.[384,385]

Is there a bottom line for all these alternative approaches?

Yes. Taking charge of one's own pain is key. The recommendation is to do it all—exercise, meditation, acupuncture, massage, omega-3 fatty acids. If each of these reduces the pain a few notches, then the combination—along with the feeling that you are somewhat more in charge of your situation, not just a victim—can make a huge difference.

8

THE WAY FORWARD

In the past few decades, people with AIDS, breast cancer, disabilities, and other conditions have managed—by banding together, shedding their shame, and taking to the streets—to put their diseases on the world's radar screen.

Haggard men with AIDS hung quilts in cities around the world to remind the still-uninfected that behind the statistics were human beings with lives worth living. Tired women in sneakers and bright T-shirts walked miles to raise money for breast cancer, some still in headscarves from chemotherapy, some holding mementos of dead mothers, daughters, sisters, wives.

People with disabilities gathered in front of the Capitol Building in Washington, DC, abandoned their crutches and wheelchairs, and crawled up all 100 of the Capitol steps—the "Capitol Crawl of 1990." The Americans with Disabilities Act was passed soon thereafter.[1]

It takes a lot of political action, it would seem, to raise the world's consciousness, pass laws and fund research. But it can pay off. Today in the United States, thanks to the vociferous efforts of people with HIV/AIDS, the government spends $2,562 for every person with the diagnosis. It spends only $4 for every person living with chronic pain.[2]

Discouraging, to be sure. But such funding disparities show that political efforts can yield change. In some pockets of the world, dogged political efforts have already led to better pain relief and palliative care.

Are there examples?

Yes, and perhaps the most striking example is Kerala state in India, where progress is due largely to one man, M. R. Rajagopal, a palliative care physician, and the colleagues he enlisted in his mission.

Rajagopal is a slight, balding gentleman—and "gentleman" is exactly the right word—with compassionate eyes that glow behind his glasses, a calm smile, and a well-trimmed mustache. Trained as an anesthesiologist, he has proven that decent pain management *is* possible, even in countries with some of the most draconian morphine restrictions on the planet.

Born nearly 70 years ago in Kerala, Rajagopal's dedication to palliative care began decades ago, when he witnessed a neighbor screaming in pain. The man was dying of cancer, with tumors all over his scalp. As a young medical student, Rajagopal had never seen anything like it, pain so bad it made a grown man cry all day and all night, unable to think of anything else. The man's family asked Rajagopal to help, but he couldn't. He was just a medical student.[3]

But the incident sparked a lifelong mission that began after medical school—a crusade for better pain relief for India's masses. Building on early progress in pain relief at Calicut Medical College, in 2003 Rajagopal founded Pallium India, a nongovernmental charitable trust.[4,5,6,7] He is now the chairman.

In 2012, Pallium's flagship program, the Trivandrum Institute of Palliative Sciences, was declared a collaborating center of the World Health Organization (WHO), a formal mechanism to help spread pain relief policies worldwide.

Today, thanks largely to the efforts of Rajagopal's group, Kerala has a thriving palliative care system with about 170 palliative care centers. By comparison, Andhra Pradesh, another state with serious pain problems because of HIV/AIDS, has only four.[8,9]

Indeed, Kerala, with 1 percent of India's land mass and 3 percent of its population, has led the way toward easing regulatory restrictions on morphine. The result is that, today, 75 to 80 percent of India's palliative care centers are in Kerala.[10,11,12]

In India as a whole, only 1 percent of people dying from cancer receive morphine and only half of regional cancer hospitals even stock it. In Kerala, 40 percent of people dying of cancer can now get morphine.[13,14,15]

How did Rajagopal do this?

Rajagopal demonstrated—and made public—how quality care could work, then relied on ethical and legal arguments to change the system. The Indian constitution guarantees the right to life with dignity. Rajagopal argued that Indians also have the right to die with dignity and that lack of access to pain relief and palliative care denies that right. He also argued that cost was not the issue since morphine is cheap—India even grows the poppies from which morphine is made. Denying morphine to people in pain, he argued, is a denial based on "ignorance or callousness."[16]

How did those arguments change India's narcotics laws?

India's 1985 law, the Narcotic Drugs and Psychotropic Substances Act, was actually a book of regulations that came to 1,642 pages. Among other things, it called for a 10-year mandatory prison sentence for violations involving narcotic drugs, prompting many pharmacies to cut their stocks to avoid potential penalties.[17] It also called for mandatory imprisonment for *any* error with an opioid prescription—even a minor, unintentional error that did not lead to any abuse.[18]

In the 1990s, working with the Wisconsin-based Pain and Policy Studies Group, Rajagopal convinced the Indian government to recommend reforms to state governments. Then, focusing on Kerala, he succeeded in prompting some changes in opioid policy, most important, creating simplified procedures for medical institutions to obtain oral morphine. Slowly, the idea that pain relief was possible spread from city to city in Kerala.

In 2005, Rajagopal pressured the state government again. By 2008, Kerala had formally declared a state palliative care policy that integrated palliative care into its primary care system. Today, most of Kerala's roughly 900 primary health centers have at least one nurse with three months of training in palliative care, a substantial step forward even though many of the changes Rajagopal wanted have still not reached major hospitals.

In 2008, Rajagopal filed a lawsuit with the Supreme Court of India, urging the Indian government to simplify opioid regulations for the country as a whole. The lawsuit asked the court to instruct the government to remove unnecessary barriers to pain treatment that had been instituted by the 1985 law, to instruct medical and nursing councils to include palliative care in medical curricula, and to have state governments include palliative care in their state health policies.[19,20,21]

In 2014, Parliament finally did amend the 1985 act, eliminating the long list of licenses required of drug makers and hospitals to obtain and store morphine.[22] Rajagopal's argument carried the day—that pain relief is a human right and that any stringent regulation against access to drugs to control pain is a violation of that right.[23]

The amended law calls for uniform regulation across states for giving out licenses to manufacture, stock, and dispense morphine-based drugs. Each medical institution, which previously needed four or five different licenses from different agencies to store morphine, now needs only one.[24] By 2015, the government had followed up on the steps outlined in the 2014 amendment, specifying the procedures for acquiring morphine, though these procedures still have to be implemented by the states and India's six union territories.[25]

Is palliative care in India now on par with Western countries?

No.

More than half of Kerala's population still does not have access to palliative care, according to Human Rights Watch. Palliative care is still inadequate or nonexistent in most health-care institutions. Most medical professionals still are inadequately trained in palliative care.[26] Countrywide, despite advances in Kerala, less than 1 percent of the Indian population has access to morphine.[27]

Perhaps that is not surprising. Generations of doctors have been practicing medicine without having even seen a tablet of morphine, a mindset that is unlikely to change overnight.

But the gains to date are worth gold to Rajagopal. He points to two pictures of the same man before and after morphine. Before, the man, who had lung cancer, couldn't lie down for more than 10 minutes at a time. He had to rest on his knees and elbows most of the day and night because he couldn't tolerate the pain in any other position. In less than an hour after morphine, he was sitting up enjoying a cup of tea. Rajagopal says it is stories like this that keep him going. It is the looks of relief on the faces of his patients and his patients' families— and the knowledge that morphine is now available to 10 million Indians who couldn't get it before.[28]

Where else have there been improvements in morphine availability?

Uganda.

As in Kerala, the improvements in morphine availability in Uganda have been sparked by a single individual, in this case, Anne Merriman, a British physician and missionary.

Uganda is an extremely poor country with very few doctors; there is approximately one doctor for every 19,000 people. Nearly 60 percent of the population has never even seen a health worker. Making matters worse, the country has faced a particularly bad chronic pain burden because of the endemic HIV/AIDS crisis. Indeed, unlike many countries, where cancer is a leading cause of death, in Uganda, 73 percent of terminally ill patients die of HIV/AIDS, according to the WHO. By contrast, 22 percent die from cancer, 3 percent from both, and only 2 percent from other diseases.[29]

Merriman, who was born in Liverpool, went to medical school in Ireland and worked for a time in Nigeria, Malaysia, and Singapore.[30] In 1990, she became the first medical director of the Nairobi Hospice in Kenya. In 1993, she moved to Uganda, where she founded Hospice Uganda, which has become the "Merriman model" for palliative care throughout Africa.[31]

Thanks to her efforts, the Ugandan government now allows hospice workers to bring oral morphine into the country. In 2002, the government changed the law so that more prescribers—including midwives and nurses—can give morphine to patients.[32,33]

What other countries have made progress?

Costa Rica has increased pain and palliative care efforts. In fact, this small country has made the most dramatic improvements of 19 countries in Latin America, according to researchers from Germany and Texas who rated the countries on such measures as the proportion of medical schools offering palliative care education, the number of accredited physicians working in palliative care, and the amount of opioids consumed per capita.[34,35] Chile, Mexico, and Argentina are also doing better than many other Latin American countries.

Greater access to morphine has also improved in Nigeria, Bangladesh, Myanmar, and Jordan, according to researchers writing in *Health Affairs*.[36] Human Rights Watch also cites progress in Colombia and Romania, thanks largely to medical leaders working with nongovernmental organizations and governments to reduce barriers to pain control.[37]

In Nepal, a single oncologist, supported by an international pain policy fellowship, was able to get three forms of oral morphine manufactured in the country, help train health-care practitioners in how to use morphine for pain relief, and help a national palliative care association develop a palliative care curriculum.[38]

In Jordan, a WHO demonstration project in Amman has begun serving as a model for pain relief elsewhere in the Middle East.[39] The program includes palliative care for inpatients, outpatients, and patients at home. As part of the program, regulations on opioid prescribing have also been eased to encourage better pain management.

In Ukraine, international pressure and media reports of people dying in pain have pushed the government to approve the manufacture and distribution of oral morphine.[40]

In Vietnam, palliative care advocates, using WHO-suggested strategies, have been able to give morphine to many more patients. By 2010, morphine consumption was nine times greater than it had been in 2003, a greater increase per capita than in many other Asian countries. The number of hospitals offering palliative care also increased from 3 to 15.[41]

In a 2013 report, researchers found that 67 countries had small increases in opioid consumption between 2006 and 2010.[42]

Is pain relief now on the world's agenda?

Not really, but there have been incremental steps.[43,44]

In 2011, the WHO published a set of 21 guidelines to help countries ensure that the needs of people in pain not be sacrificed because of efforts to control drug abuse.[45]

In 2014, the World Health Assembly (WHA) issued a landmark resolution calling for increased palliative care as part of integrated medical treatment and urging greater access to essential medicines such as morphine.[46] (The WHA is the forum through which the WHO is governed.)

The WHA resolution noted that more than 40 million people around the world now require palliative care every year. It acknowledged that the International Narcotics Control Board (INCB) should prevent diversion of narcotic drugs, but it also recognized the need to prevent unavoidable suffering. The resolution specifically urged countries to give the INCB accurate estimates of their needs for palliative care medicines and urged continuation of the WHO's Access to Controlled Medicines Programme.

In 2015, top pain physicians and researchers from many countries announced the formation of the Harvard Global Equity Initiative–Lancet Commission on global access to pain control and palliative care, a move that could bring high-level influence to policymakers in numerous countries.[47,48]

What about the United States? Is pain on the agenda there?

Not really.

Federal funding is still minuscule, and not just at the National Institutes of Health (NIH). Like the NIH, the Department of Defense and the Department of Veterans Affairs also earmark tiny percentages of their budgets to pain research. Research investment in academia is actually falling, and pharmaceutical industry support for pain research has also declined.[49]

The American Pain Society, a professional organization of pain physicians and researchers, notes that chronic pain is still substantially underfunded relative to its prevalence, disease burden, and economic toll: "It is difficult to overstate the societal impact of pain, yet pain research remains woefully underfunded in both public and private sectors," that group concluded. "Although efforts are being made to improve federal funding for pain research, these incremental measures are inadequate for the magnitude of the problem."[50]

According to the American Pain Society, we need to put money and effort into developing new pain treatments. We also need to improve prevention, diagnosis, and management of chronic pain conditions. In addition, we need to make better use of treatments already available, understand better how health policies impact pain treatment, and improve pain education.[51]

But that will take leadership, the group says: "The top-down decisions to send humans to the moon, declare a war on cancer, decode the human genome, and find a way to halt the acquired immune deficiency syndrome epidemic serve as excellent examples. Is the daily suffering of 100 million Americans less important?"[52]

Meanwhile, the media still focuses almost entirely on opioid abuse and only fleetingly on the needs of pain patients. Thus large numbers of Americans are still being denied the most effective pain treatments, according to a 2014 workshop at the NIH.[53]

And there is still a dearth of reliable data on the long-term effects—good and bad—of opioids. That means, as the 2014 NIH report put it, that there is still "insufficient evidence for every clinical decision that a provider needs to make regarding the use of opioids for chronic pain."[54]

Has anything come of the 2011 Institute of Medicine report?

Not much, and what progress has been made is mostly behind the scenes.

After that report came out—generating almost no publicity—the Inter-Agency Pain Research Coordinating Committee (IPRCC), which had been mandated as part of the Affordable Care Act in 2010, held meetings to address the recommendations of the Institute of Medicine (IOM) report.

Working with almost no budget, the IPRCC created a subcommittee to formulate what came to be called the National Pain Strategy, a kind of operational plan for the IOM report.[55]

That report was released in March 2016 by the Department of Health and Human Services.[56]

The National Pain Strategy is meant to "create a comprehensive population health level strategy for pain prevention, treatment, management and research."[57,58] The document notes that achievement of the "cultural transformation" of how pain is treated in the United States will not be possible "without sustained and indeed expanded investment" into pain research and treatments.

The committee writing the National Pain Strategy did not shy away from the "conundrum" of opioid abuse highlighted in the IOM report. It recognized

the serious problem of diversion and abuse of opioid drugs, as well as questions about their usefulness long-term, but believes that when opioids are used as prescribed and appropriately monitored, they can be safe and effective, especially for acute, post-operative and procedural pain, as well as for patients near the end of life who desire more pain relief.[59]

Negative stereotypes about pain and people in chronic pain, including the attitudes of health professionals, can also undermine care, the committee noted.[60] It is also important to refine the current reimbursement system to promote interdisciplinary, patient-centered care instead of the current fee-for-service approach and to improve education about pain in medical schools.[61,62]

Elsewhere, are there efforts to move things along?

Yes, but the going is tough, and, as Rajagopal discovered in India, progress is measured in bureaucratic baby steps.

Perhaps the most prominent US effort is through a group called PAINS—the Pain Action Alliance to Implement a

National Strategy.[63] The group is led by bioethicist Myra Christopher at the Center for Practical Bioethics in Kansas City. Christopher was on the IOM committee, the IPRCC, and the National Pain Strategy committee. Like Rajagopal, Christopher has worked for years with federal committees as well as private and academic groups to put chronic pain on the national agenda.

In June 2015, PAINS convened a conference in Washington, DC, with the Consumer Pain Advocacy Task Force, a coalition of 17 groups working to improve pain care in the United States. The groups agreed to present four core messages to the public: (a) chronic pain is real and complex and may exist by itself or in conjunction with other medical conditions, (b) chronic pain is an unrecognized and underresourced public health crisis, (c) effective pain care requires access to a wide range of treatment options, and (d) allowing people to suffer with unmanaged pain is immoral and unethical.[64]

The specific goal of that conference (which involved more than 100 representatives from professional societies, academic institutions, federal agencies, and patient advocacy groups) was to help move the National Pain Strategy from a vision to a reality.[65] But the conference attendees expressed concern that the strategy lacked specificity and accountability, it contained no timeline or funding for implementation, and the reimbursement for health care costs needed to be restructured.

The group also urged more research on pain, investigation of disparities in pain care for people of color, and expanding to the civilian sector work done by the Department of Defense to develop better pain screening tools for physicians and more continuing education in pain for practicing clinicians. Importantly, attendees also backed the politically charged idea that pain patient advocates and advocates for people with addiction problems should work together, instead of being at odds, to find ways to accomplish the goals of both groups.

The PAINS team has also been trying to make Kansas City the national model for changing the way pain is taught and treated. But, in an all-too-familiar story, the effort has recently stalled for lack of sufficient funding. On the plus side, the Patient-Centered Outcomes Research Institute, an independent, nonprofit, nongovernmental organization based in Washington, DC, whose goal is to fund research that determines what works and what doesn't in health care, has funded the Kansas City effort to a small degree.

Another active group is the American Chronic Pain Association, founded in 1980 and led by Penney Cowan, a chronic pain patient who was part of the IPRCC.[66,67] Cowan's group focuses on peer support and education in how to manage pain.

At the University of California, Los Angeles, researchers have set up a worldwide database of brain scan images for chronic pain conditions.[68] More than a dozen institutions in North America and Europe are participating. The growing database should help spur pain research.

At Stanford, the Stanford–NIH Pain Registry, now called the Collaborative Health Outcomes Information Registry (CHOIR), is an open-source, open standard, free group that provides clinicians with information on treatment outcomes.[69]

At Tufts University, anesthesiologist Daniel Carr helped found an innovative program called PREP (Pain Research, Education, and Policy) that now grants master of science degrees to future health-care leaders.[70,71]

Within the federal government, the NIH and the IPRCC have also set up a database to keep track of more than 1,200 pain research projects.[72] In addition, the NIH has established a dozen "centers of excellence" in pain education to act as hubs for better pain education for doctors and other health professionals.[73] They are in Baltimore, Seattle, Philadelphia, Edwardsville (Ill.), Rochester, Albuquerque, Boston, and Pittsburgh.

Finally, the US Food and Drug Administration is now requiring that pharmaceutical companies do additional studies and clinical trials—including postmarketing surveillance—for extended release and long-acting opioids.[74] Those studies must try to answer questions such as what the risks of addiction are among legitimate pain patients (as opposed to abusers). In addition, drug companies are instructed to look at how much "doctor-shopping" occurs and whether that means people are abusing drugs or merely trying to obtain good care. Another objective is to examine how well, if at all, medical records show whether someone is having problems with opioids. The companies are directed to attempt to ascertain whether patients are merely dependent on opioids or misusing them and becoming addicted and whether patients are developing opioid-induced hyperalgesia—an *increase* in pain caused by opioids.

That, of course, is a very tall order, and whether there is enough political will to make these goals attainable is an open question.

Will the Affordable Care Act improve pain treatment?

Possibly. The act designates chronic disease management (which ostensibly should include chronic pain) as a priority with the potential of increased support for care coordination and self-management training.[75] But it's not clear whether this will happen.

Is education on pain improving in US medical schools?

There is no data suggesting that things have improved since the 2011 Johns Hopkins study showing that American medical students receive a median of only nine hours of pain education over four years of medical school.

In 2012, the International Association for the Study of Pain, a large academic group, revised curriculum guidelines for many disciplines including medicine, nursing, pharmacy, psychology, physical therapy, and occupational therapy.[76] But pain education is still inadequate in US medical schools, and it is not clear whether these guidelines are being widely adopted.

So is there any real hope for better pain care in the United States?

Yes, but, as in India and Uganda, progress is glacial and incremental, and the burden seems to fall disproportionately on a few individuals.

In the United States, one of those individuals is Cindy Steinberg, a former product development manager for a learning technology company just outside of Harvard Square in Cambridge, Massachusetts.

Steinberg, with her short hair, dancing eyes, and quick wit, almost seems destined for the role she now plays in the ongoing pain and opioid wars of American politics, though she never dreamed her life would take this course. Her life changed at 10 AM on March 3, 1995. She was in her 30s, happily married with a two-year-old daughter. She had never missed a day of work, not even the day she went into labor.

On that fateful day in 1995, her company was moving offices. She was on the phone to a client and went outside her office to open a drawer to retrieve a file. Unbeknownst to her, moving men had dismantled the cubicles and stacked them against the back of her file cabinet.

When she opened the drawer, the whole filing cabinet and 10 cubicle walls began to fall on her. She tried to turn away but wasn't fast enough. The drawer struck her in the middle of her back and knocked her over, crushing her underneath the filing cabinet and cubicle walls.[77] The crash tore ligaments and nerves in the middle of her back. Since that accident, she has not had a minute, much less a day, without pain.

For the first five years afterward, she kept working, running meetings for staff and contractors, as well as her Fortune 500 corporate clients, lying flat on her back. At the end of many days, she would go home in tears. Eventually, the pain was so debilitating that she had to give up her career. Even today, her spine remains so unstable that she can't hold herself up long; when she tries, the muscle spasms can become unbearable. So she stays upright for an hour or so, then lies down for 25 minutes, back and forth, all day long. She still goes to concerts at Boston's Symphony Hall, but she lies down at intermission. When she flies, she buys two seats so she can lie across them.

She copes—with medications, lots of exercise, and a passionate commitment to her new career: patient advocacy. At meetings, she delivers her speech, then takes her yoga mat and pillow and retreats to a corner of the room where she can lie down and still hear the other speakers. When it's time for a panel discussion, she goes back to her seat and participates with vigor. She runs the monthly meetings of her pain patient support group from the floor, greeting each member with a warm wave and a hello.

Steinberg, long the chair of the policy council of the Massachusetts Pain Initiative, has recently taken on national roles, currently as the national director of policy and advocacy for the US Pain Foundation. She speaks at national science and medical conferences. She testifies at state and federal government meetings, including at the advisory committee for the US Food and Drug Administration.

As Rajagopal discovered in India, Steinberg's work takes tough, nitty-gritty persistence.

In 2009, she spent a year working with the Massachusetts State Department of Public Health writing guidelines to ensure that the policies of the health boards were fair to people with pain.[78] For the Boards of Registration in Dentistry, Nursing, Physician Assistants and Pharmacy, for instance, Steinberg worked to make the standards for practitioners include a pain management plan, legible entries into patient records, and recognition that "tolerance and physical dependence are normal consequences of sustained use of opioids and are not synonymous with addiction." (The policy rulings affected 140,000 health-care professionals in Massachusetts.)[79]

She worked with state legislators to require three hours of continuing education units for physicians in pain management, including safe opioid prescribing, as a condition of licensure.

That work has made Massachusetts one of the few states requiring pain management training on a recurring basis.[80]

In 2014, two days after Charlie Baker was elected as the new governor of Massachusetts, he announced he would form a task force to confront the opioid crisis in that state. Steinberg immediately wrote a piece for the local NPR station urging that Baker, in his quest to fix the opioid abuse problem, not make it harder for legitimate pain patients to obtain opioids if they need them.[81]

Steinberg was quickly appointed to that task force, the only one of the 18 members representing pain management. After holding meetings around the state, taking testimony from 1,100 people, and analyzing mountains of documents submitted by more than 150 stakeholder organizations, including health-care institutions, medical societies, district attorney's offices, and community organizations, the task force devised a credible plan to improve addiction and recovery programs for addicts.[82,83]

But that report would not have mentioned chronic pain had it not been for Steinberg, who fought repeatedly to include a statement in the report regarding access to opioids for individuals living with pain. It was taken out. She argued to put it back in. Back and forth they went. Finally, she won. That statement reads, "These recommendations aim to ensure access to pain medication for individuals with chronic pain while reducing opportunities for individuals to access and use opioids for nonmedical purposes."[84]

This was a small victory, perhaps, but a victory nonetheless, and a step on the way to recognizing the rights of people in chronic pain. Steinberg was also able to have other recommendations written into the report that could be beneficial in reducing abuse and addiction without harming legitimate access for pain sufferers. These include pain management, safe prescribing and addiction training for all prescribers as a condition of licensure, and encouraging public and private insurers to cover alternative therapies for pain.

As Steinberg discovered in the United States, Rajagopal in India, and Anne Merriman in Uganda, change is hard-won and frustratingly slow. But fixing the global pain crisis is a moral imperative. By any ethical measure, it is unacceptable for people, whether in rich countries or poor, to live and die in pain. This will take changes in government funding, changes in medical schools, and changes in laws and regulations.

Those changes will only occur when physicians like Drs. Rajagopal and Merriman can obtain morphine for their dying patients and when pain patient advocates like Steinberg, Christopher, and Cowan make their voices heard. And when the rest of the world listens.

APPENDIX I: RESOURCES

Access to Opioid Medication in Europe (ATOME): http://www.atome-project.eu

European Association for Palliative Care: http://www.eapcnet.eu

European Society for Medical Oncology: http://www.esmo.org

Global Opioid Policy Initiative: http://www.esmo.org/Policy/Global-Opioid-Policy-Initiative

Harvard Global Equity Initiative: http://hgei.harvard.edu/icb/icb.do

Human Rights Watch: http://www.hrw.org

Institute of Medicine, *Relieving Pain in America: A Blueprint for Transforming Prevention, Care, Education and Research* (Washington, DC: National Academies Press, 2011). Abstract: https://www.iom.edu/Reports/2011/Relieving-Pain-in-America-A-Blueprint-for-Transforming-Prevention-Care-Education-Research.aspx. Book: http://www.nap.edu/openbook.php?record_id=13172

Lancet Commission on Global Access to Pain Control and Palliative Care (GPCPC): http://hgei.harvard.edu/icb/icb.do?keyword=k62597&pageid=icb.page704146

Pain & Policy Studies Group (University of Wisconsin): http://www.painpolicy.wisc.edu

Treat the Pain: http://www.treatthepain.org

Union for International Cancer Control: http://www.uicc.org

World Health Organization: http://www.who.int/en

APPENDIX II: TREATMENTS FOR PAIN

In general, use no drugs at all if possible. Exercise, physical therapy, acupuncture, massage, and meditation have all been shown to ease pain. With back pain in particular, moving around—exercise—is often best. Don't stay in bed any longer than necessary—rest is rust.

There is no "best" drug for each and every pain condition. Drugs ultimately are given to individuals—what works for one person may not work for another with apparently the same condition. Sometimes the most efficacious drug may not be the safest for any particular person.[1]

Another warning: Popular over-the-counter pain pills include nonsteroidal anti-inflammatory drugs (NSAIDs) such as ibuprofen (Motrin, Advil, Aleve) and aspirin, as well as acetaminophen, the main ingredient in Tylenol.

NSAIDs are good for both inflammatory problems like arthritis or low back pain with inflammation, as well as some noninflammatory problems like headaches. Acetaminophen, which does not reduce inflammation, is also good for minor pain and is better than the stronger NSAIDs if one can't take NSAIDs because of heart disease or other problems. But both NSAIDs and acetaminophen have serious risks—thousands die yearly from NSAIDs and many thousands more are hospitalized due to liver damage from acetaminophen. Do not drink alcohol if taking acetaminophen.

With these caveats in mind, here are some medications often used for common conditions:

Arthritis: NSAIDs, acetaminophen, and capsaicin cream can all help, particularly with rheumatoid arthritis. Prescription NSAIDs such as Celebrex help with more severe pain, as can corticosteroid injections and other steroids such as Deltasone tablets and Liquid Pred. Many of these medications also help with osteoarthritis; for knee osteoarthritis specifically, hyaluronic acid may help.

Back pain: For acute (short-term) pain, use NSAIDs, acetaminophen, and hot and cold packs. (Heat brings blood to the area; cold reduces inflammation.)

For chronic back pain, all of these are used, plus, in more severe cases, opioids such as OxyContin (oxycodone) or Zohydro (hydrocodone). In some cases, injections called nerve root blocks can help.

Burns and scrapes (minor): Lidocaine Plus, Topicaine, and Numb Master (lidocaine creams) are useful.

Fibromyalgia: Lyrica, an anticonvulsant drug containing pregabalin can help, as can Cymbalta (duloxetine) and Savella, Ixel, Toledomin, and Dalcipran (minalcipran).

Gum and mouth sores: Benzocaine gels and liquids such as Benz-O-Sthetic (do not use in children under two) and Peridex or Periogard (chlorhexidine) may help. But note: common mouth sores are different from blisters caused by the herpes simplex 1 virus, for which antiviral medications can be used, including Zovirax (acyclovir), Famvir (famcyclovir), INN (valaciclovir), and USAN (valacyclovir).

Headache, tension: NSAIDs, acetaminophen, aspirin.

Headache, migraines, and cluster headaches: Imitrex (sumatriptan) and Mazalt.

Irritable bowel syndrome: Antispasmodics such as BAN (hyoscine), Dicetel (pinaverium), and Alginor (cimetropium) may help with abdominal pain.

Neuropathic (nerve) pain: Prescription medications containing gabapentin such as Neurontin and carbamazepine (Tegretol) help. Antidepressants can also reduce pain from injured nerves, among them Elavil and Cymbalta (duloxetine). For pain from damaged nerves close to the skin, a lidocaine patch can help.

Posttherpetic neuralgia: See "Shingles."

Shingles: Antivirals such as Zovirax, Famvir, INN, and USAN, as mentioned. Lyrica (pregabalin) may also help. The vaccine Zostavax can help prevent shingles.

Various types of moderate to severe pain not alleviated by other medications: Opioids (narcotics) such as Vicodin (hydrocodone plus acetaminophen), OxyContin (oxycodone), Zohydro (hydrocodone), and Methadose (methadone). These drugs can cause physical dependence and addiction and, ironically, may sometimes make pain worse, a condition called opioid-induced hyperalgesia.

NOTES

Introduction

1. US Institute of Medicine, Committee on Advancing Pain Research, Care, and Education. (2011). *Relieving pain in America: A blueprint for transforming prevention, care, education and research* (pp. 2–6). Washington, DC: National Academies Press.
2. National Institutes of Health. (2015). [Table shows appropriations of funds by the NIH for FY 1938–2014]. *Appropriations (section 2) from the NIH Almanac.* Retrieved from http://www.nih.gov/about/alma-nac/appropriations/part2.htm
3. National Institutes of Health. (2015). [Table shows the annual support level by the NIH for FY 2011–2014 and estimates for FY 2015–2016]. *Estimates of funding for various research, condition, and disease categories (RCDC).* Retrieved from http://report.nih.gov/rcdc/categories
4. R. Myles (personal communication, February 23, 2012).
5. National Institutes of Health. (n.d.). [Table shows NIH budget information for FY 2014–2016]. *All purpose table.* Retrieved from http://officeofbudget.od.nih.gov/pdfs/FY16/Executive%20Summary.pdf
6. National Institutes of Health. (2015). [Table shows the annual support level by the NIH for FY 2011–2014 and estimates for FY 2015–2016]. *Estimates of funding for various research, condition, and disease categories (RCDC).* Retrieved from http://report.nih.gov/rcdc/categories
7. L. Porter (personal communication, April 28, 2015).
8. D. Bradshaw (personal communication, April 20, 2015).
9. Gereau, R.W. III, Sluka, K.A., Maixner, W., et al. (2014). A pain research agenda for the 21st century. *Journal of Pain, 15,* 1203–1214.
10. National Institutes of Health. (2014). *Pathways to Prevention Workshop: The Role of Opioids in the Treatment of Chronic Pain.* Retrieved

from https://prevention.nih.gov/docs/programs/p2p/ODPPain PanelStatementFinal_10-02-14.pdf

11. US Institute of Medicine, Committee on Advancing Pain Research, Care, and Education. (2011). *Relieving pain in America: A blueprint for transforming prevention, care, education and research* (pp. 2–26) Washington, DC: National Academies Press.

12. Fisch, M.J., Lee, J-W., Weiss, M., et al. (2012). Prospective, observational study of pain and analgesic prescribing in medical oncology outpatients with breast, colorectal, lung, or prostate cancer. *Journal of Clinical Oncology, 30*(16), 1980–1988.

13. Ackerman, T. (2012, April 19). Pain treatment lacking for a third of cancer patients, study says. *Houston Chronicle.* Retrieved from http://www.chron.com/news/houston-texas/article/A-third-of-cancer-patients-pain-3496068.php

14. Tsang, A., Von Korff, M., Lee, S., et al. (2008). Common chronic pain conditions in developed and developing countries: Gender and age differences and comorbidity with depression-anxiety disorders. *Journal of Pain, 9*(10), 883–889.

15. F. Knaul (personal communication, January 26, 2015).

16. Cherny, N.I., Baselga, J., de Conno, F., & Radbruch, L. (2010). Formulary availability and regulatory barriers to accessibility of opioids for cancer pain in Europe: A report from the ESMO/EAPC opioid policy initiative. *Annals of Oncology, 21*(3), 615–626.

17. World Health Organization. (2011). Ensuring balance in national policies on controlled substances: Guidance for availability and accessibility of controlled medicine. Retrieved from http://www.atome-project.eu/documents/gls_ens_balance_eng.pdf

18. Human Rights Watch. (2011). *Global state of pain treatment: Access to palliative care as a human right.* Retrieved from http://www.hrw.org/sites/default/files/reports/hhr0511W.pdf

19. American Cancer Society, Treat the Pain. (2015). *Ethiopia: A country snapshot.* Retrieved from http://www.treatthepain.org/Assets/CountryReports/Ethiopia.pdf

20. M. O'Brien (personal communication, January 7, 2015).

21. American Cancer Society, Treat the Pain. (2014). *Nigeria: A country snapshot.* Retrieved from http://www.treatthepain.org/Assets/CountryReports/Nigeria.pdf

22. Human Rights Watch. (2011). *Global state of pain treatment: Access to palliative care as a human right* (p. 11). Retrieved from http://www.hrw.org/sites/default/files/reports/hhr0511W.pdf

23. American Cancer Society, Treat the Pain. (2014). *Access to essential pain medicine brief (2012 data).* Retrieved from http://www.treatthe-pain.org/Assets/Fact%20sheet%20May%202014.pdf

24. Single Convention on Narcotic Drugs. (n.d). In *Wikipedia.* Retrieved from http://en.wikipedia.org/wiki/Single_Convention_on_Narcotic_Drugs

25. United Nations, International Narcotics Review Board. (2010). *Availability of internationally controlled drugs: Ensuring adequate access for medical and scientific purposes.* Retrieved from http://www.incb.org/documents/Publications/AnnualReports/AR2010/Supplement-AR10_availability_English.pdf

26. Cleary, J.F., Hutson, P., & Joranson, D. (2010). Access to therapeutic opioid medications in Europe by 2011? Fifty years on from the Single Convention on Narcotic Drugs [Editorial]. *Palliative Medicine, 24*(2), 109–110.

27. C. Lenard (personal communication, April 16, 2015).

28. National Institutes of Health. (2014). *Pathways to Prevention workshop: The role of opioids in the treatment of chronic pain.* Retrieved from https://prevention.nih.gov/docs/programs/p2p/ODPPainPanel StatementFinal_10-02-14.pdf

29. Human Rights Watch. (2011). *Global state of pain treatment: Access to palliative care as a human right.* Retrieved from http://www.hrw.org/sites/default/files/reports/hhr0511W.pdf

30. Mezei, L., Murinson, B.B., & Johns Hopkins Pain Curriculum Development Team. (2011). Pain education in North American medical schools. *Journal of Pain, 12*(12), 1199–1208.

31. Watt-Watson, J., McGillion, M., Hunter, J., et al. (2009). A survey of prelicensure pain curricula in health science faculties in Canadian universities. *Pain Research and Management, 14*(6), 439–444.

32. Briggs, E.V., Carr, E.C.J., & Whittaker, M.S. (2011). Survey of undergraduate pain curricula for healthcare professionals in the United Kingdom. *European Journal of Pain, 15*(8), 789–795.

33. Human Rights Watch. (2011). *Global state of pain treatment: Access to palliative care as a human right.* Retrieved from http://www.hrw.org/sites/default/files/reports/hhr0511W.pdf

34. National Institutes of Health. (2014). *Pathways to Prevention workshop: The role of opioids in the treatment of chronic pain.* Retrieved from https://prevention.nih.gov/docs/programs/p2p/ODPPain PanelStatementFinal_10-02-14.pdf

Chapter 1

1. International Association for the Study of Pain. (2012). IASP taxonomy: Pain. Retrieved from http://www.iasp-pain.org/Taxonomy
2. Morales, K. (2015, May 6). Brain chemicals may offer new clues in treating chronic pain. UT Dallas News Center. Retrieved from http://www.utdallas.edu/news/2015/5/6-31524_Brain-Chemical-May-Offer-New-Clues-in-Treating-Chr-_story-wide.html
3. Costigan, M., Scholz, J., & Woolf, C.J. (2009). Neuropathic pain: A maladaptive response of the nervous system to damage. *Annual Review of Neuroscience, 32,* 1–32.
4. Scholz, J., & Woolf, C.J. (2002). Can we conquer pain? [Review]. *Nature Neuroscience, 5*(Suppl.), 1062–1067.
5. Brenner, G.J., & Woolf, C.J. (2007). Mechanisms of chronic pain. In *Anesthesiology,* ed. D.E. Longnecker, D.L. Brown, M.F. Newman, & W.M Zapol (pp. 2000–2019). New York: McGraw-Hill.
6. Ibid.
7. Costigan, M., Scholz, J., & Woolf, C.J. (2009). Neuropathic pain: A maladaptive response of the nervous system to damage. *Annual Review of Neuroscience, 32,* 1–32.
8. Haanpää, M., & Treede, R.D. (2010). Diagnosis and classification of neuropathic pain. *Pain Clinical Updates, 18*(7), 1–6.
9. Braz, J.M., Sharif-Naeini, R., Vogt, D., et al. (2012). Forebrain GABAergic neuron precursors integrate into adult spinal cord and reduce injury-induced neuropathic pain. *Neuron, 74*(4), 663–675.
10. G. Brenner (personal communication, October 28, 2010).
11. Hovaguimian, A., & Gibbons, C.H. (2011). Diagnosis and treatment of pain in small fiber neuropathy. *Current Pain and Headache Reports, 15*(3), 193–200.
12. Talkington, M. (2011, June 25). Nav 1.7 mutations move into the mainstream. Pain Research Forum. Retrieved from http://www.painresearchforum.org/news/7360-nav17-mutations-move-mainstream
13. Ibid.
14. Faber, C.G., Hoeijmakers, J.G., Ahn, H.S., et al. (2012). Gain of function Nav 1.7 mutations in idiopathic small fiber neuropathy. *Annals of Neurology, 71*(1), 26–39.
15. Woolf, C.J., & Ma, Q. (2007). Nociceptors—Noxious stimulus detectors. *Neuron Review, 55,* 353–364.
16. Brenner, G.J., & Woolf, C.J. (2007). Mechanisms of chronic pain. In *Anesthesiology,* ed. D.E. Longnecker, D.L. Brown, M.F. Newman, & W.M Zapol (pp. 2000–2019). New York: McGraw-Hill.

17. Patapoutian, A., Tate, S., & Woolf, C.J. (2009). Transient receptor potential channels: Targeting pain at the source. *Nature Reviews Drug Discovery, 8*(1), 55–68.

18. Foreman, J. (2014). *A nation in pain* (pp. 24–30). New York: Oxford University Press.

19. Talkington, M. (2011, June 30). A new chapter for sodium channels. Pain Research Forum. Retrieved from http://www.painresearchforum.org/news/7484-new-chapter-sodium-channels

20. Wortman, M. (2012). Where does it hurt? Researchers are getting to the molecular details of pain's circuitry to answer the question with real specificity. *Howard Hughes Medical Institute Bulletin, 25*(1), 33.

21. Pain Medicine News staff. (2015, February). Novel compound yields long-acting anesthetic effect. *Pain Medicine News, 13*(4). Retrieved from http://www.anesthesiologynews.com/ViewArticle.aspx?d=Pain%2BMedicine&d_id=2&i=February+2015&i_id=1145&a_id=29338

22. Porreca, F. (2011, October 17). Cancer biology seminar series: Descending modulatory circuits and cancer pain [Video file]. Retrieved from http://streaming.biocom.arizona.edu/people/?id=11499

23. Foreman, J. (2014). *A nation in pain* (pp. 24–30). New York: Oxford University Press.

24. Beecher, H.K. (1956). Relationship of significance of wound to pain experienced. *The Journal of the American Medical Association, 161*(17), 1609–1613.

25. Von Mourik, O. (2006, April 2). Penfield's homunculus and the mystery of phantom limbs. [Web log comment]. Retrieved from http://journalism.nyu.edu/publishing/archives/annotate/node/270

26. G. Brenner (personal communication, March 13, 2012).

27. NOVA Online. (n.d.). Secrets of the mind: Brain-mapping pioneers. Retrieved from http://www.pbs.org/wgbh/nova/mind/prob_pio.html

28. Blakeslee, S., & Blakeslee, M. (2007). *The body has a mind of its own: How body maps in your brain help you do (almost) everything better* (pp. 17–22). New York: Random House.

29. Ramachandran, V.S., Rogers-Ramachandran, D., & Stewart, M.I. (1992). Perceptual correlates of massive cortical reorganization. *Science, 258* (5085), 1159–1160.

30. Apkarian, A.V., Sosa, Y., Sonty, S., et al. (2004). Chronic back pain is associated with decreased prefrontal and thalamic gray matter density. *Journal of Neuroscience, 24*(46), 10410–10415.

31. Tracey, I., & Bushnell, M.C. (2009). How neuroimaging studies have challenged us to rethink: Is chronic pain a disease? *The Journal of Pain, 10*(11), 1113–1120.
32. Latremoliere, A., & Woolf, C. (2009). Central sensitization: A generator of pain hypersensitivity by central neural plasticity [Critical review]. *The Journal of Pain, 10*(9), 895–926.
33. Brenner, G.J., & Woolf, C.J. (2007). Mechanisms of chronic pain. In *Anesthesiology,* ed. D.E. Longnecker, D.L. Brown, M.F. Newman, & W.M Zapol (pp. 2000–2019). New York: McGraw-Hill.
34. Woolf, C.J. (2007). Central sensitization: Uncovering the relation between pain and plasticity. *Anesthesiology, 106*(4), 864–867.
35. Woolf, C.J. (2010, September). Central sensitization: How plasticity produces pain. Paper presented at the 13th World Congress on Pain, Montreal.
36. Apkarian, A.V., Baliki, M.N., & Geha, P.Y. (2009). Towards a theory of chronic pain. *Progress in Neurobiology, 87,* 81–97.
37. Apkarian, A.V., Bushnell, M.C., Treede, R.D., & Zubieta, J.K. (2005). Human brain mechanisms of pain perception and regulation in health and disease. *European Journal of Pain, 9*(4), 463–484.
38. Foreman, J. (2014). *A nation in pain* (pp. 31–35). New York: Oxford University Press.
39. Morales, K. (2015, May 6). Brain chemicals may offer new clues in treating chronic pain. UT Dallas News Center. Retrieved from http://www.utdallas.edu/news/2015/5/6-31524_Brain-Chemical-May-Offer-New-Clues-in-Treating-Chr-_story-wide.html
40. Gottschalk, A., Smith, D.S., Jobes, D.R., et al. (1998). Preemptive epidural analgesia and recovery from radical prostatectomy: A randomized controlled trial. *The Journal of the American Medical Association, 279*(14), 1076–1082.
41. L.R. Watkins (personal communication, October 28, 2009).
42. Ji, R.R., Kawasaki, Y., Zhuang, Z.Y., Wen, Y.R., & Decosterd, I. (2006). Possible role of spinal astrocytes in maintaining chronic pain sensitization: Review of current evidence with focus on bFGF/JNK pathway. *Neuron Glia Biology, 2*(4), 259–269.
43. Meller, S.T., Dykstra, C., Grzybycki, D., Murphy, S., & Gebhart, G.F. (1994). The possible role of glia in nociceptive processing and hyperalgesia in the spinal cord of the rat [Abstract]. *Neuropharmacology, 33*(11), 1471–1478.
44. Zhang, J.H., & Huang, Y.G. (2006). The immune system: A new look at pain. *Chinese Medical Journal, 119*(11), 930–938.

45. Watkins, L.R., Hutchinson, M.R., Ledeboer, A., Wieseler-Frank, J., Milligan, E.D., & Maier, S.F. (2007). Glia as the "bad guys": Implications for improving clinical pain control and the clinical utility of opioids. *Brain, Behavior, and Immunity, 21*(2), 131–146.

46. L.R. Watkins (personal communication, October 28, 2009).

47. Watkins, L.R., Milligan, E.D., & Maier, S.F. (2003). Glial proinflammatory cytokines mediate exaggerated pain states: Implications for clinical pain [Abstract]. *Advances in Experimental Medicine and Biology, 521*, 1–21.

48. L.R. Watkins (personal communication, November 9, 2009).

49. Ellis, A., Wieseler, J., Favret, J., et al. (2014). Systemic administration of propentofylline ibudilast, and (+)-naltrexone each reverses mechanical allodynia in a novel rat model of central neuropathic pain. *The Journal of Pain, 15*(4), 407–421.

50. Younger, J., & Mackey, S. (2009). Fibromyalgia symptoms are reduced by low-dose naltrexone: A pilot study. *Pain Medicine, 10*(4), 663–672.

51. Younger, J., Noor, N., McCue, R., & Mackey, S. (2013). Low-dose naltrexone for the treatment of fibromyalgia: Findings of a small, randomized, double-blind, placebo-controlled, counterbalanced, crossover trial accessing daily pain levels. *Arthritis & Rheumatology, 65*(2), 529–538.

52. Ibid.

53. Loggia, M.L., Chonde, D.B., Akeju, O., et al. (2015). Evidence for brain glial activation in chronic pain patients. *Brain, 138*, 604–615.

54. Tracey, I., & Bushnell, M.C. (2009). How neuroimaging studies have challenged us to rethink: Is chronic pain a disease? *The Journal of Pain, 10*(11), 1113–1120.

55. Brown, J.E., Chatterjee, N., Younger, J., & Mackey, S. (2011). Towards a physiology-based measure of pain: Patterns of human brain activity distinguish painful from non-painful thermal stimulation. *PLoS ONE, 6*(9), e24124.

56. White, T. (2011). Does that hurt? Objective way to measure pain being developed at Stanford [Press release]. Retrieved from http://med.stanford.edu/ism/2011/september/pain.html

57. Wager, T.D., Atlas, L.Y., Lindquist, M.A., Roy, M., Woo, C., & Kross, E. (2013). An fMRI-based neurologic signature of physical pain. *The New England Journal of Medicine, 368*, 1388–1397.

58. Apkarian, A.V., Bushnell, M.C., Treede, R.D., & Zubieta, J.K. (2005). Human brain mechanisms of pain perception and regulation in health and disease. *European Journal of Pain, 9*(4), 463–484.

59. Schweinhardt, P., Glynn, C., Brooks, J., et al. (2006). An fMRI study of cerebral processing of brush-evoked allodynia in neuropathic pain patients. *NeuroImage, 32*(1), 256–265.

60. Apkarian, A.V., Baliki, M.N., & Geha, P.Y. (2009). Towards a theory of chronic pain. *Progress in Neurobiology, 87,* 81–97.

61. S. Mackey (personal communication, April 14, 2012).

62. Miller, G. (2009). Brain scans of pain raise questions for the law. *Science, 323*(5911), 195.

63. White, T. (2011, September 13). Does that hurt? Objective way to measure pain being developed at Stanford [Press release]. Retrieved from http://med.stanford.edu/ism/2011/september/pain.html

64. Apkarian, A.V., Sosa, Y., Sonty, S., et al. (2004). Chronic back pain is associated with decreased prefrontal and thalamic gray matter density. *Journal of Neuroscience, 24*(46), 10410–10415.

65. Kuchinad, A., Schweinhardt, P., Seminowicz, D.A., Wood, P.B., Chizh, B.A., & Bushnell, M.C. (2007). Accelerated brain gray matter loss in fibromyalgia patients: Premature aging of the brain? *Journal of Neuroscience, 27*(15), 4004–4007.

66. Seminowicz, D.A., Labus, J.S., Bueller, J.A., Tillisch, K., Naliboff, B.D., & Bushnell, M.C. (2010). Regional gray matter density changes in brains of patients with irritable bowel syndrome. *Gastroenterology, 139*(1), 48–57.

67. Schmidt-Wilcke, T., Leinisch, E., Straube, A., et al. (2005). Gray matter decrease in patients with chronic tension type headache. *Neurology, 65,* 1483–1486.

68. Da Silva, A.F., Becerra, L., Pendse, G., Chizh, B., Tully, S., & Borsook, D. (2008). Colocalized structural and functional changes in the cortex of patients with trigeminal neuropathic pain. *PLoS ONE, 3*(10), e3396.

69. Draganski, B., Moser, T., Lummel, N., Ganssbauer, S., Bogdahn, U., Haas, F., & May, A. (2006). Decrease of thalamic gray matter following limb amputation. *NeuroImage, 31*(3), 951–957.

70. Wrigley, P.J., Gustin, S.M., Macey, P.M., et al. (2009). Anatomical changes in human motor cortex and motor pathways following complete thoracic spinal cord injury. *Cerebral Cortex, 19*(1), 224–232.

71. Rodriguez-Raecke, R., Niemeier, A., Ihle, K., Ruether, W., & May, A. (2009). Brain gray matter decrease in chronic pain is the consequence and not the cause of pain. *Journal of Neuroscience, 29*(44), 13746–13750.

72. Gwilym, S.E., Fillipini, N., Douaud, G., Carr, A.J., & Tracey, I. (2010). Thalamic atrophy associated with painful osteoarthritis of the hip is

reversible after arthroplasty: A longitudinal voxel-based-morphometric study. *Arthritis & Rheumatism, 62*(10), 2930–2940.

73. Seminowicz, D.A., Wideman, T.H., Naso, L., et al. (2011). Effective treatment of chronic low back pain in humans reverses abnormal brain anatomy and function. *Journal of Neuroscience, 31*(20), 7540–7550.

74. D. Borsook (personal communication, July 1, 2010).

75. Da Silva, A.F., Becerra, L., Pendse, G., Chizh, B., Tully, S., & Borsook, D. (2008). Colocalized structural and functional changes in the cortex of patients with trigeminal neuropathic pain. *PLoS ONE, 3*(10), e3396.

76. Borras, M.C., Becerra, L., Ploghaus, A., Gostic, J.M., DaSilva, A., Gonzalez, R.G., & Borsook, D. (2004). fMRI measurement of CNS responses to naloxone infusion and subsequent mild noxious thermal stimuli in healthy volunteers. *Journal of Neurophysiology, 91*(6), 2723–2733.

77. Borsook, D. (2012, August). Imaging opioid effects on the brain— From preclinical to postclinical [Abstract]. Paper presented at the International Association for the Study of Pain's 14th World Congress on Pain, Milan, Italy. Retrieved from http://www.abstracts2view.com/iasp/sessionindex.php

78. Alpkarian, A.V., Baliki, M.N., & Farmer, M.A. (2013). Predicting transition to chronic pain. *Current Opinion in Neurology, 26*(4), 360–367.

79. Ahmed, A. (2013, October 8). Brain activity shifts as pain becomes chronic. Pain Research Forum. Retrieved from http://painresearchforum.org/news/32409-brain-activity-shifts-pain-becomes-chronic

80. Mansour, A.R., Baliki, M.N., Huang, L., et al. (2013). Brain white matter structural properties predict transition to chronic pain. *PAIN, 154*(10), 2160–2168.

81. Ahmed, A. (2013, October 8). Brain activity shifts as pain becomes chronic. Pain Research Forum. Retrieved from http://painresearchforum.org/news/32409-brain-activity-shifts-pain-becomes-chronic

82. Foreman, J. (2015, July). A new kind of brain scan can see your pain, literally. *Popular Science.*

83. Loggia, M.L., Chonde, D.B., Akeju, O., et al. (2015). Evidence for brain glial activation in chronic pain patients. *Brain, 38*(Pt. 3), 604–615.

84. Melzack, R. (n.d.). The McGill Pain Questionnaire. Retrieved from http://www.cebp.nl/vault_public/filesystem/?ID=1400

85. D. Price (personal communication, November 1, 2010).

86. R. Staud (personal communication, October 21, 2010).

87. R. Jamison (personal communication, February 14, 2011).

88. Marceau, L.D., Link, C., Jamison R.N., & Carolan, S. (2007). Electronic diaries as a tool to improve pain management: Is there any evidence? *Pain Medicine, 8,* S101–S109.

89. Jamison, R.N., Raymond, S.A., Levine, J.G., Slawsby, E.A., Nedeljkovic, S.S., & Katz, N.P. (2001). Electronic diaries for monitoring chronic pain: 1-year validation study. *PAIN, 91*(3), 277–285.

90. Scholz, J., Mannion, R.J., Hord, D.E., et al. (2009). A novel tool for the assessment of pain: Validation in low back pain. *PLoS Medicine, 6*(4), e1000047.

91. Prkachin, K.M., & Craig, K.D. (1995). Expressing pain: The communication and interpretation of facial pain signals. *Journal of Nonverbal Behavior, 19*(4), 191–205.

92. Ashraf, A.B., Lucey, S., Cohn, J.F., et al. (2009). The painful face— Pain expression recognition using active appearance models. *Image and Vision Computing, 27*(12), 1788–1796.

93. K. Prkachin (personal communication, October 21, 2010).

94. Kappesser, J., Williams, A.C., & Prkachin, K. (2006). Testing two accounts of pain underestimation. *PAIN, 124*(1–2), 109–116.

95. Prkachin, K.M., Solomon, P., Hwang, T., & Mercer, S.R. (2001). Does experience influence judgments of pain behaviour? Evidence from relatives of pain patients and therapists. *Pain Research and Management, 6*(2), 105–112.

96. K. Prkachin (personal communication, October 21, 2010).

97. Kappesser, J., Williams, A.C., & Prkachin, K. (2006). Testing two accounts of pain underestimation. *PAIN, 124*(1–2), 109–116.

98. K. Craig (personal communication, October 26, 2010).

99. Bufano, P. (2014). Computer detects fake expressions of pain better than people. *Current Biology, 24,* 738–743.

100. Nielsen, C.S., Staud, R., & Price, D.D. (2009). Individual differences in pain sensitivity: Measurement, causation and consequences. *The Journal of Pain, 10*(3), 231–237.

101. M. Rowbotham (personal communication, November 11, 2010).

102. Thyregod, H.G., Rowbotham, M.C., Peters, M., Possehn, J., Berro, M., & Petersen, K.L. (2007). Natural history of pain following herpes zoster. *PAIN, 128,* 148–156.

103. National Diabetes Information Clearinghouse. (2009). What are diabetic neuropathies? Retrieved from http://diabetes.niddk.nih.gov/dm/pubs/neuropathies/index.aspx

104. O'Hare, J.A., Abuaisha, F., & Geoghegan, M. (1994). Prevalence and forms of neuropathic morbidity in 800 diabetics [Abstract]. *Irish Journal of Medical Science, 163*(3), 132–135.
105. J. Mogil (personal communication, June 12, 2015).
106. Ibid.
107. Foreman, J. (2014). *A nation in pain* (pp. 45–52). New York: Oxford University Press.
108. Weiss, J., Pyrski, M., Jacobi, E., Bufe, B., Willnecker, V., & Schick, B. (2011). Loss-of-function mutations in channel Nav1.7 cause anosmia. *Nature, 472,* 186–190.
109. S. Waxman (personal communication, September 25, 2012).
110. Faber, C.G., Hoeijmakers, J.G., Ahn, H.S., et al.,(2012). Gain of function Nav 1.7 mutations in idiopathic small fiber neuropathy. *Annals of Neurology, 71*(1), 26–39.
111. Reimann, F., Cox, J.J., Belfer, A., et al. (2010). Pain perception is altered by a nucleotide polymorphism in *SCN9A. Proceedings of the National Academy of Sciences, 107*(11), 5148–5153.
112. Drenth, J. te Morsche, R. Guillet, G., Taieb, A., Kirby, R. & Jansen, J. (2005). SCN9A mutations define primary erythermalgia as a neuropathic disorder of voltage gated sodium channels. *Journal of Investigative Dermatology, 124,* 1333–1338.
113. Legroux-Crespel, E., Sassolas, B., Guillet, G., Kupfer, I., Dupre, D., & Misery, L. (2003). Treatment of familial erythermalgia with the association of lidocaine and mexiletine. *Annales de dermatologie et de vénéréologie, 130*(4), 429–433.
114. Fischer, T.A., Gilmore, E.S., Estacion, M., et al. (2009). A novel Na$_v$1.7 mutation producing carbamazepine-responsive erythromelalgia. *Annals of Neurology, 65*(6), 733–741.
115. Cummins, T.R., Dib-Hajj, S.D., & Waxman, S.G. (2004). Electrophysiological properties of mutant Na$_v$1.7 sodium channels in a painful inherited neuropathy. *Journal of Neuroscience, 24*(38), 8232–8236.
116. Dib-Hajj, S.D., Cummins, T.R., Black, J.A., & Waxman, S.G. (2010). Sodium channels in normal and pathological pain. *Annual Review of Neuroscience, 33,* 325–347.
117. Dib-Hajj, S.D., Cummins, T.R., Black, J.A., & Waxman, S.G. (2007). From genes to pain: Na$_v$1.7. and human pain disorders. *Trends in Neuroscience, 30*(11), 555–563.
118. Black, J.A., Nikolajsen, L., Kroner, K., Jensen, T.S., & Waxman, S.G. (2008). Multiple sodium channel isoforms and mitogen-activated

protein kinases are present in painful human neuromas. *Annals of Neurology, 64*(6), 644–653.

119. S. Waxman (personal communication, September 25, 2012).

120. Mogil, J.S., Wilson, S.G., Bon, K., et al. (1999). Heritability of nociception I: Responses of 11 inbred mouse strains on 12 measures of nociception. *PAIN, 80*(1), 67–82.

121. Mogil, J.S. (1999). The genetic mediation of individual differences in sensitivity to pain and its inhibition. *Proceedings of the National Academy of Sciences, 96*, 7744–7751.

122. MacGregor, A.J., Andrew, T., Sambrook, P.N., & Spector, T.D. (2004). Structural, psychological and genetic influences on low back and neck pain: A study of adult female twins. *Arthritis Care & Research, 51*(2), 160–167.

123. Norbury, T.A., MacGregor, A.J., Urwin, J., Spector, T.D., & McMahon, S.B. (2007). Heritability of responses to painful stimuli in women: A classical twin study. *Brain, 130,* 3041–3049.

124. Nielsen, C.S., Stubhaug, A., Price, D.D., Vassend, O., Czajkowski, N., & Harris, J.R. (2008). Individual differences in pain sensitivity: Genetic and environmental contributions. *PAIN, 136*(1), 21–29.

125. Hartvigsen, J., Nielsen, J., Kyvik, K.O., et al. (2009). Heritability of spinal pain and consequences of spinal pain: A comprehensive genetic epidemiologic analysis using a population-based sample of 15,328 twins ages 20–71 years. *Arthritis Care & Research, 61*(10), 1343–1351.

126. Markkula, R., Jarvinen, P., Leino-Arjas, P., Koskenvuo, M., Kalso, E., & Kaprio, J. (2009). Clustering of symptoms associated with fibromyalgia in a Finnish twin cohort. *European Journal of Pain, 13*(7), 744–750.

127. Mogil, J.S. (1999). The genetic mediation of individual differences in sensitivity to pain and its inhibition. *Proceedings of the National Academy of Sciences, 96*, 7744–7751.

128. Spector, T.D., & MacGregor, A.J. (2004). Risk factors for osteoarthritis: Genetics. *Osteoarthritis and Cartilage, 12*, S39–S44.

129. Solis, M. (2014, June 23). Human brain mechanisms of pain perception and regulation in health and disease: Same genes? Pain Research Forum. Retrieved from http://www.painresearchforum.org/news/42352-different-pain-same-genes

130. Vehof, J., Zavos, J.M., Lachance, G., Hammond, C.J., & Williams, F.M. (2014). Shared genetic factors underlie chronic pain syndromes. *PAIN, 155*(8), 1562–1568.

131. J. Mogil (personal communication, June 12, 2015).

132. Langford, D.J., Bailey, A.L., Chanda, M.L., et al. (2010). Coding of facial expressions of pain in the laboratory mouse. *Nature Methods, 7,* 447–449.

133. Mogil, J. (2012, February). The nature and nurture of pain. Paper presented at the International Association for the Study of Pain Research Symposium, Miami Beach, FL.

134. J. Mogil (personal communication, June 12, 2015).

135. Costigan, M., Belfer, I., Griffin, R.S., et al. (2010). Multiple chronic pain states are associated with a common amino acid-changing allele in KCNS1. *Brain, 133*(9), 2519–2527.

136. Neely, G.G., Hess, A., Costigan, M., et al. (2010). A genome-wide *Drosophila* screen for heat nociception identifies α2δ3 as an evolutionarily conserved pain gene. *Cell, 143*(4), 628–638.

137. M. Moskowitz (personal communication, November 29, 2010).

138. Gardner, K.L. (2006). Genetics of migraine: An update. *Headache: The Journal of Head and Face Pain, 46,* S19–S24.

139. Anttila, V., Stefansson, H., Kallela, M., et al. (2010). Genome-wide association study of migraine implicates a common susceptibility variant on 8q22.1 [Letter]. *Nature Genetics, 42,* 869–873.

140. Tegeder, I., Costigan, M., Griffin, R.S., et al. (2006). GTP cyclohydrolase and tetrahydrobiopterin regulate pain sensitivity and persistence. *Nature Medicine, 12*(11), 1269–1277.

141. Tegeder, I., Adolph, J., Schmidt, H., Woolf, C.J., Geisslinger, G., & Lotsch, J. (2008). Reduced hyperalgesia in homozygous carriers of a GTP cyclohydrolase 1 haplotype. *European Journal of Pain, 12*(8), 1069–1077.

142. Cromie, W.J. (2006, November 16). Sensitivity to pain explained. *Harvard University Gazette.* Retrieved from http://news.harvard.edu/gazette/story/2006/11/sensitivity-to-pain-explained

143. Lotsch, J., Belfer, I., Kirchhof, A., et al. (2007). Reliable screening for a pain-protective haplotype in the GTP cyclohydrolase 1 gene (GCH1) through the use of 3 or fewer single nucleotide polymorphisms. *Clinical Chemistry, 53*(6), 1010–1015.

144. L. Diatchenko (personal communication, November 1, 2010).

145. Maixner, W. (2012, February). Unraveling persistent pain conditions with genetic and phenotypic biomarkers. Paper presented at the International Association for the Study of Pain Research Symposium, Miami Beach, FL.

146. Tchivileva, I.E., Lim, P.F., Smith, S.B., et al. (2010). Effect of catechol-O-methyltransferase polymorphism on response to propranolol

therapy in chronic musculoskeletal pain: A randomized, double-blind, placebo-controlled, crossover pilot study. *Pharmacogenetics and Genomics, 20*(4), 239–248.

147. Light, K.C., Bragdon, E.E., Grewen, K.M., Brownley, K.A., Girdler, S.S., & Maixner, W. (2009). Adrenergic dysregulation and pain with and without acute beta-blockage in women with fibromyalgia and temporomandibular disorder. *The Journal of Pain, 10*(5), 542–552.

148. Emery, E.C., Young, G.T., Berrocoso, E.M., Chen, L., & McNaughton, P.A. (2011). HCN2 ion channels play a central role in inflammatory and neuropathic pain. *Science, 333*(6048), 1462–1466.

149. McNaughton, P. (2011, September 9). Gene that controls chronic pain identified. [Press release]. University of Cambridge. Retrieved from http://www.bbsrc.ac.uk/news/health/2011/110909-pr-gene-that-controls-pain.aspx

150. Bond, C., LaForge, K.S., Tian, M., et al. (1998). Single-nucleotide polymorphism in the human mu opioid receptor gene alters B-endorphin binding and activity: Possible implications for opiate addiction. *Proceedings of the National Academy of Sciences, 95*(16), 9608–9613.

151. Pan, Y. (2005). Diversity and complexity of the mu opioid receptor gene: Alternative pre-mRNA splicing and promoters. *DNA and Cell Biology, 24*(11), 736–750.

152. Walter, C., & Lotsch, J. (2009). Meta-analysis of the relevance of the OPRM1 118A> G genetic variant for pain treatment. *PAIN, 146,* 270–275.

153. University of North Carolina at Chapel Hill. (2011, November 10). Large-scale jaw pain study sheds light on pain disorders [Press release]. *EurekAlert!* Retrieved from http://uncnews.unc.edu/content/view/4910/71/

154. Slade, G.D., Bair, E., By, K., et al. (2011). Study methods, recruitment, sociodemographic findings, and demographic representativeness in OPPERA study. *The Journal of Pain, 12*(11), 12–26.

155. Lamas, D., & Rosenbaum, L. (2012). Painful inequities: Palliative care in developing countries. *The New England Journal of Medicine, 366*(3), 200.

156. Watt-Watson, J., McGillion, M., Hunter, J., et al. (2009). A survey of prelicensure pain curricula in health science faculties in Canadian universities. *Pain Research and Management, 14*(6), 439–444.

157. Briggs, E.V., Carr, E.C.J., & Whittaker, M.S. (2011). Survey of undergraduate pain curricula for healthcare professionals in the United Kingdom. *European Journal of Pain, 15*(8), 789–795.

158. Mezei, L., Murinson, B.B., & Johns Hopkins Pain Curriculum Development Team. (2011). Pain education in North American medical schools. *The Journal of Pain, 12*(12), 1199–1208.

159. US Institute of Medicine, Committee on Advancing Pain Research, Care, and Education. (2011). *Relieving pain in America: A blueprint for transforming prevention, care, education and research* (pp. 4–14). Washington, DC: National Academies Press.

Chapter 2

1. Ayroles, J.F., Carbone, M.A., Stone, E.A., et al. (2009). Systems of genetics of complex traits in *Drosophila melanogaster*. *Nature Genetics, 41*(3), 305.

2. I. Belfer (personal communication, March 7, 2012).

3. Unruh, A.M. (1996). Gender variations in clinical pain experience [Abstract]. *PAIN, 65*(2–3), 123–167.

4. LeResche, L. (2011). Defining gender disparities in pain management. *Clinical Orthopaedics and Related Research, 469*(7), 1871–1877.

5. Fillingim, R.B., King, C.D., Ribeiro-Dasilva, M.C., Rahim-Williams, B., & Riley, J.L. III. (2009). Sex, gender, and pain: A review of recent clinical and experimental findings. *The Journal of Pain, 10*(5), 447–485.

6. Aubrun, F., Salvi, N., Coriat, P., & Riou, B. (2005). Sex-and age-related differences in morphine requirements for postoperative pain relief [Abstract]. *Anesthesiology, 103*(1), 156–160.

7. Tsang, A., Von Korff, M., Lee, S., et al. (2008). Common chronic pain conditions in developed and developing countries: Gender and age differences and comorbidity with depression-anxiety disorders. *The Journal of Pain, 9*(10), 883–891.

8. Fillingim, R.B., King, C.D., Ribeiro-Dasilva, M.C., Rahim-Williams, B., & Riley, J.L. III. (2009). Sex, gender, and pain: A review of recent clinical and experimental findings. *The Journal of Pain, 10*(5), 447–485.

9. Bennett, M.I., Lee, A.J., Smith, B.H., & Torrance, N. (2006). The epidemiology of chronic pain of predominantly neuropathic origin. Results from a general population survey [Abstract]. *The Journal of Pain, 7*(4), 281–289.

10. National Institute of Neurological Disorders and Stroke. (n.d.). NINDS complex regional pain syndrome. Retrieved from http://www.ninds.nih.gov/disorders/reflex_sympathetic_dystrophy/reflex_sympathetic_dystrophy.htm

11. de Mos, M., De Bruijn, A.G.J., Huygen, F., Dieleman, J.P., Stricker, B.H., & Sturkenboom, M. (2007). The incidence of complex regional

pain syndrome: A population-based study [Abstract]. *PAIN, 129* (1–2), 12–20.

12. Hall, G.C., Carroll, D., Parry, D., & McQuay, H.J. (2006). Epidemiology and treatment of neuropathic pain: The UK primary care perspective. *PAIN, 122*(1–2), 156–162.

13. Fillingim, R.B., King, C.D., Ribeiro-Dasilva, M.C., Rahim-Williams, B., & Riley, J.L III. (2009). Sex, gender, and pain: A review of recent clinical and experimental findings. *The Journal of Pain, 10*(5), 447–485.

14. Srikanth, V.K., Fryer, J.L., Zhai, G., Winzenberg, T.M., Hosmer, D., & Jones, G. (2005). A meta-analysis of sex differences prevalence, incidence and severity of osteoarthritis [Abstract]. *Osteoarthritis and Cartilage, 13*(9), 769–781.

15. Christmas, C., Crespo, C.J., Franckowiak, S.C., Bathon, J.M., Bartlett, S.J., & Andersen, R.E. (2002). How common is hip pain among older adults? Results from the Third National Health and Nutrition Examination Survey. *The Journal of Family Practice, 51*(4), 345–348.

16. Fillingim, R.B., King, C.D., Ribeiro-Dasilva, M.C., Rahim-Williams, B., & Riley, J.L. III. (2009). Sex, gender, and pain: A review of recent clinical and experimental findings. *The Journal of Pain, 10*(5), 447–485.

17. Ibid.

18. Ibid.

19. Sandler, R.S. (1990). Epidemiology of irritable bowel syndrome in the United States [Abstract]. *Gastroenterology, 99*(2), 409–415.

20. M. Gold (personal communication, April 25, 2012).

21. Fillingim, R.B., King, C.D., Ribeiro-Dasilva, M.C., Rahim-Williams, B., & Riley, J.L. III. (2009). Sex, gender, and pain: A review of recent clinical and experimental findings. *The Journal of Pain, 10*(5), 447–485.

22. Ruau, D., Liu, L.Y., Clark, J.D., Angst, M.S., & Butte, A.J. (2012). Sex differences in reported pain across 11,000 patients captured in electronic medical records. *The Journal of Pain, 13*(3), 228–234.

23. B. Maixner (personal communication, November 1, 2010).

24. H. Bursztajn (personal communication, October 20, 2010).

25. Mogil, J.S., & Chanda, M.L. (2005). The case for the inclusion of female subjects in basic science studies of pain. *PAIN, 117*(1–2), 1–5.

26. Clayton, J.A. & Collins, F.S. (2014). Policy: NIH to balance sex in cell and animal studies. *Nature, 509*(7500), 282–283.

27. Sorge, R.E., Mapplebeck, J.C., Rosen, S., et al. (2015). Different immune cells mediate mechanical pain hypersensitivity in male and female mice. *Nature Neuroscience, 18*, 1081–1083.

28. Wizemann, T.M., & Pardue, M-L. (2001). *Exploring the biological contributions to human health: Does sex matter?* Washington, DC: National Academies Press.

29. Fillingim, R.B., King, C.D., Ribeiro-Dasilva, M.C., Rahim-Williams, B., & Riley, J.L. III. (2009). Sex, gender, and pain: A review of recent clinical and experimental findings. *The Journal of Pain, 10*(5), 447–485.

30. Greenspan, J.D., Craft, R.M., LeResche, L., et al. (2007). Studying sex and gender differences in pain and analgesia: A consensus report. *PAIN, 132,* S26–S45.

31. Clayton, J.A. & Collins, F.S. (2014). Policy: NIH to balance sex in cell and animal studies. *Nature, 509*(7500), 282–283.

32. Sutherland, S. (2014, May 28). A move toward sex equality in preclinical research. Pain Research Forum. Retrieved from http://www.painresearchforum.org/news/41234-move-toward-sex-equality-preclinical-research

33. K. Berkley (personal communication, October 5, 2010).

34. Levine, F.M., & De Simone, L.L. (1991). The effects of experimenter gender on pain report in male and female subjects [Abstract]. *PAIN, 44*(1), 69–72.

35. Gijsbers, K., & Nicholson, F. (2005). Experimental pain thresholds influenced by sex of experimenter. *Perceptual and Motor Skills, 101*(3), 803–807.

36. Fillingim, R.B., Browning, A.D., Powell, T., & Wright, R.A. (2002). Sex differences in perceptual and cardiovascular responses to pain: The influence of a perceived ability manipulation [Abstract]. *The Journal of Pain, 3*(6), 439–445.

37. R. Fillingim (personal communication, July 31, 2015).

38. Kallai, I., Barke, A., & Voss, U. (2004). The effects of experimenter characteristics on pain reports in women and men. *PAIN, 112,* 142–147.

39. Weisse C.S., Foster, K.K., & Fisher, E.A. (2005). The influence of experimenter gender and race on pain reporting: Does racial or gender concordance matter? *Pain Medicine, 6*(1), 80–87.

40. Vigil, J.M., DiDominico, J., Strenth, C., et al. (2015). Experimenter effects on pain reporting in women vary across the menstrual cycle. *International Journal of Endocrinology, 2015,* 1–8.

41. Katsnelson, A. (2014, April 28). Male researchers stress out rodents. *Nature.* Retrieved from http://www.nature.com/news/male-researchers-stress-out-rodents-1.15106

42. Sorge, R.E., Martin, L.J., Isbester, K.A., et al. (2014). Olfactory exposure to males, including men, causes stress and related analgesia in rodents. *Nature Method, 11,* 629–632.

43. R. Fillingim (personal communication, July 31, 2015).

44. Racine, M., Tousignant-Laflamme, Y., Kloda, L.A., Dion, D., Dupuis, G., & Choiniere, M. (2012). A systematic literature review of 10 years of research on sex/gender and experimental pain perception—Part I: Are there really differences between men and women? *PAIN, 153*(3), 602–618.

45. Fillingim, R.B., King, C.D., Ribeiro-Dasilva, M.C., Rahim-Williams, B., & Riley, J.L. III. (2009). Sex, gender, and pain: A review of recent clinical and experimental findings. *The Journal of Pain, 10*(5), 447–485.

46. Ibid.

47. Ibid.

48. Sarlani, E., Grace, E.G., Reynolds, M.A., & Greenspan, J.D. (2004). Sex differences in temporal summation of pain and aftersensations following repetitive noxious mechanical stimulation. *PAIN, 109*(1), 115–123.

49. Sarlani, E., & Greenspan, J.D. (2002). Gender differences in temporal summation of mechanically evoked pain [Abstract]. *PAIN, 97*(1), 163–169.

50. Racine, M., Tousignant-Laflamme, Y., Kloda, L.A., Dion, D., Dupuis, G., & Choiniere, M. (2012). A systematic literature review of 10 years of research on sex/gender and experimental pain perception—Part 2: Do biopsychosocial factors alter pain sensitivity differently in women and men? *PAIN, 153*(3), 619–635.

51. J. Greenspan (personal communication, October 20, 2010).

52. Paulson, P.E., Minoshima, S., Morrow, T.J., & Casey, K.L. (1998). Gender differences in pain perception and patterns of cerebral activation during noxious heat stimulation in humans [Abstract]. *PAIN, 76*(1–2), 223–229.

53. Naliboff, B.D., Berman, S., Chang, L., et al. (2003). Sex-related differences in IBS patients: Central processing of visceral stimuli. *Gastroenterology, 124*(7), 1738–1747.

54. Maleki, N., Linnman, C., Brawn, J., Burstein, R., Becerra, L., & Borsook, D. (2012). Her versus his migraine: Multiple sex differences in brain function and structure. *Brain, 135*(8), 2546–2559.

55. J. Levine (personal communication, September 21, 2010).

56. Klein, M.M., Downs, H.M., & Oaklander, A.L. (2010, September). Normal innervation in distal-leg skin biopsies: Evidence of

superabundance in youth, subsequent axonal pruning, plus new diagnostic recommendations. Paper presented at the 135th annual meeting of the American Neurological Association, San Francisco, CA.

57. Racine, M., Tousignant-Laflamme, Y., Kloda, L.A., Dion, D., Dupuis, G., & Choiniere, M. (2012). A systematic literature review of 10 years of research on sex/gender and experimental pain perception—Part 2: Do biopsychosocial factors alter pain sensitivity differently in women and men? *PAIN, 153*(3), 619–635.

58. Lipton, R.B., Stewart, W.F., Diamond, S., Diamond, M.L., & Reed, M. (2001). Prevalence and burden of migraine in the United States: Data from the American migraine study II [Abstract]. *Headache: The Journal of Head and Face Pain, 41*(7), 646–657.

59. Stewart, W.F., Lipton, R.B., Celentano, D.D., & Reed, M.L. (1992). Prevalence of migraine headache in the United States—Relation to age, income, race, and other sociodemographic factors [Abstract]. *The Journal of the American Medical Association, 267*(1), 64–69.

60. LeResche, L. (1997). Epidemiology of temporomandibular disorders: Implications for the investigation of etiologic factors [Abstract]. *Critical Reviews in Oral Biology & Medicine, 8*(3), 291–305.

61. LeResche, L., Mancl, L.A., Drangsholt, M.T., Saunders, K., & Korff, M.V. (2005). Relationship of pain and symptoms to pubertal development in adolescents [Abstract]. *PAIN, 118*(1–2), 201–209.

62. Ibid.

63. Cicero, T.J., Nock, B., O'Connor, L., & Meyer, E.R. (2002). Role of steroids in sex differences in morphine-induced analgesia: Activational and organizational effects. *Journal of Pharmacology and Experimental Therapeutics, 300*(2), 695–70.

64. L. Zeltzer (personal communication, August 31, 2010).

65. LeResche, L., Mancl, L., Sherman, J.J., Gandara, B., & Dworkin, S.F. (2003). Changes in temporomandibular pain and other symptoms across the menstrual cycle. *PAIN, 106*(3), 253–61.

66. W. Maixner (personal communication, February 8, 2012).

67. Ji, Y., Murphy, A.Z., & Traub, R.J. (2003). Estrogen modulates the visceromotor reflex and responses of spinal dorsal horn neurons to colorectal stimulation in the rat [Abstract]. *The Journal of Neuroscience, 23*(9), 3908–3915.

68. LeResche, L., Saunders, K., Von Korff, M.R., Barlow, W., & Dworkin, S.F. (1997). Use of exogenous hormones and risk of temporomandibular disorder pain [Abstract]. *PAIN, 69*(1–2), 153–160.

69. Musgrave, D.S., Vogt, M.T., Nevitt, M.C., & Cauley, J.A. (2001). Back problems among postmenopausal women taking estrogen

replacement therapy: The study of osteoporotic fractures [Abstract]. *Spine, 26*(14), 1606–1612.

70. Brynhildsen, J.O., Björs, E., Skarsgård, C., & Hammar, M.L. (1998). Is hormone replacement therapy a risk factor for low back pain among postmenopausal women? [Abstract]. *Spine, 23*(7), 809–813.

71. Fillingim, R.B., & Edwards, R.R. (2001). The association of hormone replacement therapy with experimental pain responses in post-menopausal women. *PAIN, 92*(1–2), 229–234.

72. Ockene, J.K., Barad, D.H., Cochrane, B.B., et al. (2005). Symptom experience after discontinuing use of estrogen plus progestin. *The Journal of the American Medical Association, 294*(2), 183–193.

73. Lichten, E.M., Lichten, J.B., Whitty, A., & Pieper, D. (1996). The confirmation of a biochemical marker for women's hormonal migraine: The Depo-Estradiol challenge test [Abstract]. *Headache: The Journal of Head and Face Pain, 36*(6), 367–371.

74. M. Gold (personal communication, April 25, 2012).

75. Aloisi, A.M., Bachiocco, V., Costantino, A., et al. (2007). Cross-sex hormone administration changes pain in transsexual women and men [Abstract]. *PAIN, 132*, S60–S67.

76. LeResche, L., Mancl, L., Sherman, J.J., Gandara, B., & Dworkin, S.F. (2003). Changes in temporomandibular pain and other symptoms across the menstrual cycle [Abstract]. *PAIN, 106*(3), 253–261.

77. Di Cecco, R., Patel, U., & Upshur, R.E. (2002). Is there a clinically significant gender bias in post-myocardial infarction pharmacological management in the older (>60) population of a primary care practice? *BMC Family Practice, 3*, 8.

78. Fowler, R.A., Sabur, N., Li, P., et al. (2007). Sex- and age-based differences in the delivery and outcomes of critical care. *Canadian Medical Association Journal, 177*(12), 1513–1519.

79. Weisse, C.S., Sorum, P.C., & Dominguez, R.E. (2003). The influence of gender and race on physicians' pain management decisions. *The Journal of Pain, 4*(9), 505–510.

80. Leresche, L. (2011). Defining gender disparities in pain management. *Clinical Orthopedics and Related Research, 469*(7), 1871–1877.

81. Raftery, K.A., Smith-Coggins, R., & Chen, A.H.M. (1995). Gender-associated differences in emergency department pain management [Abstract]. *Annals of Emergency Medicine, 26*(4), 414–421.

82. Hoffmann, D.E., & Tarzian, A.J. (2001). The girl who cried pain: A bias against women in the treatment of pain. *The Journal of Law, Medicine & Ethics, 28*, 13–27.

83. Fishbain, D.A., Goldberg, M., Meagher, B.R., Steele, R., & Rosomoff, H. (1986). Male and female chronic pain patients categorized by DSM-III psychiatric diagnostic criteria [Abstract]. *PAIN, 26*(2), 181–197.

84. Schulman, K.A., Berlin, J.A., Harless, W., et al. (1999). The effect of race and sex on physicians' recommendations for cardiac catheterization [Abstract]. *The New England Journal of Medicine, 340*(8), 618–626.

85. Daly, C., Clemens, F., Lopez Sendon, J.L., et al. (2006). Gender differences in the management and clinical outcome of stable angina [Abstract]. *Circulation, 113*(4), 490–498.

86. Roger, V.L., Farkouh, M.E., Weston, S.A., et al. (2000). Sex differences in evaluation and outcome of unstable angina [Abstract]. *The Journal of the American Medical Association, 283*(5), 646–652.

87. M. O'Connor (personal communication, April 6, 2012).

88. O'Connor, M.I. (2011). Implant survival, knee function and pain relief after TKA. *Clinical Orthopaedics and Related Research, 469*, 1846–1851.

89. Borkhoff, C.M., Hawker, G.A., Kreder, H.J., Glazier, R.H., Mahomed, N.N., & Wright, J.G. (2008). The effect of patients' sex on physicians' recommendations for total knee arthroplasty. *Canadian Medical Association Journal, 178*(6), 681–687.

90. Chen, E.H., Shofer, F.S., Dean, A.J., et al. (2008). Gender disparity in analgesic treatment of emergency department patients with acute abdominal pain. *Academic Emergency Medicine, 15*(5), 414–418.

91. Cleeland, C.S., Gonin, R., Hatfield, A.K., & Edmonson, J.H. (1994). Pain and its treatment in outpatients with metastatic cancer. [Abstract]. *The New England Journal of Medicine, 330*(9), 592–596.

92. Breitbart, W., Rosenfeld, B.D., Passik, S.D., McDonald, M.V., Thaler, H., & Portenoy, R.K. (1996). The undertreatment of pain in ambulatory AIDS patients [Abstract]. *PAIN, 65*(2–3), 243–249.

93. Hamberg, K., Risberg, G., Johansson, E.E., & Westman, G. (2002). Gender bias in physicians' management of neck pain: A study of the answers in a Swedish national examination [Abstract]. *Journal of Women's Health & Gender-Based Medicine, 11*(7), 653–666.

94. Fillingim, R.B., & Gear, R.W. (2004). Sex differences in opioid analgesia: Clinical and experimental findings. *European Journal of Pain, 8*(5), 413–42.

95. Sarton, E., Olofsen, E., Romberg, R., et al. (2000). Sex differences in morphine analgesia: An experimental study in healthy volunteers [Abstract]. *Anesthesiology, 93*(5), 1245–1254.

96. Stoffel, E.C., Ulibarri, C.M., Folk, J.E., Rice, K.C., & Craft, R.M. (2005). Gonadal hormone modulation of mu, kappa, and delta opioid

antinociception in male and female rats [Abstract]. *The Journal of Pain, 6*(4), 261–274.

97. Niesters, M., Dahan, A., Kest, B., Zacny, J., Stijnen, T., Aarts, L., & Sarton, E. (2010). Do sex differences exist in opioid analgesia? A systematic review and meta-analysis of human experimental and clinical studies. *PAIN, 151*(1), 61–68.

98. M. Gold (personal communication, April 25, 2012).

99. J. Mogil (personal communication, April 5, 2012).

100. Fillingim, R. B., & Gear, R. W. (2004). Sex differences in opioid analgesia: Clinical and experimental findings. *European Journal of Pain, 8*(5), 413–42.

101. Loyd, D.R., Wang, X., & Murphy, A.Z. (2008). Sex differences in μ-opioid receptor expression in the rat midbrain periaqueductal gray are essential for eliciting sex differences in morphine analgesia. *The Journal of Neuroscience, 28*(52), 14007–14017.

102. Wang, X., Traub, R.J., & Murphy, A.Z. (2006). Persistent pain model reveals sex difference in morphine potency. *American Journal of Physiology: Regulatory, Integrative and Comparative Physiology, 291,* r300–r306.

103. Cepeda, M.S., & Carr, D.B. (2003). Women experience more pain and require more morphine than men to achieve a similar degree of analgesia. *Anesthesia & Analgesia, 97*(5), 1464–1468.

104. R.W. Gear (personal communication, September 22, 2010).

105. Smith, Y.R., Stohler, C.S., Nichols, T.E., Bueller, J.A., Koeppe, R.A., & Zubieta, J-K. (2006). Pronociceptive and antinociceptive effects of estradiol through endogenous opioid neurotransmission in women [Abstract]. *The Journal of Neuroscience, 26*(21), 5777–5785.

106. Niesters, M., Dahan, A., Kest, B., Zacny, J., Stijnen, T., Aarts, L., & Sarton, E. (2010). Do sex differences exist in opioid analgesia? A systematic review and meta-analysis of human experimental and clinical studies. *PAIN, 151*(1), 61–68.

107. Ibid.

108. J. Mogil (personal communication, April 5, 2012).

109. Anderson, K.O., Green, C.R., & Payne, R. (2009). Racial and ethnic disparities in pain: Causes and consequences of unequal care. *The Journal of Pain, 10*(12), 1187–1204.

110. Ibid.

111. Vallerand, A.H., Hasenau, S., Templin, T., & Collins-Bohler, D. (2005). Disparities between black and white patients with cancer

pain: The effect of perception of control over pain. *Pain Medicine*, 6(3), 242–250.

112. Reyes-Gibby, C.C., Aday, L.A., Todd, K.H., Cleeland, C.S., & Anderson, K.O. (2007). Pain in aging community-dwelling adults in the United States: Non-Hispanic whites, non-Hispanic blacks, and Hispanics. *The Journal of Pain, 8*, 75–84.

113. Weisse C.S., Foster, K.K., & Fisher, E.A. (2005). The influence of experimenter gender and race on pain reporting: Does racial or gender concordance matter? *Pain Medicine, 6*(1), 80–87.

114. Anderson, K.O., Green, C.R., & Payne, R. (2009). Racial and ethnic disparities in pain: Causes and consequences of unequal care. *The Journal of Pain, 10*(12), 1187–1204.

115. Rahim-Williams, B., Riley, J.L, Williams, A.K., & Fillingim, R.B. (2012). A quantitative review of ethnic group differences in experimental pain response: Do biology, psychology and culture matter? *Pain Medicine, 13*, 522–540.

116. Cruz-Almeida, Y., Sibille, K.T., Goodin, B.R., et al. (2014). Racial and ethnic differences in older adults with knee osteoarthritis. *Arthritis & Rheumatology, 66*(7), 1800–1810.

117. Graham, R. (2014, June 15). I don't feel your pain—Men and women appear to suffer pain differently. So do blacks and whites. Modern medicine has trouble even talking about it. *Boston Globe*. Retrieved from http://www.bostonglobe.com/ideas/2014/06/14/don-feel-your-pain/cIrKD5czM0pgZQv7PgCmxI/story.html

118. US Institute of Medicine, Committee on Advancing Pain Research, Care, and Education. (2011). *Relieving pain in America: A blueprint for transforming prevention, care, education and research* (pp. 67–71). Washington, DC: National Academies Press.

119. Trawalter, S., Hoffman, K.M., & Waytz, A. (2012, November 14). Racial bias in perceptions of others' pain. *PLoS ONE*. Retrieved from http://journals.plos.org/plosone/article?id=10.1371/journal.pone.0048546

120. Morrison, R.S., Wallenstein, S., Natale, D.K., Senzel, R.S. & Huang, L. (2000, April 6). "We don't carry that"—Failure of pharmacies in predominantly nonwhite neighborhoods to stock opioid analgesics. *The New England Journal of Medicine*. Retrieved from http://www.nejm.org/doi/full/10.1056/NEJM200004063421406#t=article

121. Tamayo-Sarver, J.H., Hinze, S.W., Cydulka, R.K., & Baker, D.W. (2003). Racial and ethnic disparities in emergency department analgesic prescription. *American Journal of Public Health, 93*(12), 2067–2073.

122. Society of Behavioral Medicine. (2010). Racial/ethnic disparities in the management of cancer pain [Press release]. Retrieved from http://www.sbm.org/emails/message/Racial%20Disparities%20in%20Pain.html

123. Jimenez, N., Seidel, K., Martin, L.D., Rivara, F.P., & Lynn, A.M. (2010). Perioperative analgesic treatment in Latino and non-Latino pediatric patients. *Journal of Healthcare for the Poor and Underserved, 21*(1), 229–236.

124. Becker, W.C., Starrels, J.L., Heo, M., Li, X., Weiner, M.G., & Turner, B.J. (2011). Racial differences in primary care opioid risk reduction strategies. *Annals of Family Medicine, 9*(3), 219–225.

125. Anderson, K.O., Green, C.R., & Payne, R. (2009). Racial and ethnic disparities in pain: Causes and consequences of unequal care. *The Journal of Pain, 10*(12), 1187–1204.

126. Ibid.

127. Ibid.

128. Weiner, D.K., Karp, J.F., Bernstein, C.D., & Morone, N.E. (2013). Pain medicine in older adults: How should it differ? In *Comprehensive treatment of chronic pain by medical, interventional, and integrative approaches,* ed. T.R. Deer, S. Leong, A. Buvanendran, et al. New York: Springer.

129. Ibid.

130. Ibid.

131. US Institute of Medicine, Committee on Advancing Pain Research, Care, and Education. (2011). *Relieving pain in America: A blueprint for transforming prevention, care, education and research* (pp. 79–80). Washington, DC: National Academies Press.

132. Fillingim, R.B., Yezierski, R.P. & Turk, D.C. (2016). Pain in the elderly. In *Advances in geroscience,* ed. F. Sierra & R. Kohanski. Cham: Springer.

133. Ibid.

134. Ibid.

135. Ibid.

136. Ibid.

137. Bernabei, R., Gambassi, G., Lapane, K., et al. (1998). Management of pain in elderly patients with cancer. SAGE study group. Systematic assessment of geriatric drug use via epidemiology. *The Journal of the American Medical Association, 279*(23), 1877–1882.

138. Schechter, N.L., & Allen, D. (1986). Physicians' attitudes toward pain in children [Abstract]. *Journal of Developmental and Behavioral Pediatrics, 7*(6), 350–354.

139. Chamberlain, D.B. (1991, May). Babies don't feel pain: A century of denial in medicine. Paper presented at the Second International Symposium on Circumcision, San Francisco, CA.

140. Eland, J.M., & Anderson, M.J. (1977). The experience of pain in children. In *Pain: A sourcebook for nurses and other health professionals*, ed. A. Jacox (pp. 453–476). Boston: Little, Brown.

141. Perry, S., & Heidrich, G. (1982). Management of pain during debridement: A survey of US burn units [Abstract]. *PAIN, 13*(3), 267–280.

142. Beyer, J.E., DeGood, D.E., Ashley, L.C., & Russell, G.A. (1983). Patterns of postoperative analgesic use with adults and children following cardiac surgery [Abstract]. *PAIN, 17*(1), 71–81.

143. Mather, L., & Mackie, J. (1983). The incidence of postoperative pain in children [Abstract]. *PAIN, 15*(1–4), 271–282.

144. Schechter, N.L., Allen, D.A., & Hanson, K. (1986). Status of pediatric pain control: A comparison of hospital analgesic usage in children and adults [Abstract]. *Pediatrics, 77*(1), 11–15.

145. Fitzgerald, M., & Beggs, S. (2001). The neurobiology of pain: Developmental aspects [Abstract]. *The Neuroscientist, 7*(3), 246–257.

146. Fitzgerald, M., Millard, C., & McIntosh, N. (1989). Cutaneous hypersensitivity following peripheral tissue damage in newborn infants and its reversal with topical anaesthesia [Abstract]. *PAIN, 39*(1), 31–36.

147. Slater, R., Fabrizi, L., Worley, A., Meek, J., Boyd, S., & Fitzgerald, M. (2010). Premature infants display increased noxious-evoked neuronal activity in the brain compared to healthy age-matched term-born infants [Abstract]. *NeuroImage, 52*(2), 583–589.

148. Slater, R., Worley, A., Fabrizi, L., et al. (2010). Evoked potentials generated by noxious stimulation in the human infant brain [Abstract]. *European Journal of Pain, 14*(3), 321–326.

149. Andrews, K., & Fitzgerald, M. (1994). The cutaneous withdrawal reflex in human neonates: Sensitization, receptive fields, and the effects of contralateral stimulation [Abstract]. *PAIN, 56*(1), 95–101.

150. Fitzgerald, M., & Jennings, E. (1999). The postnatal development of spinal sensory processing. *Proceedings of the National Academy of Sciences, 96*(14), 7719–7722.

151. Marsh, D., Dickenson, A., Hatch, D., & Fitzgerald, M. (1999). Epidural opioid analgesia in infant rats II: Responses to carrageenan and capsaicin. *PAIN, 82*(1), 33–38.

152. Fitzgerald, M. (1991). Development of pain mechanisms. *British Medical Bulletin, 47*(3), 667–675.

153. Fitzgerald, M., & Walker, S.M. (2009). Infant pain management: A developmental neurobiological approach. *Nature Clinical Practice Neurology, 5*(1), 35–50.

154. Anand, K.J., & Hickey, P.R. (1987). Pain and its effects in the human neonate and fetus. *The New England Journal of Medicine, 317*(21), 1323.

155. Anand, K.J. (2001). Consensus statement for the prevention and management of pain in the newborn [Abstract]. *Archives of Pediatrics and Adolescent Medicine, 155*(2), 173–180.

156. Anand, K.J. (1998). Clinical importance of pain and stress in preterm neonates [Abstract]. *Biology of the Neonate, 73*(1), 1–9.

157. Anand, K.J., & Carr, D.B. (1989). The neuroanatomy, neurophysiology, and neurochemistry of pain, stress, and analgesia in newborns and children [Abstract]. *Pediatric Clinics of North America, 36*(4), 795–822.

158. Anand, K.J., Hall, R., Desai, N., et al. (2004). Effects of morphine analgesia in ventilated preterm neonates: Primary outcomes from the NEOPAIN randomised trial. *The Lancet, 363*(9422), 1673–1682.

159. Anand, K.J., Aranda, J.V., Berde, C. B. et al. (2006). Summary proceedings from the neonatal pain-control group [Abstract]. *Pediatrics, 117*(3), S9–S22.

160. Anand, K.J., Johnston, C.C., Oberlander, T.F., Taddio, A., Tutag Lehr, V., & Walco, G.A. (2005). Analgesia and local anesthesia during invasive procedures in the neonate [Abstract]. *Clinical Therapeutics, 27*(6), 844–876.

161. Carbajal, R., & Anand, K, J. (2008). Prevention of pain in neonates—Reply. *The Journal of the American Medical Association, 300*(19), 2248–2249.

162. Fabrizi, L., Slater, R., Worley, A., et al.(2011). A shift in sensory processing that enables the developing human brain to discriminate touch from pain. *Current Biology, 21*(18), 1552–1558.

163. Johnston, C. (2010). From the mouths of babes: What have we learned from studies of pain in neonates? Paper presented at the International Association of Pain's 13th World Congress on Pain, Montreal, Canada.

164. Emde, R.N, Harmon, R.J., Metcalf, D., Koenig, K.L., & Wagonfeld, S. (1971). Stress and neonatal sleep [Abstract]. *Psychosomatic Medicine, 33*(6), 491–497.

165. Talbert, L.M., Kraybill, E.N., & Potter, H.D. (1976). Adrenal cortical response to circumcision in the neonate [Abstract]. *Obstetrics & Gynecology, 48*(2), 208–210.

166. Williamson, P.S., & Williamson, M.L. (1983). Physiologic stress reduction by a local anesthetic during newborn circumcision. *Pediatrics, 71*(1), 36–40.
167. Taddio, A., Katz, J., Ilersich, A.L., & Koren, G. (1997). Effect of neonatal circumcision on pain response during subsequent routine vaccination [Abstract]. *The Lancet, 349*(9052), 599–603.
168. Taddio, A., Stevens, B., Craig, K., et al. (1997). Efficacy and safety of lidocaine–prilocaine cream for pain during circumcision [Abstract]. *The New England Journal of Medicine, 336*(17), 1197–1201.
169. Weisman, S.J., Bernstein, B., & Schechter, N.L. (1998). Consequences of inadequate analgesia during painful procedures in children [Abstract]. *Archives of Pediatrics and Adolescent Medicine, 152*(2), 147–149.
170. Zeltzer, L.K., & Krane, E.J. (2011). Pediatric pain management. In *Nelson's textbook of pediatrics* (19th ed.), ed. R.M. Kliegman, R.E. Behrmen, B.F. Stanton, N. Schor, & J. St. Geme (p. 7). New York: Elsevier.
171. Cohen, M.M., Cameron, C.B., & Duncan, P.G. (1990). Pediatric anesthesia morbidity and mortality in the perioperative period [Abstract]. *Anesthesia & Analgesia, 70*(2), 160–167.
172. Zeltzer, L.K., & Krane, E.J. (2011). Pediatric pain management. In *Nelson's textbook of pediatrics* (19th ed.), ed. R.M. Kliegman, R.E. Behrmen, B.F. Stanton, N. Schor, & J. St. Geme (p. 5). New York: Elsevier.
173. Schechter, N. (2014). Pediatric pain management and opioids—The baby and the bathwater. *Journal of the American Medical Association Pediatrics, 168*(11), 987–988.
174. Rappaport, B., Mellon, R.D., Simone, A. & Woodcock, J. (2011). Defining safe use of anesthesia in children. *The New England Journal of Medicine, 364*, 1387–1390.
175. Anand, K.J., & Arnold, J.H. (1994). Opioid tolerance and dependence in infants and children [Abstract]. *Critical Care Medicine, 22*(2), 334–342.
176. Suresh, S., & Anand, K.J. (1998). Opioid tolerance in neonates: Mechanisms, diagnosis, assessment, and management [Abstract]. *Seminars in Perinatology, 22*(5), 425–433.
177. Anand, K.J., Sippell, W.G., & Aynsley-Green, A. (1987). Randomised trial of fentanyl anaesthesia in preterm babies undergoing surgery: Effects on the stress response. [Abstract]. *The Lancet, 1*(8524), 62–66.

178. Anand, K.J., Carr, D.B., & Mickey, P.R. (1987). Randomised trial of high-dose sufentanil anesthesia in neonates undergoing cardiac surgery: Hormonal and hemodynamic stress responses [Abstract]. *Anesthesiology, 67*(3), a501.

179. Berde, C.B., & Sethna, N.F. (2002). Analgesics for the treatment of pain in children. *The New England Journal of Medicine, 347*(14), 1094–1103.

180. Ibid.

181. Berde, C.B., Lehn, B.M., Yee, J.D., Sethna, N.F., & Russo, D. (1991). Patient-controlled analgesia in children and adolescents: A randomized, prospective comparison with intramuscular administration of morphine for postoperative analgesia [Abstract]. *The Journal of Pediatrics, 118*(3), 460–466.

182. Zeltzer, L.K., & Krane, E.J. (2011). Pediatric pain management. In *Nelson's textbook of pediatrics* (19th ed.), ed. R.M. Kliegman, R.E. Behrmen, B.F. Stanton, N. Schor, & J. St. Geme (p. 8). New York: Elsevier.

183. N. Schechter (personal communication, July 21, 2015).

184. Ibid.

185. Carbajal, R., Chauvet, X., Couderc, S., & Olivier-Martin, M. (1999). Randomised trial of analgesic effects of sucrose, glucose, and pacifiers in term neonates. *British Medical Journal, 319*(7222), 1393–1397.

186. Gray, L., Miller, L.W., Philipp, B.L., & Blass, E.M. (2002). Breastfeeding is analgesic in healthy newborns [Abstract]. *Pediatrics, 109*(4), 590–593.

187. Carbajal, R., Veerapen, S., Couderc, S., Jugie, M., & Ville, Y. (2003). Analgesic effect of breast feeding in term neonates: Randomised controlled trial. *British Medical Journal, 326*(7379), 1–5.

188. Johnston, C. (2010). From the mouths of babes: What have we learned from studies of pain in neonates? Paper presented at the International Association of Pain's 13th World Congress on Pain, Montreal, Canada.

189. Barr, R.G., Pantel, M.S., Young, S.N., Wright, J.H., Hendricks, L.A., & Gravel, R. (1999). The response of crying newborns to sucrose: Is it a "sweetness effect?" *Physiology & Behavior, 66*(3), 409–417.

190. Stevens, B., Yamada, J., & Ohlsson, A. (2010). Sucrose for analgesia in newborn infants undergoing painful procedures [Review]. *The Cochrane Library, 1,* 1–114.

191. Akman, I. (2002). Sweet solutions and pacifiers for pain relief in newborn infants [Abstract]. *The Journal of Pain, 3*(3), 199–202.

192. Barr, R.G., Young, S.N., Wright, J.H., Gravel, R., & Alkawaf, R. (1999). Differential calming responses to sucrose taste in crying infants with and without colic [Abstract]. *Pediatrics, 103*(5), e68.

193. Johnston, C.C., Filion, F., Campbell-Yeo, M., et al. (2009). Enhanced kangaroo mother care for heel lance in preterm neonates: A cross-over trial [Abstract]. *Journal of Perinatology, 29*(1), 51–56.

194. Johnston, C.C., Filion, F., Campbell-Yeo, M., et al. (2008). Kangaroo mother care diminishes pain from heel lance in very preterm neonates: A crossover trial. *BMC Pediatrics, 8*(1), 13.

195. Gray, L., Watt, L., & Blass, E.M. (2000). Skin-to-skin contact is analgesic in healthy newborns [Abstract]. *Pediatrics, 105*(1), e14.

196. Johnston, C.C., Abbott, F. V., Gray-Donald, K., & Jeans, M. E. (1992). A survey of pain in hospitalized patients aged 4–14 years [Abstract]. *The Clinical Journal of Pain, 8*(2), 154–163.

197. Jacob, E., & Puntillo, K.A. (2000). Variability of analgesic practices for hospitalized children on different pediatric specialty units [Abstract]. *Journal of Pain and Symptom Management, 20*(1), 59–67.

198. Ellis, J.A., O'Connor, B.V., Cappelli, M., Goodman, J.T., Blouin, R., & Reid, C.W. (2002). Pain in hospitalized pediatric patients: How are we doing? [Abstract]. *The Clinical Journal of Pain, 18*(4), 262–269.

199. Karling, M., Renström, M., & Ljungman, G. (2002). Acute and postoperative pain in children: A Swedish nationwide survey [Abstract]. *Acta Paediatrica, 91*(6), 660–666.

200. Alexander, J., & Manno, M. (2003). Underuse of analgesia in very young pediatric patients with isolated painful injuries [Abstract]. *Annals of Emergency Medicine, 41*(5), 617–622.

201. Simons, S.H., van Dijk, M., Anand, K.J., Roofthooft, D., van Lingen, R.A., & Tibboel, D. (2003). Do we still hurt newborn babies? A prospective study of procedural pain and analgesia in neonates [Abstract]. *Archives of Pediatrics and Adolescent Medicine, 157*(11), 1058–1064.

202. Carbajal, R., Rousset, A., Danan, C., et al. (2008). Epidemiology and treatment of painful procedures in neonates in intensive care units. *The Journal of the American Medical Association, 300*(1), 60–70.

203. Carbajal, R., Nguyen-Bourgain, C., & Armengaud, J.B. (2008). How can we improve pain relief in neonates? *Expert Review of Neurotherapeutics, 8*(11), 1617–1620.

204. Taylor, E.M., Boyer, K., & Campbell, F.A. (2008). Pain in hospitalized children: A prospective cross-sectional survey of pain prevalence, intensity, assessment and management in a Canadian pediatric teaching hospital. *Pain Research & Management, 13*(1), 25–32.

205. N. Schechter (personal communication, December 3, 2010).
206. Schechter, N.L., Allen, D.A., & Hanson, K. (1986). Status of pediatric pain control: A comparison of hospital analgesic usage in children and adults [Abstract]. *Pediatrics, 77*(1), 11–15.
207. Schechter, N.L., Zempsky, W.T., Cohen, L.L., McGrath, P.J., McMurtry, C.M., & Bright, N.S. (2007). Pain reduction during pediatric immunizations: Evidence-based review and recommendations. *Pediatrics, 119*(5), e1184–e1198.
208. Schechter, N.L., Bernstein, B.A., Zempsky, W.T., Bright, N.S., & Willard, A.K. (2010). Educational outreach to reduce immunization pain in office settings. *Pediatrics, 126*(6), e1514–e1521.
209. Schechter, N.L. (1989). The undertreatment of pain in children: An overview. *Pediatric Clinics of North America, 36*(4), 781–794.
210. Schechter, N.L. (2008). From the ouchless place to comfort central: The evolution of a concept. *Pediatrics, 122*(3), s154–s160.
211. Harrison, D., Loughnan, P., & Johnston, L. (2006). Pain assessment and procedural pain management practices in neonatal units in Australia [Abstract]. *Journal of Paediatrics and Child Health, 42*(1–2), 6–9.
212. Wolfe, J., Grier, H.E., Klar, N., et al. (2000). Symptoms and suffering at the end of life in children with cancer [Abstract]. *The New England Journal of Medicine, 342*(5), 326–333.
213. Wolfe, J., Hammel, J.F., Edwards, K.E., et al. (2008). Easing of suffering in children with cancer at the end of life: Is care changing? *Journal of Clinical Oncology, 26*(10), 1717–1723.
214. Schechter, N.L., Finley, G.A., Bright, N.S., Laycock, M., & Forgeron, P. (2010). ChildKind: A global initiative to reduce pain in children. *Pediatric Pain Letter, 12*(3), 26–30.

Chapter 3

1. National Institutes of Health. (2014). *Pathways to prevention workshop: The role of opioids in the treatment of chronic pain* (p. 34). Retrieved from https://prevention.nih.gov/docs/programs/p2p/ODPPain PanelStatementFinal_10-02-14.pdf
2. Ibid., p. 34.
3. Chapman, C.R. (2013). Opioid pharmacotherapy for chronic non-cancer pain: The American experience. *Korean Journal of Pain, 26*(1), 3–13.
4. Thomas, D., Frascella, J., Hall, T., et al. (2015). Reflections on the role of opioids in the treatment of chronic pain: A shared solution for prescription opioid abuse and pain. *Journal of Internal Medicine, 278*(1), 92–94.

5. Musto, D.F. (1999). *The American disease: Origins of narcotic control* (3rd ed.). Oxford: Oxford University Press.

6. Ballantyne, J.C., & Shin, N.S. (2008). Efficacy of opioids for chronic pain: A review of the evidence. *The Clinical Journal of Pain, 24*(6), 469–478.

7. Ballantyne, J.C. (2009). U.S. opioid risk management initiatives. *Pain Clinical Updates, 17*(6), 1–5.

8. Eban, K. (2011). Painful medicine: What the strange saga of Purdue Pharma—and its $3 billion drug, OxyContin—tells us about our national dependence on painkillers. *Fortune, 164*(8), 144.

9. US Food and Drug Administration. (2013). FDA approves abuse-deterrent labeling for reformulated OxyContin [Press release]. Retrieved from http://www.fda.gov/NewsEvents/Newsroom/PressAnnouncements/ucm348252.htm

10. Lexchin, J., & Kohler, J.C. (2011). The danger of imperfect regulation: OxyContin use in the United States and Canada. *The International Journal of Risk & Safety in Medicine, 23*(4), 233–240.

11. R. Chou (personal communication, May 14, 2015).

12. US General Accounting Office. (2003). *Prescription drugs: OxyContin abuse and diversion and efforts to address the problem* (Report to Congressional Requesters). Retrieved from http://www.gao.gov/new.items/d04110.pdf

13. CBC News Canada. (2012, March 8). OxyContin marketing blamed for addiction epidemic. Retrieved from http://www.cbc.ca/news/canada/story/2012/03/08/oxycontin-marketing.html

14. Meier, B. (2007, May 10). In guilty plea: OxyContin maker to pay $600 million. *The New York Times.* Retrieved from http://www.nytimes.com/2007/05/10/business/11drug-web.html?pagewanted=all

15. CNN Money. (2007). Purdue in $634 million settlement over OxyContin [Press release]. Retrieved from http://money.cnn.com/2007/07/20/news/companies/purdue/index.htm

16. Purdue Pharma. (2007). Statement of Purdue Pharma regarding resolution of the federal investigation in the western district of Virginia [Press release]. Retrieved from http://www.evaluatepharma.com/Universal/View.aspx?type=Story&id=126370

17. T. Constantino (personal communication, Aug. 30, 2016).

18. N. Gill (personal communication, September 25, 2015).

19. Ballantyne, J.C. (2009). U.S. opioid risk management initiatives [Table 1: Summary of U.S. retail drug purchases, 1997–2005]. *Pain Clinical Updates, 17*(6), 2.

20. Ibid.
21. Frenk, S.M., Porter, K.S., & Paulozzi, L.J. (2015). *Prescription opioid analgesic use among adults: United States, 1999–2012* (National Center for Health Statistics data brief). Retrieved from http://www.cdc.gov/nchs/data/dataBriefs/db189.pdf
22. J. Dahl (personal communication, April 13, 2015).
23. Dart, R.C., Surratt, H.L., Cicero, T.J. et al. (2015). Trends in opioid analgesic abuse and mortality in the United States. *The New England Journal of Medicine, 372,* 241–248.
24. D. Thomas (personal communication, May 12, 2015).
25. Ornstein, C., & Weber, T. (2012, May 8). American Pain Foundation shuts down as senators launch investigation of prescription narcotics. Retrieved from http://www.propublica.org/article/senate-panel-investigates-drug-company-ties-to-pain-groups
26. American Pain Foundation. (2010). *2010 annual report* (p. 16). Retrieved from http://s3.documentcloud.org/documents/277604/apf-2010-annual-report.pdf
27. Jones, C.M., Mack, K.A., & Paulozzi, L.J. (2013). Pharmaceutical overdose deaths, United States, 2010. *The Journal of the American Medical Association, 309*(7), 657–659.
28. C. Lenard (personal communication, January 21, 2015).
29. Thomas, D. (2015). Centers for Excellence in Pain Education & the role of opioids in the treatment of chronic pain [PowerPoint slides].Retrievedfromhttp://iprcc.nih.gov/meetings/4-17-2015%20Meeting%20Presentations/6_Thomas_CoEPEs_OpioidChronic Pain.pdf
30. Jones, C.M., Mack, K.A. & Paulozzi, L.J. (2013). Pharmaceutical overdose deaths, United States, 2010. *The Journal of the American Medical Association, 309*(7), 657–659.
31. Centers for Disease Control and Prevention. (2015). Injury prevention & control: Prescription drug overdose. Retrieved from http://www.cdc.gov/drugoverdose/
32. Jones, C.M., Mack, K.A. & Paulozzi, L.J. (2013). Pharmaceutical overdose deaths, United States, 2010. *The Journal of the American Medical Association, 309*(7), 657–659.
33. C. Lenard (personal communication, April 16, 2015).
34. Chen, L.H., Hedegaard, H., & Warner, M. (September 2014). Drug-poisoning deaths involving opioid analgesics: United States, 1999–2011. Center for Disease Control and Prevention. Retrieved from http://www.cdc.gov/nchs/data/databriefs/db166.htm

35. Centers for Disease Control and Prevention. (2015). Injury prevention & control: Prescription drug overdose. Retrieved from http://www.cdc.gov/drugoverdose

36. Centers for Disease Control and Prevention. (2014). Smoking & tobacco use, Fast facts (Diseases and deaths). Retrieved from http://www.cdc.gov/tobacco/data_statistics/fact_sheets/fast_facts

37. Centers for Disease Control and Prevention. (2014). Fact sheets—Alcohol and your health. Retrieved from http://www.cdc.gov/alcohol/fact-sheets/alcohol-use.htm

38. Wiegand, T. (2015, March 11). Nonsteroidal anti-inflammatory agent toxicity. Medscape. Retrieved from http://emedicine.medscape.com/article/816117-overview

39. Wiegand, T.J., Wax, P.M., Schwartz, T., Finkelstein, Y., Gorodetsky, R., & Brent, J. (2013). The Toxicology Investigators Consortium case registry—The 2011 experience. *Journal of Medical Toxicology, 8*(4), 360–377.

40. Institute of Medicine, Committee on Advancing Pain Research, Care, and Education. (2011). *Relieving pain in America: A blueprint for transforming prevention, care, education and research* (pp. 2–29). Washington, DC: National Academies Press.

41. Breslau, N., Schultz, L., Lipton, R., Peterson, E., & Welch, K.M.A. (2012). Migraine headaches and suicide attempt. *Headache: The Journal of Head and Face Pain, 52*(5), 723–731.

42. Cheatle, M.D. (2011). Depression, chronic pain, and suicide by overdose: On the edge. *Pain Medicine, 12,* S43–S48.

43. National Institutes of Health. (2014). *Pathways to prevention workshop: The role of opioids in the treatment of chronic pain.* Retrieved from https://prevention.nih.gov/docs/programs/p2p/ODPPainPanelStatementFinal_10-02-14.pdf

44. Mayday Fund. (2009). *A call to revolutionize chronic pain care in America: An opportunity in health care reform.* Retrieved from http://www.maydaypainreport.org/docs/A%20Call%20to%20Revolutionize%20Chronic%20Pain%20Care%20in%20America%2003.04.10.pdf

45. Shi Q., Langer, G., Cohen, J., & Cleeland, C.S. (2007). People in pain: How do they seek relief? *The Journal of Pain, 8*(8), 624–636.

46. Jonas, W.B., & Schoomaker, E.B. (2014). Pain and opioids in the military: We must do better. *The Journal of the American Medical Association, 174*(8), 1402–1403.

47. Volkow, N.D. (2012). Realities of Rx drug abuse. General Session at the National Drug Abuse Summit, Atlanta, GA.

48. Chapman, C.R., Lipschitz, D.L., Angst, M.S., et al. (2010). Opioid pharmacotherapy for chronic non-cancer pain in the United States: A research guideline for developing an evidence-base. *The Journal of Pain, 11*(9), 807–829.

49. Degenhart, L., Bruno, R., Lintzeris, N., et al. (2015). Agreement between definitions of pharmaceutical opioid use disorders and dependence in people taking opioids for chronic non-cancer pain (POINT): A cohort study. *The Lancet Psychiatry, 2*(4), 314–322.

50. Ibid.

51. Ross, E.L., Holcomb, C., & Jamison, R.N. (2009). Addressing abuse and misuse of opioid analgesics. *Drug Benefit Trends, 21*(2), 54–63.

52. Institute of Medicine, Committee on Advancing Pain Research, Care, and Education. (2011). *Relieving pain in America: A blueprint for transforming prevention, care, education and research* (p. GL-1). Washington, DC: National Academies Press.

53. American Society of Addiction Medicine. (2011). Public policy statement: Definition of addiction. Retrieved from http://www.asam.org/for-the-public/definition-of-addiction

54. American Society of Addiction Medicine. (2011, August 15). ASAM releases new definition of addiction. *EurekAlert!* Retrieved from http://www.eurekalert.org/pub_releases/2011-08/asoa-arn072111.php

55. Szalavitz, M. (2011, August 16). Why the new definition of addiction, as "brain disease," falls short. *Time.* Retrieved from http://healthland.time.com/2011/08/16/why-the-new-definition-of-addiction-as-brain-disease-falls-short

56. American Society of Addiction Medicine. (2011). Public policy statement: Definition of addiction. Retrieved from http://www.asam.org/for-the-public/definition-of-addiction

57. J. Dahl (personal communication, March 17, 2013).

58. Ballantyne, J.C., Sullivan, M.D., & Kolodny, A. (2012). Opioid dependence vs. addiction—A distinction without a difference? *Archives of Internal Medicine, 172*(17), 1342–1343.

59. Physicians for Responsible Opioid Prescribing. (2012, July 25). Citizen petition (Document ID: FDA-2012-P-0818-0001). Retrieved from http://www.regulations.gov/#!documentDetail;D=FDA-2012-P-0818-0001

60. Public Citizen. (2012). Doctors, researchers and health officials call on FDA to change labels on opioid painkillers to deter misprescribing [Press release]. Retrieved from http://www.citizen.org/pressroom/pressroomredirect.cfm?ID=3674

61. Bono Mack, M. (2012, July 26). Letter to Margaret Hamburg, M.D., Commissioner, Food and Drug Administration. Retrieved from http://www.hpm.com/pdf/blog/Hamburg-Adolescent-Use-of-E-Cigarette-2013-9-16.pdf

62. US Food and Drug Administration. (2013). FDA announces safety labeling changes and postmarket study requirements for extended-release and long-acting opioid analgesics [Press release]. Retrieved from http://www.fda.gov/NewsEvents/Newsroom/PressAnnouncements/ucm367726.htm

63. M. von Korff (personal communication, April 16, 2015).

64. S. Simson (personal communication, April 24, 2015).

65. National Institutes of Health. (2014). *Pathways to prevention workshop: The role of opioids in the treatment of chronic pain* (p. 34). Retrieved from https://prevention.nih.gov/docs/programs/p2p/ODPPainPanel StatementFinal_10-02-14.pdf

66. Vowles, K.E., McEntee, M.L., Julnes, P.S., Forhe, T., Ney, J.P., & van der Goes, D.N. (2015). Rates of opioid misuse, abuse and addiction in chronic pain: A systematic review and data synthesis, *PAIN, 156*(4), 569–576.

67. Ballantyne, J.C. (2015). Assessing the prevalence of opioid misuse, abuse, and addiction in chronic pain. *PAIN, 156*(4), 567–568.

68. Minozzi, S., Amato, L., & Davoli, M. (2013). Development of dependence following treatment with opioid analgesics for pain relief: A systematic review. *Addiction, 108*(4), 688–698.

69. Fishbain, D.A., Rosomoff, H.L., & Rosomoff, R.S. (1992). Drug abuse, dependence, and addiction in chronic pain patients. *The Clinical Journal of Pain, 8*(2), 77–85.

70. Fishbain, D.A., Cole, B., Lewis, J., Rosomoff, H.L., & Rosomoff, R.S. (2008). What percentage of chronic nonmalignant pain patients exposed to chronic opioid analgesic therapy develop abuse/addiction and/or aberrant drug-related behaviors? A structured evidence-based review. *Pain Medicine, 9*(4), 444–459.

71. Chapman, C.R., Lipschitz, D.L., Angst, M.S., et al. (2010). Opioid pharmacotherapy for chronic non-cancer pain in the United States: A research guideline for developing an evidence-base. *The Journal of Pain, 11*(9), 807–829.

72. Noble, M., Treadwell, J.R., Tregear, S.J., et al. (2010). Long-term opioid management for chronic noncancer pain. *Cochrane Database of Systematic Reviews, 2010*(1), CD006605.

73. Banta-Green, C.J., Merrill, J.O., Doyle, S.R., Boudreau, D.M., & Calsyn, D.A. (2009). Opioid use behaviors, mental health and

pain—Development of a typology of chronic pain patients. *Drug and Alcohol Dependence, 104*(1–2), 34–42.

74. J. Kauffman (personal communication, February 23, 2011).
75. Von Korff, M. (2010). Commentary on Boscarino et al.: Understanding the spectrum of opioid abuse, misuse and harms among chronic opioid therapy patients. *Addiction, 105*(10), 1783–1784.
76. Wasan, A., Butler, S.F., Budman, S.H., Benoit, C., Fernandez, K., & Jamison, R.N. (2007). Psychiatric history and psychologic adjustment as risk factors for aberrant drug-related behavior among patients with chronic pain. *The Clinical Journal of Pain, 23*(4), 307–315.
77. Jamison, R.N., Link, C.L., & Marceau, L.D. (2009). Do pain patients at high risk for substance misuse experience more pain? A longitudinal outcomes study. *Pain Medicine, 10*(6), 1084–1094.
78. Jamison, R.N., Ross, E.L., Michna, E., Chen, L.Q., Holcomb, C., & Wasan A.D. (2010). Substance misuse treatment for high-risk chronic pain patients on opioid therapy: A randomized trial. *PAIN, 150*(3), 390–400.
79. R. Chou (personal communication, May 14, 2015).
80. L. Webster (personal communication, May 17, 2012).
81. Gelernter, J., Panhuysen, C., Wilcox, M., et al. (2006). Genomewide linkage scan for opioid dependence and related traits. *American Journal of Human Genetics, 78*(5), 759–769.
82. D. Carr (personal communication, April 23, 2012).
83. D. Carr (personal communication, October 4, 2012).
84. Ibid.
85. J. Dahl (personal communication, March 27, 2013).
86. L. Webster (personal communication, May 25, 2011).
87. J. Kauffman (personal communication, February 23, 2011).
88. J. Kauffman (personal communication, May 13, 2012).
89. J. Dahl (personal communication, May 25, 2011).
90. J. Kauffman (personal communication, May 13, 2012).
91. MacArthur, G.J., Minozzi, S., Martin, N., et al. (2012). Opiate substitution treatment and HIV transmission in people who inject drugs: Systematic review and meta-analysis. *British Medical Journal, 345*, e5945.
92. Arbuck, D.M. (2011, April 6). Is buprenorphine effective for chronic pain? Pain Treatment Topics. Retrieved from http://updates.pain-topics.org/2011/04/is-buprenorphine-effective-for-chronic.html
93. US Food and Drug Administration. (2014). Subutex and Suboxone questions and answers. Retrieved from http://www.fda.gov/Drugs/

DrugSafety/PostmarketDrugSafetyInformationforPatientsand
Providers/ucm191523.htm

94. D. Carr (personal communication, April 23, 2012).

95. Arbuck, D.M. (2011, April 6). Is buprenorphine effective for chronic
    pain? Pain Treatment Topics. Retrieved from http://updates.pain-
    topics.org/2011/04/is-buprenorphine-effective-for-chronic.html

96. L. Webster (personal communication, May 25, 2011).

97. S. Leavitt (personal communication, May 10, 2011).

98. Weiss, R.D., Potter, J.S., Fiellin, D.A., et al. (2011). Adjunctive
    counseling during brief and extended buprenorphine-naloxone
    treatment for prescription opioid dependence. *Archives of General
    Psychiatry, 68*(12), 1238–1246.

99. Drugs.com. (n.d.). Butrans approval history. Retrieved from http://
    www.drugs.com/history/butrans.html

100. Ling, W., Casadonte, P., Bigelow, G., et al. (2010). Buprenorphine
     implants for treatment of opioid dependence: A randomized clini-
     cal trial. *The Journal of the American Medical Association, 304*(14),
     1576–1583.

101. O'Connor, P.G. (2010). Advances in the treatment of opioid depen-
     dence: Continued progress and ongoing challenges. *The Journal of
     the American Medical Association, 304*(14), 1612–1614.

102. Steiner, D., Munera, C., Hale, M., Ripa, S., & Landau, C. (2011).
     Efficacy and safety of buprenorphine transdermal system (BTDS)
     for chronic moderate to severe low back pain: A randomized,
     double-blind study. *The Journal of Pain, 12*(11), 1163–1172.

103. Arbuck, D.M. (2011, April 6). Is buprenorphine effective for chronic
     pain? Pain Treatment Topics. Retrieved from http://updates.pain-
     topics.org/2011/04/is-buprenorphine-effective-for-chronic.html

104. Sontag, D. (2013, November 16). Addiction treatment with a dark
     side. *The New York Times.* Retrieved from http://www.nytimes.
     com/2013/11/17/health/in-demand-in-clinics-and-on-the-street-
     bupe-can-be-savior-or-menace.html?_r=0

105. Hitt, E. (2010, October 14). Once-monthly naltrexone approved for
     treatment of opioid addiction. Medscape. Retrieved from http://
     www.medscape.com/viewarticle/730457?src=rss

106. Chapman, C.R., Lipschitz, D.L., Angst, M.S., et al. (2010). Opioid
     pharmacotherapy for chronic non-cancer pain in the United
     States: A research guideline for developing an evidence-base. *The
     Journal of Pain, 11*(9), 807–829.

107. Saunders, K.W., Dunn, K.M., Merrill, J.O., et al. (2010). Relationship of opioid use and dosage levels to fractures in older chronic pain patients. *Journal of General Internal Medicine, 25*(4), 310–315.
108. National Osteoporosis Foundation. (2011). Fast facts. Retrieved from http://www.nof.org/node/40
109. Rajagopal, A., Vassilopoulou-Sellin, R., Palmer, J.L., Kaur, G., & Bruera, E. (2003). Hypogonadism and sexual dysfunction in male cancer survivors receiving chronic opioid therapy. *Journal of Pain and Symptom Management, 26*(5), 1055–1061.
110. Rubinstein, A., Carpenter, D.M., & Minkoff, J. (2013). Hypogonadism in men with chronic pain linked to the use of long-acting rather than short-acting opioids. *The Clinical Journal of Pain, 29*(10), 840–845.
111. J. Dahl (personal communication, March 17, 2013).
112. Katz, M.H. (2010). Long-term opioid treatment of nonmalignant pain—A believer loses his faith [Editorial]. *Archives of General Medicine, 170*(16), 1422–1423.
113. Von Korff, M. (2010). Commentary on Boscarino et al. (2010). Understanding the spectrum of opioid abuse, misuse and harms among chronic opioid therapy patients. *Addiction, 105*(10), 1783–1784.
114. Chapman, C.R., Lipschitz, D.L., Angst, M.S., et al. (2010). Opioid pharmacotherapy for chronic non-cancer pain in the United States: A research guideline for developing an evidence-base. *The Journal of Pain, 11*(9), 807–829.
115. Dunn, K.M., Saunders, K.W., Rutter, C.M., et al. (2010). Opioid prescriptions for chronic pain and overdose. *Annals of Internal Medicine, 152*, 85–92.
116. Bohnert, A.S.B., Valenstein, M., Bair, M.J., et al. (2011). Association between opioid prescribing patterns and opioid overdose-related deaths. *The Journal of the American Medical Association, 305*(13), 1315–1321.
117. Gomes, T., Mamdani, M.M., Dhalla, I.A., Paterson, J.M., & Juurlink, D.N. (2011). Opioid dose and drug-related mortality in patients with nonmalignant pain. *Archives of Internal Medicine, 171*(7), 686–691.
118. Hall, A.J., Logan, J.E., Toblin, R.L., et al. (2008). Patterns of abuse among unintentional pharmaceutical overdose fatalities. *The Journal of the American Medical Association, 300*(22), 2613–2620.
119. Arria, A.M., Garnier-Dykstra, L.M., Caldeira, K.M., Vincent, K.B., & O'Grady, K.E. (2001). Prescription analgesic use among young adults: Adherence to physician instructions and diversion. *Pain Medicine, 12*(6), 898–903.

120. Cruciani, R., Fine, P., & January, C. (2010, May 8). Methadone prescribing: Everything you wanted to know but were afraid to ask. Paper presented at the 29th annual meeting of the American Pain Society Meeting, Baltimore, MD.

121. J. Dahl (personal communication, May 24, 2011).

122. H. Heit (personal communication, May 18, 2012).

123. D. Carr (personal communication, April 23, 2012).

124. L. Webster (personal communication, May 17, 2012).

125. US Food and Drug Administration. (2006). Public health advisory: Methadone use for pain control may result in death and life-threatening changes in breathing and heart beat [Press release]. Retrieved from http://www.fda.gov/Drugs/DrugSafety/PostmarketDrugSafetyInformationforPatientsandProviders/DrugSafetyInformationforHeathcareProfessionals/PublicH

126. J. Kauffman (personal communication, February 23, 2011).

127. National Institutes of Health. (2014). *Pathways to prevention workshop: The role of opioids in the treatment of chronic pain* (p. 15). Retrieved from https://prevention.nih.gov/docs/programs/p2p/ODPPainPanelStatementFinal_10–02-14.pdf

128. Leavitt, S.B. (2010, October 1). Intranasal naloxone for at-home opioid rescue. *Practical Pain Management.* Retrieved from http://www.practicalpainmanagement.com/treatments/pharmacological/opioids/intranasal-naloxone-home-opioid-rescue

129. Szalavitz, M. (2011, September 27). Drugs, risk and the myth of the "evil" addict [Blog post]. Retrieved from http://opinionator.blogs.nytimes.com/2011/09/27/drugs-risk-and-the-myth-of-the-evil-addict

130. Project Lazarus. (n.d.). Project Lazarus results for Wilkes County. Retrieved from http://www.projectlazarus.org/project-lazarus-results-wilkes-county

131. Albert, S., Brason, F.W. II, Sanford, C.K., Dasgupta, N., Graham, J., & Lovette, B. (2011). Project Lazarus: Community-based overdose prevention in rural North Carolina. *Pain Medicine, 12*, s77–s85.

132. Lazar, K. (2011, August 31). Progress seen in fight on heroin. *The Boston Globe.* Retrieved from http://articles.boston.com/2011-08-31/news/29949874_1_narcan-overdose-deaths-addicts

133. Massachusetts Department of Public Health. (2012, April 25). Opioid overdose prevention & reversal [Information sheet]. Retrieved from http://www.mass.gov/eohhs/docs/dph/substance-abuse/naloxone-info.pdf

134. Centers for Disease Control and Prevention. (2012). Community-based opioid overdose prevention programs providing naloxone— United States, 2010. *Morbidity and Mortality Weekly Report, 61*(6), 101–105.

135. Department of Justice, Drug Enforcement of Administration. (2014). Schedules of controlled substances: Rescheduling of hydrocodone combination products from Schedule III to Schedule II. Retrieved from https://www.federalregister.gov/articles/2014/08/22/ 2014-19922/schedules-of-controlled-substances-rescheduling-of-hydrocodone-combination-products-from-schedule

136. Chou, R., Turner, J.A., Devine, E.B., et al. (2015). The effectiveness and risks of long-term opioid therapy for chronic pain: A systematic review for a National Institutes of Health Pathways to Prevention Workshop. *Annals of Internal Medicine, 162*(4), 276–286.

137. National Institutes of Health. (2014). *Pathways to prevention workshop: The role of opioids in the treatment of chronic pain.* Retrieved from https://prevention.nih.gov/docs/programs/p2p/ODPPain PanelStatementFinal_10-02-14.pdf

138. Tennant, F. (2010, January 1). Opioid treatment 10-year longevity survey final report. *Practical Pain Management.* Retrieved from http://www.practicalpainmanagement.com/treatments/pharmacological/opioids/opioid-treatment-10-year-longevity-survey-final-report

139. National Institutes of Health. (2014). *Pathways to prevention workshop: The role of opioids in the treatment of chronic pain.* Retrieved from https://prevention.nih.gov/docs/programs/p2p/ODPPain PanelStatementFinal_10-02-14.pdf

140. R. Chou (personal communication, May 14, 2015).

141. Noble, M., Tregear, S.J., Treadwell, J.R., & Schoelles, K. (2008). Long-term opioid management for chronic noncancer pain: A systematic review and meta-analysis of efficacy and safety. *Journal of Pain and Symptom Management, 35*(2), 214–228.

142. Noble, M., Treadwell, J.R., Tregear, S.J., et al. (2010). Long-term opioid management for chronic noncancer pain [Intervention review]. *Cochrane Database of Systematic Reviews, 2010*(1), CD006605.

143. Chapman, C.R., Lipschitz, D.L., Angst, M.S., et al. (2010). Opioid pharmacotherapy for chronic non-cancer pain in the United States: A research guideline for developing an evidence-base. *The Journal of Pain, 11*(9), 807–829.

144. Eriksen, J., Sjogren, P., Bruera, E., Ekhold, O., & Rasmussen, N.K. (2006). Critical issues on opioids in chronic non-cancer pain: An epidemiological study. *PAIN, 125*, 172–179.

145. Sjogren, P., Gronbaek, M., Peuckmann, V., & Ekholm, O. (2010). A population-based cohort study on chronic pain: The role of opioids. *The Clinical Journal of Pain, 26*(9), 763–769.

146. Franklin, G.M. (2014). Opioids for chronic noncancer pain. *Neurology, 83*(14), 1277–1284.

147. Chu, L.F., Angst, M.S., & Clark, D. (2008). Opioid-induced hyperalgesia in humans: Molecular mechanisms and clinical considerations. *The Clinical Journal of Pain, 24*(6), 479–496.

148. L. Watkins (personal communication, October 28, 2009).

149. Chu, L.F., Angst, M.S., & Clark, D. (2008). Opioid-induced hyperalgesia in humans: Molecular mechanisms and clinical considerations. *The Clinical Journal of Pain, 24*(6), 479–496.

150. Chapman, C.R., Lipschitz, D.L., Angst, M.S., et al. (2010). Opioid pharmacotherapy for chronic non-cancer pain in the United States: A research guideline for developing an evidence-base. *The Journal of Pain, 11*(9), 807–829.

151. R. Chou (personal communication, May 14, 2015).

152. R. Jamison (personal communication, February 14, 2011).

153. Chou, R., Fanciullo, G.J., Fine, P.G., et al. (2009). Clinical guidelines for the use of chronic opioid therapy in chronic noncancer pain. *The Journal of Pain, 10*(2), 113–130.

154. National Institutes of Health. (2014). *Pathways to prevention workshop: The role of opioids in the treatment of chronic pain*. Retrieved from https://prevention.nih.gov/docs/programs/p2p/ODPPain PanelStatementFinal_10-02-14.pdf

155. R. Chou (personal communication, May 14, 2015).

156. Institute of Medicine, Committee on Advancing Pain Research, Care, and Education. (2011). *Relieving pain in America: A blueprint for transforming prevention, care, education and research* (pp. 2–26). Washington, DC: National Academies Press.

157. Fisch, M.J., Lee, J-W., Weiss, M., et al. (2012). Prospective, observational study of pain and analgesic prescribing in medical oncology outpatients with breast, colorectal, lung, or prostate cancer. *Journal of Clinical Oncology, 30*(16), 1980–1988.

158. Ackerman, T. (2012, April 19). Pain treatment lacking for a third of cancer patients, study says. *Houston Chronicle*. Retrieved from

http://www.chron.com/news/houston-texas/article/A-third-of-cancer-patients-pain-3496068.php

159. Von Korff, M. (2015, May). Opioid dosing and strategies to reduce dose. Paper presented at the American Pain Society annual meeting, Palm Springs, CA.

160. National Institutes of Health. (2014). *Pathways to prevention workshop: The role of opioids in the treatment of chronic pain.* Retrieved from https://prevention.nih.gov/docs/programs/p2p/ODPPain PanelStatementFinal_10-02-14.pdf

161. Hariharan, J., Lamb, G.C., & Neuner, J.M. (2007). Long-term opioid contract use for chronic pain management in primary care practice: A five year experience. *Journal of General Internal Medicine, 22*(4), 485–490.

162. Starrels, J.L., Becker, W.C., Alford, D.P., Kapoor, A., Williams, A.R., & Turner, B.J. (2010). Systematic review: Treatment agreements and urine drug testing to reduce opioid misuse in patients with chronic pain. *Annals of Internal Medicine, 152*(11), 712–720.

163. Katz, M.H. (2010). Long-term opioid treatment of nonmalignant pain—A believer loses his faith [Editorial]. *Archives of General Medicine, 170*(16), 1422–1423.

164. R. Chou (personal communication, May 14, 2015).

165. Payne, R., Anderson, E., Arnold, R., et al. (2010). A rose by any other name: Pain contracts/agreements. *American Journal of Bioethics, 10*(11), 5–12.

166. Andrews, M. (2011, April 4). Some doctors require patients to sign contracts get opioid painkillers. *The Washington Post.* Retrieved from http://www.washingtonpost.com/national/health/some-doctors-require-patients-to-sign-contracts-get-opioid-painkillers/2011/03/29/AF7D31dC_story.html

167. Pergolizzi, J., Pappagallo, M., Stauffer, J., et al. (2010). The role of urine drug testing for patients on opioid therapy. *Pain Practice, 10*(6), 497–507.

168. Centers for Disease Control and Prevention. (2010, July). *Unintentional drug poisoning in the United States.* Retrieved from http://www.cdc.gov/HomeandRecreationalSafety/pdf/poison-issue-brief.pdf

169. R. Chou (personal communication, May 14, 2015).

170. R. Twillman (personal communication, June 2, 2011).

171. Quest Diagnostics. (2012, April 27). Three in five Americans misuse their prescription drugs, finds national study of prescription medication lab testing [Press release]. *The New York Times.* Retrieved from http://markets.on.nytimes.com/research/stocks/news/press_

release.asp?docTag=201204271507PR_NEWS_USPRX____
NY95661&feedID=600&press_symbol=89411

172. Quest Diagnostics. (2012). *Prescription drug misuse in America: Laboratory insights into the new drug epidemic.* Retrieved from http://www.questdiagnostics.com/dms/Documents/health-trends/PDF-MI3040_PDM-Report_24638_FIN_Digital_4-20-12/PDF%20MI3040_PDM%20Report_24638_FIN_Digital_4-20-12.pdf

173. West, R., Pesce, A., West, C., et al. (2010). Observations of medication compliance by measurement of urinary drug concentrations in a pain management population. *Journal of Opioid Management, 6*(4), 253–257.

174. Collen, M. (2009). Opioid contracts and random drug testing for people with chronic pain—Think twice. *Journal of Law, Medicine & Ethics, 37*(4), 841–845.

175. R. Twillman (personal communication, April 13, 2015).

176. Wang, J., & Christo, P.J. (2009). The influence of prescription monitoring programs on chronic pain management. *Pain Physician, 12,* 507–515.

177. Pain & Policy Studies Group. (n.d.). Prescription monitoring programs (PMPs). Retrieved from http://www.painpolicy.wisc.edu/domestic/pmp.htm

178. Leavitt, S.B. (2011, February 24). Rx monitoring doesn't stem opioid overdose deaths. Pain Treatment Topics. Retrieved from http://updates.pain-topics.org/2011/02/rx-monitoring-doesnt-stem-opioid.html

179. Gilson, A., Twillman, R., Dahl, J., & Fishman, S. (2010, May 7). Prescription monitoring programs' impact on medication diversion and availability: What do we know and where should we go? Paper presented at the 29th annual meeting of the American Pain Society, Baltimore, MD.

180. Ibid.

181. Simeone, R., & Holland, L. (2006, September 1). *An evaluation of prescription drug monitoring programs* [Executive summary]. Retrieved from https://www.bja.gov/publications/pdmpexecsumm.pdf

182. Katz, N., Panas, L., Kim, M., et al. (2010). Usefulness of prescription monitoring programs for surveillance—Analysis of Schedule II opioid prescription data in Massachusetts, 1996–2006. *Pharmacoepidemiology and Drug Safety, 19*(2), 115–123.

183. Paulozzi, L.J., Kilbourne, E.M., & Desai, H.A. (2011). Prescription drug monitoring programs and death rates from drug overdose. *Pain Medicine, 12*(5), 747–754.

184. Kerlikowske, G., Jones, C.M., LaBelle, R.M., & Condon, T.P. (2011). Prescription drug monitoring programs—Lack of effectiveness or a call to action? [Editorial]. *Pain Medicine, 12*, 687–689.

185. Reifler, L.M., Droz, D., Bailey, J.E., et al. (2012). Do prescription monitoring programs impact state trends in opioid abuse/misuse? *Pain Medicine, 13*(3), 434–442.

186. Passik, S.D., Kirsh, K.L., & Twillman, R.K. (2015). FDA/DEA/ PDMP/ UDT: Alphabet soup or sensible and integrated risk management? *Journal of Opioid Management, 11*(1), 77–81.

187. Passik, S. (2015, March 29). New research points to reduced access, patient suffering due to hydrocodone rescheduling. PR Newswire. Retrieved from http://www.prnewswire.com/news-releases/ new-research-points-to-reduced-access-patient-suffering-due-to-hydrocodone-rescheduling-300053505.html#

188. Ibid.

189. Patrick, S.W., Schumacher, R.E., Benneyworth, B.D., Krans, E.E., McAllister, J.M., & Davis, M.M. (2012). Neonatal abstinence syndrome and associated health care expenditures—United States 2000–2009. *The Journal of the American Medical Association, 307*(18), 1934–1940.

190. US Food and Drug Administration. (2013). FDA announces safety labeling changes and postmarket study requirements for extended-release and long-acting opioid analgesics. Retrieved from http:// www.fda.gov/NewsEvents/Newsroom/PressAnnouncements/ ucm367726.htm

191. C. Lenard (personal communication, January 21, 2015).

192. D. Thomas. (2015). Centers for Excellence in Pain Education and the role of opioids in the treatment of chronic pain [PowerPoint slides]. Retrieved from http://iprcc.nih.gov/meetings/4-17-2015%20 Meeting%20Presentations/6_Thomas_CoEPEs_OpioidChronic Pain.pdf

193. D. Thomas (personal communication, March 17, 2014).

194. National Institute of Drug Abuse. (2014). Abuse of prescription pain medications risks heroin use. Retrieved from http://www. drugabuse.gov/related-topics/trends-statistics/infographics/ abuse-prescription-pain-medications-risks-

195. D. Thomas (personal communication, March 17, 2014).

196. National Institutes of Health. (2014). *Pathways to prevention workshop: The role of opioids in the treatment of chronic pain.* Retrieved from https://prevention.nih.gov/docs/programs/p2p/ODPPainPanel StatementFinal_10-02-14.pdf

197. Cicero, T.J., & Ellis, M.S. (2015). Abuse-deterrent formulations and the prescription opioid abuse epidemic in the United States: Lessons learned from OxyContin. *The Journal of the American Medical Association, 72*(5), 424–430.

198. Cicero, T.J., Ellis, M.S., Surratt, H.L., & Kurtz, S.P. (2014). The changing face of heroin use in the United States: A retrospective analysis of the past 50 years. *The Journal of the American Medical Association, 71*(7), 821–826.

199. Centers for Disease Control and Prevention. (2015). Today's heroin epidemic. Retrieved from http://www.cdc.gov/vitalsigns/heroin/index.html

200. Schlosberg, J.E., Vendruscolo, L.F., Bremer, P.T., et al. (2013). Dynamic vaccine blocks relapse to compulsive intake of heroin. *Proceedings of the National Academy of Sciences, 110*(22), 9036–9041.

201. Sifferlin, A. (2015, January 9). Why you've never heard of the vaccine for heroin addiction. *Time.* Retrieved from http://time.com/3654784/why-youve-never-heard-of-the-vaccine-for-heroin-addiction

202. Ehrenberg, R. (2015, May 18). Engineered yeast paves the way for home-brew heroin. *Nature.* Retrieved from http://www.nature.com/news/engineered-yeast-paves-way-for-home-brew-heroin-1.17566?WT.mc_id=TWT_NatureNews

203. D. Thomas (2015). Centers for Excellence in Pain Education and the role of opioids in the treatment of chronic pain [PowerPoint slides]. Retrieved from http://iprcc.nih.gov/meetings/4-17-2015%20Meeting%20Presentations/6_Thomas_CoEPEs_OpioidChronicPain.pdf

204. National Institutes of Health. (2014). *Pathways to prevention workshop: The role of opioids in the treatment of chronic pain.* Retrieved from https://prevention.nih.gov/docs/programs/p2p/ODPPainPanelStatementFinal_10-02-14.pdf

205. Ibid.

206. Van Zeller, M. (2009, October 15). The OxyContin express [Webisode]. In *Vanguard.* Retrieved from http://current.com/groups/vanguard-the-oxycontin-express

207. Anderson, C. (2011, April 20). Deadly abuse puts focus on "pill mills." *The Boston Globe.* Retrieved from http://articles.boston.com/2011-04-20/news/29451932_1_cocaine-deaths-oxycodone-pills-prescription-drugs

208. LaMendola, B., & Campbell, A. (2011, February 23). Feds, police raid 11 south Florida pill mills. *South Florida Sun-Sentinel.* Retrieved

from http://articles.sun-sentinel.com/2011-02-23/health/fl-pill-mill-raids-20110223_1_pain-clinics-pill-mills-pain-pill

209. US Drug Enforcement Administration. (2011, October 28). DEA administrator, attorney general announce enforcement efforts against illegal prescription drug distributors in Florida [Press release]. Retrieved from http://www.justice.gov/dea/pubs/pressrel/pr102811.html

210. Hoffmann, D. (2008). Treating pain v. reducing drug diversion and abuse: Recalibrating the balance in our drug control laws and policies. *St. Louis University Journal of Health Law and Policy, 1*(2), 256.

211. Atluri, S., Sudarshan, G., & Manchikanti, L. (2014). Assessment of the trends in medical use and misuse of opioid analgesics from 2004 to 2011. *Health Policy Research, 17*(2), e119–e128.

212. Centers for Disease Control and Prevention. (2015). Injury prevention & control: Prescription drug overdose. Retrieved from http://www.cdc.gov/drugoverdose/data/index.html

213. D. Thomas (2015). Centers for Excellence in Pain Education and the role of opioids in the treatment of chronic pain [PowerPoint slides]. Retrieved from http://iprcc.nih.gov/meetings/4-17-2015%20Meeting%20Presentations/6_Thomas_CoEPEs_OpioidChronicPain.pdf

214. Centers for Disease Control and Prevention. (2014). Opioid painkiller prescribing. Retrieved from http://www.cdc.gov/vitalsigns/opioid-prescribing

215. Paulozzi, L.J. (2012). Prescription drug overdoses: A review. *Journal of Safety Research, 43*(4), 283–289.

216. Roland, C.L., Joshi, A.V., Mardekian, J., Walden, S.C., & Harnett, J. (2013). Prevalence and cost of diagnosed opioid abuse in a privately insured population in the United States. *Journal of Opioid Management, 9*(3), 161–175.

217. Institute of Medicine, Committee on Advancing Pain Research, Care, and Education. (2011). *Relieving pain in America: A blueprint for transforming prevention, care, education and research* (p. S-3). Washington, DC: National Academies Press.

218. National Institutes of Health. (2014). *Pathways to prevention workshop: The role of opioids in the treatment of chronic pain.* Retrieved from https://prevention.nih.gov/docs/programs/p2p/ODPPainPanelStatementFinal_10-02-14.pdf

219. Ibid.

220. Fishbain, D.A., Cole, B., Lewis, J., Rosomoff, H.L., & Rosomoff, R.S. (2008). What percentage of chronic nonmalignant pain patients

exposed to chronic opioid analgesic therapy develop abuse/addiction and/or aberrant drug-related behaviors? A structured evidence-based review. *Pain Medicine, 9*(4), 444–459.

221. National Institutes of Health. (2014). *Pathways to prevention workshop: The role of opioids in the treatment of chronic pain.* Retrieved from https://prevention.nih.gov/docs/programs/p2p/ODPPain PanelStatementFinal_10-02-14.pdf

222. National Institutes of Health. (2015). [Table shows appropriations of funds by the NIH for FY 1938–2014]. Appropriations (section 2) from the NIH Almanac. Retrieved from http://www.nih.gov/about/almanac/appropriations/part2.htm

223. National Institutes of Health. (2015). [Table shows the annual support level by the NIH for FY 2011–2014 and estimates for FY 2015–2016]. Estimates of funding for various research, condition, and disease categories (RCDC). Retrieved from http://report.nih.gov/rcdc/categories

224. D. Bradshaw (personal communication, April 20, 2015).

225. National Institutes of Health. (n.d). [Table shows NIH budget information for FY 2014–2016]. All purpose table. Retrieved from http://officeofbudget.od.nih.gov/pdfs/FY16/Executive%20Summary.pdf

226. National Institutes of Health. (2015). [Table shows the annual support level by the NIH for FY 2011–2014 and estimates for FY 2015–2016]. Estimates of funding for various research, condition, and disease categories (RCDC). Retrieved from http://report.nih.gov/rcdc/categories

227. L. Porter (personal communication, April 28, 2015).

228. D. Bradshaw (personal communication, April 20, 2015).

229. B. Saner (personal communication, April 21, 2015).

230. P. Pizzo (personal communication, September 22, 2011).

231. R. Saner (personal communication, September 22, 2011).

232. S. Rep. No. 112-84. (2012). Retrieved from the Library of Congress Database: https://www.congress.gov/congressional-report/112/senate-report/84

233. National Institutes of Health. (2015). National Pain Strategy. Retrieved from http://iprcc.nih.gov/National_Pain_Strategy/NPS_Main.htm

234. M. Christopher (personal communication, April 15, 2015).

235. B. Saner (personal communication, April 21, 2015).

236. National Institutes of Health. (2015). NINDS Office of Pain Policy. Retrieved from http://painconsortium.nih.gov/News_Other_Resources/officepainpolicy_paininfo.html

237. K. Bush (personal communication, April 25, 2011).
238. Global Commission on Drug Policy. (2011). *War on drugs: Report of the Global Commission on Drug Policy* (p. 4). Retrieved from http://www.globalcommissionondrugs.org/wp-content/themes/gcdp_v1/pdf/Global_Commission_Report_English.pdf
239. Katz, J.M. (2011, June 2). Commission declares drug war failure, urges legalization. *The Boston Globe*. Retrieved from http://www.boston.com/news/nation/articles/2011/06/02/commission_de-clares_drug_war_a_failure_urges_legalization
240. Global Commission on Drug Policy. (2011). *War on drugs: Report of the Global Commission on Drug Policy* (p. 4). Retrieved from http://www.globalcommissionondrugs.org/wp-content/themes/gcdp_v1/pdf/Global_Commission_Report_English.pdf
241. Ibid.

Chapter 4

1. M.R. Rajagopal (personal communication, June 17, 2015).
2. Tsang, A., Von Korff, M., Lee, S., et al. (2008). Common chronic pain conditions in developed and developing countries: Gender and age differences and comorbidity with depression-anxiety disorders. *The Journal of Pain, 9*(10), 883–891.
3. Degenhart, L., Bruno, R., Lintzernis, N., et al. (2015). Agreements between definitions of pharmaceutical opioid use disorders and dependence in people taking opioids for chronic non-cancer pain (POINT): A cohort study. *The Lancet Psychiatry, 2*(4), 314–322.
4. M.R. Rajagopal. (2015, March 3). How do you treat pain when most of the world's population can't get opioids? *Los Angeles Times*. Retrieved from http://www.latimes.com/opinion/op-ed/la-oe-rajagopal-pain-opioids-20150304-story.html
5. Ibid.
6. M. O'Brien (personal communication, January 7, 2015).
7. Ibid.
8. F. Knaul (personal communication, January 26, 2015).
9. Knaul, F.M., Farmer, P.E., & Bhadelia, A. (2015). Closing the divide: The Harvard Global Equity Initiative–*Lancet* Commission on global access to pain control and palliative care, Comment, *The Lancet, 386*(9995), 722–744.
10. Cherny, N.I., Baselga, J., de Conno, F., & Radbruch, L. (2010). Formulary availability and regulatory barriers to accessibility of opioids for

cancer pain in Europe: A report from the ESMO/EAPC opioid policy initiative. *Annals of Oncology, 21*(3), 615–626.

11. Joranson, D.E., Ryan, K.M., & Maurer, M.A. (2010). Opioid policy, availability and access in developing and nonindustrialized countries. In *Bonica's management of pain* (4th ed.), ed. S.M. Fishman, J.C. Ballantyne, & J.P., Rathmell (pp. 194–208). Baltimore, MD: Lippincott Williams & Wilkins.

12. Human Rights Watch. (2011). *Global state of pain treatment: Access to palliative care as a human right* (p. 2). Retrieved from http://www.hrw.org/sites/default/files/reports/hhr0511W.pdf

13. Ibid.

14. Human Rights Watch. (2009). *Unbearable pain—India's obligation to ensure palliative care.* Retrieved from http://www.hrw.org/sites/default/files/reports/health1009web.pdf

15. World Health Organization. (2009). *Access to Controlled Medications Programme: Improving access to medications controlled under international drug conventions.* Retrieved from http://www.who.int/medicines/areas/quality_safety/ACMP_BrNoteGenrl_EN_Feb09.pdf

16. Seya, M.J., Gelders, S.F., Achara, O.U., Milani, B. & Scholten, W.K. (2011). A first comparison between the consumption of and the need for opioid analgesics at country, regional and global levels. *Journal of Pain & Palliative Care Pharmacotherapy, 25*(1), 6–18.

17. Ibid.

18. Pain & Policy Studies Group. (2012). Opioid consumption maps—Morphine. Retrieved from https://ppsg.medicine.wisc.edu

19. World Health Organization. (2011). *Ensuring balance in national policies on controlled substances: Guidance for availability and accessibility of controlled medicine.* Retrieved from http://www.atome-project.eu/documents/gls_ens_balance_eng.pdf

20. Joranson, D.E., Ryan, K.M., & Maurer, M.A. (2010). Opioid policy, availability and access in developing and nonindustrialized countries. In *Bonica's management of pain* (4th ed.), ed. S.M. Fishman, J.C. Ballantyne, & J.P., Rathmell (pp. 194–208). Baltimore, MD: Lippincott Williams & Wilkins.

21. Harvard Global Equity Initiative. (2015). *10 facts about pain and palliation.* Retrieved from http://hgei.harvard.edu/fs/docs/icb.topic662843.files/Pain_and_palliation_fact_sheet_rev3.pdf

22. Harvard Global Equity Initiative. (2015). Closing the pain divide. Retrieved from http://hgei.harvard.edu/icb/icb.do?keyword=k62597&pageid=icb.page662285

23. Krakauer, E.L., Cham, N.T., Husain, S.A., et al. (2015). Toward safe accessibility of opioid medicines in Vietnam and other developing countries: A balanced policy model. *Journal of Pain and Symptom Management, 49*(5), 916–922.

24. A.R. Marx (personal communication, July 21, 2015).

25. Treat the Pain. (2015). Country reports. Retrieved from http://www.treatthepain.org/country_reports.html

26. Krakauer, E.L., Cham, N.T., Husain, S.A., et al. (2015). Toward safe accessibility of opioid medicines in Vietnam and other developing countries: A balanced policy model. *Journal of Pain and Symptom Management, 49*(5), 916–922.

27. Ibid.

28. M. O'Brien (personal communication, January 7, 2015).

29. Ibid.

30. J. Cleary (personal communication, June 5, 2015).

31. Krakauer, E.L., Cham, N.T., Husain, S.A., et al. (2015). Toward safe accessibility of opioid medicines in Vietnam and other developing countries: A balanced policy model. *Journal of Pain and Symptom Management, 49*(5), 916–922.

32. Ibid.

33. Human Rights Watch. (2011). *Global state of pain treatment: Access to palliative care as a human right* (p. 7) Retrieved from http://www.hrw.org/sites/default/files/reports/hhr0511W.pdf

34. Harvard Global Equity Initiative. (2015). About the Harvard Global Equity Initiative. Retrieved from http://isites.harvard.edu/icb/icb.do?keyword=k62597&tabgroupid=icb.tabgroup88307

35. F. Knaul (personal communication, January 26, 2015).

36. Harvard Global Equity Initiative. (2015). Closing the pain divide. Retrieved from http://hgei.harvard.edu/icb/icb.do?keyword=k62597&pageid=icb.page662285

37. Knaul, F.M., Farmer, P.E., & Bhadelia, A. (2015). Closing the divide: The Harvard Global Equity Initiative–*Lancet* Commission on global access to pain control and palliative care, Comment. *The Lancet, 386*(9995), 722–744.

38. Harvard Global Equity Initiative. (2015). Closing the pain divide. Retrieved from http://hgei.harvard.edu/icb/icb.do?keyword=k62597&pageid=icb.page662285

39. Krakauer, E.L., Cham, N.T., Husain, S.A., et al. (2015). Toward safe accessibility of opioid medicines in Vietnam and other developing

countries: A balanced policy model. *Journal of Pain and Symptom Management, 49*(5), 916–922.

40. De Lima, L., Pastrana, T., Radbruch, L., & Wenk, R. (2014). Cross-sectional pilot study to monitor the availability, dispensed prices and affordability of opioids around the globe. *Journal of Pain and Symptom Management, 48*(4), 649–659.

41. World Health Organization. (2015). *Essential medicines.* Retrieved from http://www.who.int/topics/essential_medicines/en/. See also Joranson, D.E., Ryan, K.M., & Maurer, M.A. (2010). Opioid policy, availability and access in developing and nonindustrialized countries. In *Bonica's management of pain* (4th ed.), ed. S.M. Fishman, J.C. Ballantyne, & J.P., Rathmell (pp. 194–208). Baltimore, MD: Lippincott Williams & Wilkins.

42. Cherny, N.I., Cleary, J., Scholten, W., Radbruch, L., & Torode, J. (2013). The Global Opioid Policy Initiative (GOPI) to evaluate the availability and accessibility of opioids for the management of cancer pain in Africa, Asia, Latin America and the Caribbean, and the Middle East: Introduction and methodology. *Annals of Oncology, 24*(11), xi7–xi13.

43. Ibid.

44. Ibid.

45. Human Rights Watch. (2009). India: Provide access to pain treatment. Retrieved from http://www.hrw.org/news/2009/10/28/india-provide-access-pain-treatment

46. Human Rights Watch. (2011). *Global palliative* (p. 3). Retrieved from http://www.hrw.org/reports/2011/06/02/global-state-pain-treatment-0

47. Cleary, J., Simha, N., Panieri, A., et al. (2013). Formulary availability and regulatory barriers to accessibility of opioids for cancer pain in India: A report from the Global Opioid Policy Initiative (GOPI). *Annals of Oncology, 24*(11), xi33–xi40.

48. Human Rights Watch. (2009). India: Provide access to pain treatment. Retrieved from http://www.hrw.org/news/2009/10/28/india-provide-access-pain-treatment

49. Ibid.

50. Cleary, J., Simha, N., Panieri, A., et al. (2013). Formulary availability and regulatory barriers to accessibility of opioids for cancer pain in India: A report from the Global Opioid Policy Initiative (GOPI). *Annals of Oncology, 24*(11), xi33–xi40.

51. Rajagopal, M.R. (2015, March 3). How do you treat pain when most of the world's population can't get opioids? *Los Angeles Times*. Retrieved from http://www.latimes.com/opinion/op-ed/la-oe-rajagopal-pain-opioids-20150304-story.html

52. McNeil, D.G. (2007, September 11). In India, a quest to ease the pain of the dying. *The New York Times*. Retrieved from http://www.nytimes.com/2007/09/11/health/11pain.html?pagewanted=all

53. Rajagopal, M.R. (2015, March 3). How do you treat pain when most of the world's population can't get opioids? *Los Angeles Times*. Retrieved from http://www.latimes.com/opinion/op-ed/la-oe-rajagopal-pain-opioids-20150304-story.html

54. Cleary, J., Simha, N., Panieri, A., et al. (2013). Formulary availability and regulatory barriers to accessibility of opioids for cancer pain in India: A report from the Global Opioid Policy Initiative (GOPI). *Annals of Oncology, 24*(11), xi33–xi40.

55. Ibid.

56. Maya, C. (2014, February 23). Passing of NDPS Act Amendment Bill will make morphine more accessible. *The Hindu*. Retrieved from http://www.thehindu.com/todays-paper/tp-national/passing-of-ndps-act-amendment-bill-will-make-morphine-more-accessible/article5718188.ece

57. Rajagopal, M.R. (2015, March 3). How do you treat pain when most of the world's population can't get opioids? *Los Angeles Times*. Retrieved from http://www.latimes.com/opinion/op-ed/la-oe-rajagopal-pain-opioids-20150304-story.html

58. Human Rights Watch. (2009). *Unbearable pain—India's obligation to ensure palliative care* (p. 3). Retrieved from http://www.hrw.org/reports/2009/10/28/unbearable-pain-0

59. Cleary, J., Simha, N., Panieri, A., et al. (2013). Formulary availability and regulatory barriers to accessibility of opioids for cancer pain in India: A report from the Global Opioid Policy Initiative (GOPI). *Annals of Oncology, 24*(11), xi33–xi40.

60. Ibid.

61. Ibid.

62. Human Rights Watch. (2009). *Unbearable pain—India's obligation to ensure palliative care* (pp. 4–5). Retrieved from http://www.hrw.org/reports/2009/10/28/unbearable-pain-0

63. Human Rights Watch. (2009). India: Provide access to pain treatment. Retrieved from http://www.hrw.org/news/2009/10/28/india-provide-access-pain-treatment

64. McNeil, D.G. (2007, September 10). Drugs banned, many of the world's poor suffer in pain. *The New York Times.* Retrieved from http://www.nytimes.com/2007/09/10/health/10pain.html? pagewanted=all

65. Cleary, J., Powell, R.A., Munene, C., et al. (2013). Formulary availability and regulatory barriers to accessibility of opioids for cancer pain in Africa: A report from the Global Opioid Policy Initiative (GOPI). *Annals of Oncology, 24*(11), xi14–xi23.

66. Ibid.

67. Nzimiro, C.R., Nkurikiyimfura, J.L., Mukeshimana, O., Ngizwe Nao, S., Mukasahana, D., & Clancy, C. (2014). Palliative care in Africa: A global challenge. *Ecancermedicalscience, 8,* 493.

68. Cleary, J., Powell, R.A., Munene, C., et al. (2013). Formulary availability and regulatory barriers to accessibility of opioids for cancer pain in Africa: A report from the Global Opioid Policy Initiative (GOPI). *Annals of Oncology, 24*(11), xi14–xi23.

69. Ibid.

70. Ibid.

71. Ibid.

72. Krakauer, E.L., Cham, N.T., Husain, S.A., et al. (2015). Toward safe accessibility of opioid medicines in Vietnam and other developing countries: A balanced policy model. *Journal of Pain and Symptom Management, 49*(5), 916–922.

73. Ibid.

74. Cleary, J., De Lima, L., Eisenchlas, J., Radbruch, L., Torode, J. & Cherny N.I. (2013). Formulary availability and regulatory barriers to accessibility of opioids for cancer pain in Latin America and the Caribbean: A report from the Global Opioid Policy Initiative (GOPI). *Annals of Oncology, 24*(11), xi41–xi50.

75. Ibid.

76. Ibid.

77. Ibid.

78. Human Rights Watch. (2011). *Global palliative care* (p. 2). Retrieved from http://www.hrw.org/reports/2011/06/02/global-state-pain-treatment-0

79. Ibid., p. 12.

80. Ibid., p. 2.

81. Joranson, D.E., Ryan, K.M., & Maurer, M.A. (2010). Opioid policy, availability and access in developing and nonindustrialized countries. In *Bonica's management of pain* (4th ed.), ed. S.M. Fishman, J.C.

Ballantyne, & J.P., Rathmell (pp. 194–208). Baltimore, MD: Lippincott Williams & Wilkins.

82. Human Rights Watch. (2011). *Global palliative care* (p. 2). Retrieved from http://www.hrw.org/reports/2011/06/02/global-state-pain-treatment-0

83. Cherny, N.I., Cleary, J., Scholten, W., Radbruch, L., & Torode, J. (2013). The Global Opioid Policy Initiative (GOPI) to evaluate the availability and accessibility of opioids for the management of cancer pain in Africa, Asia, Latin America and the Caribbean, and the Middle East: Introduction and methodology. *Annals of Oncology, 24*(11), xi7–xi13.

84. Ibid.

85. Knaul, F.M., Farmer, P.E., Bhadelia, A., Berman, P. & Horton, R. (2015). Closing the divide: The Harvard Global Equity Initiative-*Lancet* Commission on global access to pain control and palliative care. *The Lancet, 386*(9995), 722–724.

Chapter 5

1. National Institute on Drug Abuse. (2015). Is marijuana medicine? Retrieved from http://www.drugabuse.gov/publications/drug-facts/marijuana-medicine

2. Huestis, M.A. (2007). Human cannabinoid pharmacokinetics. *Chemistry & Biodiversity, 4*(8), 1770–1804.

3. D. Abrams (personal communication, May 20, 2015).

4. R. Merchoulam (personal communication, April 16, 2010).

5. National Institute on Drug Abuse. (2015). Drug facts: Nationwide trends. Retrieved from http://www.drugabuse.gov/publications/drugfacts/nationwide-trends

6. National Institute on Drug Abuse. (2015). Is marijuana medicine? Retrieved from http://www.drugabuse.gov/publications/drug-facts/marijuana-medicine

7. Abrams, D.I. (2010). Cannabis in pain and palliative care. *The Pain Practitioner, 20*(4), 35–45.

8. Russo, E.B. (2007). History of cannabis and its preparations in saga, science, and sobriquet. *Chemistry & Biodiversity, 4*(8), 1614–1648.

9. Eadie, M.J. (2007). The neurological legacy of John Russell Reynolds (1828–1896). *Journal of Clinical Neuroscience, 14*(4), 309–316.

10. Russo, E. (2001). Hemp for headache: An in-depth historical and scientific review of cannabis in migraine treatment. *Journal of Cannabis Therapy, 1*(2), 21–92.

11. Russo, E. (1998). Cannabis for migraine treatment: The once and future prescription? An historical and scientific review. *PAIN, 76*(1–2), 3–8.

12. Huestis, M.A. (2007). Human cannabinoid pharmacokinetics. *Chemistry & Biodiversity, 4*(8), 1770–1804.

13. Abrams, D.I. (2010). Cannabis in pain and palliative care. *The Pain Practitioner, 20*(4), 35–45.

14. Di Marzo, V., Melck, D., Bisogno, T., & De Petrocellis, L. (1998). Endocannabinoids: Endogenous cannabinoid receptor ligands with neuromodulatory action. *Trends in Neuroscience, 21*(12), 521–528.

15. Russo, E.B., & Hohmann, A. (2013). Role of cannabinoids in pain management. In *Comprehensive treatment of chronic pain by medical, interventional, and behavioral approaches: The American Academy of Pain Medicine textbook on patient management,* ed. T.R. Deer, M.S. Leong, & A.L. Ray (pp. 181–198). New York: Springer.

16. Dinacheva, I., Drysdale, A.T., Hartley, C.A., et al. (2015). FAAH genetic variation enhances fronto-amygdala function in mouse and human. *Nature Communications, 6,* 6395.

17. Friedman, R.A. (2015, March 6). The feel-good gene. *The New York Times.* Retrieved from http://www.nytimes.com/2015/03/08/opinion/sunday/the-feel-good-gene.html?_r=0

18. E.A. Romero-Sandoval (personal communication, August 29, 2011).

19. Riachlen, D.A., Foster, A.D., Gerdeman, G.L., Seillier, A., & Giuffrida, A. (2012). Wired to run: Exercise-induced endocannabinoid signaling in humans and cursorial mammals with implications for the "runner's high." *Journal of Experimental Biology, 215*(Pt. 8), 1331–136.

20. Rossi, C., Pini, L.A., Cupini, M.L., Calabresi, P., & Sarchielli, P. (2008). Endocannabinoids in platelets of chronic migraine patients and medication-overuse headache patients: Relation with serotonin levels. *European Journal of Clinical Pharmacology, 64*(1), 1–8.

21. Russo, E.B. (2004). Clinical endocannabinoid deficiency (CECD): Can this concept explain therapeutic benefits of cannabis in migraine, fibromyalgia, irritable bowel syndrome and other treatment-resistant conditions? *Neuroendocrinology Letters, 25*(1–2), 31–39.

22. Juhasz, G., Lazary, J., Chase, D., et al. (2009). Variations in the cannabinoid receptor 1 gene predispose to migraine. *Neuroscience Letters, 461*(2), 116–120.

23. Talkington, M. (2011, December 1). FLAT-tening pain: Blocking transporter boosts endocannabinoid levels in mice. Pain Research Forum. Retrieved from http://www.painresearchforum.org/news/11548-flat-tening-pain?search_term=FLAT-tening%20Pain

24. Duggan, K.C., Hermanson, D.J., Musee, L., et al. (2011). (R)-Profens are substrate-selective inhibitors of endocannabinoid oxygenation by COX-2. *Nature Chemical Biology, 7*(11), 803–809.
25. E.A. Romero-Sandoval (personal communication, June 20, 2011).
26. Abrams, D.I. (2010). Cannabis in pain and palliative care. *The Pain Practitioner, 20*(4), 35–45.
27. Martin, M., Ledent, C., Parmentier, M., Maldonado, R., & Valverde, O. (2002). Involvement of CB1 cannabinoid receptors in emotional behaviour. *Psychopharmacology, 159*(4), 379–387.
28. Poncelet, M., Maruani, J., Calassi, R., & Soubrie, P. (2003). Overeating, alcohol and sucrose consumption decrease in CB1 receptor deleted mice. *Neuroscience Letters, 343*(3), 216–218.
29. Cota, D., Marsicano, G., Tschop, M., et al. (2003). The endogenous cannabinoid system affects energy balance via central orexigenic drive and peripheral lipogenesis. *Journal of Clinical Investigation, 112*(3), 423–431.
30. Benedetti, F., Amanzio, M., Rosato, R., & Blanchard, C. (2011). Nonopioid placebo analgesia is mediated by CB1 cannabinoid receptors. *Nature Medicine, 17*(10), 1228–1230.
31. Society for Nuclear Medicine. (2011, June 6). Molecular imaging shows chronic marijuana smoking affects brain chemistry [Press release]. Retrieved from http://www.eurekalert.org/pub_releases/2011-06/sonm-mis060211.php
32. E. Russo (personal communication, August 16, 2011).
33. Beltramo, M. (2009). Cannabinoid type 2 receptor as a target for chronic pain. *Mini-Reviews in Medicinal Chemistry, 9*(1), 11–25.
34. Abrams, D.I. (2010). Cannabis in pain and palliative care. *The Pain Practitioner, 20*(4), 35–45.
35. Russo, E.B. (2011). Taming THC: Potential cannabis synergy and phytocannabinoid-terpenoid entourage effects. *British Journal of Pharmacology, 163*(7), 1344–1364.
36. Lee, M.C., Ploner, M., Wiech, K., et al. (2013). Amygdala activity contributes to the dissociative effect of cannabis on pain perception. *PAIN, 154*(1), 124–134.
37. Ware, M.A., & Tawfik, V.L. (2005). Safety issues concerning the medical use of cannabis and cannabinoids. *Pain Research & Management: The Journal of the Canadian Pain Society, 10*(Suppl. A), 32A.
38. Hazekamp, A. (2010). Review on clinical studies with cannabis and cannabinoids 2005-2009. *Cannabinoids, 5*(Special issue), 1–21.
39. Ben Amar, M. (2006). Cannabinoids in medicine: A review of their therapeutic potential. *Journal of Ethnopharmacology, 105*(1–2), 1–25.

40. D. Abrams (personal communication, May 20, 2015).
41. Amtmann, D., Weydt, P., Johnson, K.L., Jensen, M.P., & Carter, G.T. (2004). Survey of cannabis use in patients with amyotrophic lateral sclerosis. *American Journal of Hospice and Palliative Medicine, 21*(2), 95–104.
42. Lago, E.D., & Fernandez-Ruiz, J. (2007). Cannabinoids and neuroprotection in motor-related disorders. *CNS & Neurological Disorders— Drug Targets, 6*(6), 377–387.
43. Carter, G.T. (2001). Marijuana in the management of amyotrophic lateral sclerosis. *American Journal of Hospice and Palliative Care, 18*(4), 264–270.
44. Marijuana Policy Project. (n.d.). *Medical marijuana research.* Retrieved from http://www.mpp.org/assets/pdfs/library/MedConditions Handout.pdf
45. International Association for Cannabinoid Medicines. (n.d.). General remarks. Retrieved from http://www.cannabis-med.org/index. php?tpl=page&id=21&lng=en
46. D. Abrams (personal communication, May 15, 2015).
47. Abrams, D.I., & Guzman, M. (2015). Cannabis in cancer care. *Clinical Pharmacology and Therapeutics, 97*(6), 575–586.
48. Guzman, M. (2003). Cannabinoids: Potential anticancer agents. *Nature Reviews, 3,* 745–755.
49. Sarfaraz, S., Adhami, V.M., Syed, D.N., Afaq, F., & Mukhtar, H. (2008). Cannabinoids for cancer treatment: Progress and promise. *Cancer Research, 68*(2), 339- 342.
50. Marcu, J.P., Christian, R.T., Lau, D., et al. (2010). Cannabidiol enhances the inhibitory effects of delta-9-tetrahydrocanabinol on human glioblastoma cell proliferation and survival. *Molecular Cancer Therapeutics, 9*(1), 180–189.
51. Nagarkatti, P. (n.d.). Research focus: Cannabinoid-induced immunosuppression and use of cannabinoids in cancer therapy. University of South Carolina School of Medicine. Retrieved from http://pmi.med. sc.edu/PNagarkatti.asp
52. McAllister, S.D., Christian, S.D., Horowitz, M.P., Garcia, A., & Desprez, P. (2007). Cannabidiol as novel inhibitor of Ld-1 gene expression in aggressive breast cancer cells. *Molecular Cancer Therapeutics, 6,* 2921.
53. Abrams, D., Jay, C.A., Shade, S.B., et al. (2007). Cannabis in painful HIV-associated sensory neuropathy: A randomized placebo-controlled trial. *Neurology, 68*(7), 515–521.
54. Russo, E.B. (2008). Cannabinoids in the management of difficult to treat pain. *Therapeutics and Clinical Risk Management, 4*(1), 245–259.

55. Turcotte, D., Le Dorze, J.-A., Esfahani, F., Frost, E., Gomori, A., & Namaka, M. (2010). Examining the roles of cannabinoids in pain and other therapeutic indications: A review. *Expert Opinion on Pharmacotherapy, 11*(1), 17–31.
56. Lynch, M.E., & Campbell, F. (2011). Cannabinoids for treatment of chronic non-cancer pain: A systematic review of randomized trials. *British Journal of Clinical Pharmacology, 72*(5), 735–744.
57. Abrams, D.I. (2010). Cannabis in pain and palliative care. *The Pain Practitioner, 20*(4), 35–45.
58. Narang, S., Gibson, D., Wasan, A.D., et al. (2008). Efficacy of dronabinol as an adjuvant treatment for chronic pain patients on opioid therapy. *The Journal of Pain, 9*(3), 254–264.
59. Cichewicz, D.L. (2004). Synergistic interactions between cannabinoid and opioid analgesics. *Life Sciences, 74*(11), 1317–1324.
60. Hazekamp, A. (2010). Review on clinical studies with cannabis and cannabinoids 2005–2009. *Cannabinoids, 5*(Special issue), 1–21.
61. Holdcroft, A., Maze, M., Tebbs, S., & Thompson, S. (2006). A multicenter dose-escalation study of analgesic and adverse effects of an oral cannabis extract (cannador) for postoperative pain management. *Anesthesiology, 104*(5), 1040–1046.
62. Wallace, M., Schulteis, G., Atkinson, J.H., et al. (2007). Dose-dependent effects of smoked cannabis on capsaicin-induced pain and hyperalgesia in healthy volunteers. *Anesthesiology, 107*(5), 785–796.
63. Center for Medicinal Cannabis Research, University of California. (2010). *Report to the legislature and governor of the state of California presenting findings pursuant to SB847 which created the CMCR and provided state funding* (p. 4). Retrieved from http://www.cmcr.ucsd.edu/images/pdfs/CMCR_REPORT_FEB17.pdf
64. Canadian Consortium for the Investigation of Cannabinoids. (n.d.). Completed clinical research on cannabinoids. Retrieved from http://www.ccic.net/index.php?id=212,685,0,0,1,0
65. Abrams, D., Jay, C.A., Shade, S.B., et al. (2007). Cannabis in painful HIV-associated sensory neuropathy: A randomized placebo-controlled trial. *Neurology, 68*(7), 515–521.
66. Wilsey, B., Marcotte, T., Tsodikov, A., et al. (2008). A randomized, placebo-controlled, crossover trial of cannabis cigarettes in neuropathic pain. *The Journal of Pain, 9*(6), 506–521.
67. Ellis, R.J., Toperoff, W., Vaida, F., et al. (2009). Smoked medicinal cannabis for neuropathic pain in HIV: A randomized, crossover clinical trial. *Neuropsychopharmacology, 34*, 672–680.

68. Ware, M.A., Wang, T., Shapiro, S., et al. (2010). Smoked cannabis for chronic neuropathic pain: A randomized controlled trial. *Canadian Medical Association Journal, 182*, E694–E701.

69. Leavitt, S. (2010, September 4). Is smoking "pot" helpful for neuropathic pain? Pain Treatment Topics. Retrieved from http://updates. pain-topics.org/2010/09/is-smoking-pot-helpful-for-neuropathic. html

70. Skrabek, R.Q., Galimova, L., Ethans, K., & Perry, K. (2008). Nabilone for the treatment of pain in fibromyalgia. *The Journal of Pain, 9*(2), 164–178.

71. Fiz, J., Duran, M., Capella, D., Carbonell, J., & Farre, M. (2011). Cannabis use in patients with fibromyalgia: Effect on symptoms relief and health-related quality of life. *PLoS ONE, 6*(4), e18440.

72. Rog, D.J., Nurmikko, T.J., Friede, T., & Young, C.A. (2005). Randomized, controlled trial of cannabis-based medicine in central pain in multiple sclerosis. *Neurology, 65*(6), 812–819.

73. Russo, E. (1998). Cannabis for migraine treatment: The once and future prescription? An historical and scientific review. *PAIN, 76*(1–2), 3–8.

74. Akerman, S., Holland, P.R., & Goadsby, P.J. (2007). Cannabinoid (CB1) receptor activation inhibits trigeminovascular neurons. *Journal of Pharmacology and Experimental Therapeutics, 320*(1), 64–77.

75. Juhasz, G., Lazary, J., Chase, D., et al. (2009). Variations in the cannabinoid receptor 1 gene predispose to migraine. *Neuroscience Letters, 461*(2), 116–120.

76. Wang, T., Collet, J-P., Shapiro, S., & Ware, M.A. (2008). Adverse effects of medical cannabinoids: A systematic review. *Journal of the Canadian Medical Association, 178*(13), 1669–1678.

77. Degenhardt, L., & Hall, W.D. (2008). The adverse effects of cannabinoids: Implications for use of medicinal marijuana. *Journal of the Canadian Medical Association, 178*(13), 1685–1686.

78. K.S. DiFonzo (personal communication, February 27, 2015).

79. American Society of Addiction Medicine. (2011). Definition of addiction. Retrieved from http://www.asam.org/for-the-public/ definition-of-addiction

80. Vandrey, R., Budney, A.J., Kamon, J.L., & Stanger, C. (2005). Cannabis withdrawal in adolescent treatment seekers. *Drug and Alcohol Dependence, 78*(2), 205–210.

81. Grant, I. (2010, October 22). Medical marijuana: The science behind the smoke and fears. *San Diego Union Tribune*. Retrieved from http://

www.utsandiego.com/news/2010/oct/22/medical-marijuana-science-behind-smoke-and-fears/

82. National Institute on Drug Abuse. (n.d.). Research reports: Marijuana abuse—Is marijuana addictive? Retrieved from http://www.drugabuse.gov/publications/research-reports/marijuana-abuse/marijuana-addictive

83. National Institute on Drug Abuse. (2011). Topics in brief: Marijuana: Marijuana and addiction. Retrieved from http://www.drugabuse.gov/publications/topics-in-brief/marijuana

84. S. Weiss (personal communication, March 22, 2012).

85. Ware, M.A., & Tawfik, V.L. (2005). Safety issues concerning the medical use of cannabis and cannabinoids. *Pain Research & Management: The Journal of the Canadian Pain Society, 10*(Suppl. A), 33A–37A.

86. S. Weiss (personal communication, February 26, 2015).

87. Anthony, J.C., Warner, L.A., & Kessler, R.C. (1994). Comparative epidemiology of dependence on tobacco, alcohol, controlled substances, and inhalants: Basic findings from the national comorbidity study. *Experimental and Clinical Psychopharmacology, 2*(3), 244–268.

88. National Institute on Drug Abuse. (2015). Is marijuana addictive? Retrieved from http://www.drugabuse.gov/publications/research-reports/marijuana/marijuana-addictive

89. Singh, R., Sandhu, J., Kaur, B., et al. (2009). Evaluation of the DNA damaging potential of cannabis cigarette smoke by the determination of acetaldehyde derived N2-ethyl-2-deoxyguanosine adducts. *Chemical Research in Toxicology, 22*(6), 1181–1188.

90. Hashibe, M., Morgenstern, H., Cui, Y., et al. (2006). Marijuana use and the risk of lung and upper aerodigestive tract cancers: Results of a population-based case-control study. *Cancer Epidemiology, Biomarkers and Prevention, 15*(10), 1829–1834.

91. Foreman, J. (2009, July 13). Evil weed or useful drug? *The Boston Globe.* Retrieved from http://articles.boston.com/2009-07-13/news/29262455_1_medical-marijuana-marinol-marijuana-policy-project

92. National Institute on Drug Abuse. (2015). What is marijuana? Retrieved from http://www.drugabuse.gov/publications/drug-facts/marijuana

93. Berthiller, J., Yuan-chin, A.L., Boffetta, P., et al. (2009). Marijuana smoking and the risk of head and neck cancer: Pooled analysis in the INHANCE consortium. *Cancer Epidemiology, Biomarkers and Prevention, 18*(5), 1544–1551.

94. National Cancer Institute. (2014). Cannabis and cannabinoids: Human/clinical studies. Retrieved from http://www.cancer.gov/cancertopics/pdq/cam/cannabis/healthprofessional/page5#_105_toc

95. Lacson, J.C., Carroll, J.D., Tuazon, E., Castelao, E.J., Bernstein, L., & Cortessis, V.K. (2012). Population-based case-control study of recreational drug use and testis cancer confirms an association between marijuana use and nonseminoma risk, *Cancer, 118*(21), 5374–5383.

96. Zammit, S., Allebeck, P., Andreasson, S., Lundberg, I., & Lewis, G. (2002). Self-reported cannabis use as a risk factor for schizophrenia in Swedish conscripts of 1969: Historical cohort. *British Medical Journal, 325,* 1199.

97. Arseneault, L., Cannon, M., Poulton, R., Murray, R., Caspi, A., & Moffitt, T.E. (2002). Cannabis use in adolescence and risk for adult psychosis: Longitudinal prospective study. *British Medical Journal, 325*(7374), 1212.

98. van Os, J., Bak, M., Hanssen, M., Bijl, R.V., de Graaf, R., & Verdoux, H. (2002). Cannabis use and psychosis: A longitudinal population-based study. *American Journal of Epidemiology, 156,* 319–327.

99. Smit, F., Bolier, L., & Cuijpers, P. (2004). Cannabis use and the risk of later schizophrenia: A review. *Addiction, 99,* 425–430.

100. Moore, T.H., Zammit, S., Lingford-Hughes, A., et al. (2007). Cannabis use and risk of psychotic or affective mental health outcomes: A systematic review. *The Lancet, 370*(9584), 319–328.

101. McGrath, J., Welham, J., Scott, J., et al. (2010). Association between cannabis use and psychosis-related outcomes using sibling pair analysis in a cohort of young adults. *Archives of General Psychiatry, 67*(5), 440–447.

102. Large, M., Sharma, S., Compton, M.T., Slade, T., & Nielssen, O. (2011). Cannabis use and earlier onset of psychosis. *Archives of General Psychiatry, 68*(6), 555–561.

103. D. Abrams (personal communication, May 20, 2015).

104. Frisher, M., Crome, I., Martino, O., & Croft, P. (2009). Assessing the impact of cannabis use on trends in diagnosed schizophrenia in the United Kingdom from 1996 to 2005. *Schizophrenia Research, 113*(2–3), 123–128.

105. van Winkel, R. (2011). Family-based analysis of genetic variation underlying psychosis-inducing effects of cannabis. *Archives of General Psychiatry, 68*(2), 148–157.

106. Di Forti, M., Iyegbe, C., Sallis, H., et al. (2012). Confirmation that the AKT1 (rs2494732) genotype influences the risk of psychosis in cannabis users. *Biological Psychiatry, 72*(10), 811–816.

107. Caspi, A., Moffitt, T.E., Cannon, M., et al. (2005). Moderation of the effect of adolescent-onset cannabis use on adult psychosis by a functional polymorphism in the catechol-o-methyltransferase gene: Longitudinal evidence of a gene X environment interaction. *Biological Psychiatry, 57*(10), 1117–1127.
108. Proal, A.C., Fleming, J., Galvez-Buccollini, J.A. & Delisi, L.E. (2014). A controlled family study of cannabis users with and without psychosis, *Schizophrenia Research, 152*(1), 283–288.
109. Pierre, J.M. (2011). Cannabis, synthetic cannabinoids, and psychosis risk: What the evidence says. *Current Psychiatry, 10*(9), 49–57.
110. Stern, V. (2014, August 14). Can marijuana cause psychosis? *Scientific American.* Retrieved from http://www.scientificamerican.com/article/can-marijuana-cause-psychosis/
111. Ware, M.A., & Tawfik, V.L. (2005). Safety issues concerning the medical use of cannabis and cannabinoids. *Pain Research & Management: The Journal of the Canadian Pain Society, 10*(Suppl. A), 34A.
112. Patton, G.C., Coffey, C., Carlin, J.B., Degenhardt, L., Lynskey, M., & Hall, W. (2002). Cannabis use and mental health in young people: Cohort study. *British Medical Journal, 325*(7374), 1195.
113. Ware, M.A., & Tawfik, V.L. (2005). Safety issues concerning the medical use of cannabis and cannabinoids. *Pain Research & Management: The Journal of the Canadian Pain Society, 10*(Suppl. A), 34A.
114. National Institute on Drug Abuse. (2015). Is there a link between marijuana use and mental illness? Retrieved from http://www.drugabuse.gov/publications/research-reports/marijuana/there-link-between-marijuana-use-mental-illness
115. Pope, H.G., Gruber, A.J., Hudson, J.I., Cohane, G., Huestis, M.A., & Yurgelun-Todd, D. (2003). Early-onset cannabis use and cognitive deficits: What is the nature of the association? *Drug and Alcohol Dependence, 69,* 303–310.
116. Gruber, A.J., Pope, H.G., Hudson, J.I., & Yurgelun-Todd, D. (2003). Attributes of long-term heavy cannabis users: A case-control study. *Psychological Medicine, 33,* 1415–1422.
117. Yucel, M., Solowij, N., Respondek, C., et al. (2008). Regional brain abnormalities associated with long-term heavy cannabis use. *Archives of General Psychiatry, 65*(6), 694–701.
118. Hester, R., Nestor, L., & Garavan, H. (2009). Impaired error awareness and anterior cingulate cortex hypoactivity in chronic cannabis users. *Neuropsychopharmacology, 34,* 2450–2458.

119. Gruber, S.A., Dahlgren, M.K., Sagar, K.A., Gonec, A., & Lukas, S.E. (2014). Worth the wait: Effects of age of onset of marijuana use on white matter and impulsivity. *Psychopharmacology, 231*(8), 1455–1465.

120. Meier, M.H., Caspi, A., Ambler, A., et al. (2012). Persistent cannabis users show neuropsychological decline from childhood to midlife. *Proceedings of the National Academy of Sciences, 109*(40), e2657–e2664.

121. National Institute on Drug Abuse. (2014). Drug facts: Marijuana. Retrieved from http://www.drugabuse.gov/publications/drug-facts/marijuana

122. Ware, M.A., & Tawfik, V.L. (2005). Safety issues concerning the medical use of cannabis and cannabinoids. *Pain Research & Management: The Journal of the Canadian Pain Society, 10*(Suppl. A), 32A.

123. Pope, H.G., Gruber, A.J., Hudson, J.I., Huestis, M.A., & Yurgelun-Todd, D. (2001). Neuropsychological performance in long-term cannabis users. *Archives of General Psychiatry, 58*, 909–915.

124. Grant, I., Gonzalez, R., Carey, C.L., Natarajan, L., & Wolfson, T. (2003). Non-acute (residual) neurocognitive effects of cannabis use: A meta-analytic study. *Journal of the International Neuropsychological Society, 9*(5), 679–689.

125. Iverson, L. (2005). Long-term effects of exposure to cannabis. *Current Opinion in Pharmocology, 1*, 69–72.

126. Ware, M.A., & Tawfik, V.L. (2005). Safety issues concerning the medical use of cannabis and cannabinoids. *Pain Research & Management: The Journal of the Canadian Pain Society, 10*(Suppl. A), 34A.

127. Clark, A.J., Lynch, M.E., Beaulieu, P., McGilveray, I.J., & Gourlay, D. (2005). Guidelines for the use of cannabinoid compounds for chronic pain. *Pain Research Management, 10*(Suppl. A), 44A–46A.

128. Sidney, S. (2002). Cardiovascular consequences of marijuana use. *Journal of Clinical Pharmacology, 42*(Suppl. 11), 64S–70S.

129. Aldington, S., Williams, M., Nowitz, M., et al. (2007). Effects of cannabis on pulmonary structure, function and symptoms. *Thorax, 62*, 1058–1063.

130. R. Doblin (personal communication, August 9, 2011).

131. Pletcher, M.J., Vittinghoff, E., Kalhan, R., et al. (2012). Association between marijuana exposure and pulmonary function over 20 years. *The Journal of the American Medical Association, 307*(2), 173–181.

132. Moir, D., Rickert, W.S., Levasseur, G., et al. (2008). A comparison of mainstream and sidestream marijuana and tobacco cigarette

smoke produced under two machine smoking conditions. *Chemical Research in Toxicology, 21*(2), 494–502.

133. Ware, M.A., & Tawfik, V.L. (2005). Safety issues concerning the medical use of cannabis and cannabinoids. *Pain Research & Management: The Journal of the Canadian Pain Society, 10*(Suppl. A), 32A.

134. Abrams, D.I., Vizoso, H.P., Shade, S.B., Jay, C., Kelly, M.E., & Benowitz, N.L. (2007). Vaporization as a smokeless cannabis delivery system: A pilot study. *Clinical Pharmacology & Therapeutics, 82,* 572–578.

135. Van Dam, N.T., & Earleywine, M. (2010). Pulmonary function in cannabis users: Support for a clinical trial of the vaporizer. *The International Journal of Drug Policy, 21*(6), 511–513.

136. B. Behm (personal communication, February 9, 2015).

137. Centers for Disease Control and Prevention. (2014). Surgeon General's reports on smoking and tobacco use. Retrieved from http://www.cdc.gov/tobacco/data_statistics/sgr/index.htm

138. Center for Diseases Control and Prevention. (2014). Fact sheets—Alcohol use and your health. Retrieved from http://www.cdc.gov/alcohol/fact-sheets/alcohol-use.htm

139. American Nutrition Association. (2010). Deadly NSAIDS. *Nutrition Digest, 37*(3). Retrieved from http://americannutritionassociation.org/newsletter/deadly-nsaids

140. Ware, M.A., & Tawfik, V.L. (2005). Safety issues concerning the medical use of cannabis and cannabinoids. *Pain Research & Management: The Journal of the Canadian Pain Society, 10*(Suppl. A), 33A.

141. Sidney, S. (2003). Comparing cannabis with tobacco–again. *British Medical Journal, 327*(7416), 635.

142. Young, F.L. (1988, September 6). In the matter of marijuana rescheduling petition—Opinion and recommended ruling, findings of fact, conclusions of law and decision of administrative law judge (Docket No. 86-22, Part VIII). Retrieved from http://iowamedicalmarijuana.org/pdfs/young.pdf

143. S. Gust (personal communication, March 22, 2012).

144. Joy, J.E., & Benson, J.A., eds. (1999). *Marijuana and medicine: Assessing the science base* (p. 6). Washington, DC: National Academies Press.

145. Fergusson, D.M., Boden, J.M., & Horwood, L.J. (2006). Cannabis use and other illicit drug use: Testing the cannabis gateway hypothesis, *Addiction, 101*(4), 556–559.

146. Scharff, C. (2014, August 26). The gateway drug myth. *Psychology Today.* Retrieved from https://www.psychologytoday.com/blog/

ending-addiction-good/201408/marijuana-the-gateway-drug-myth

147. Morral, A.R., McCaffrey, D.F., & Paddock, S.M. (2002). Reassessing the marijuana gateway effect. *Addiction, 97*(12), 1493–1504.

148. National Institute on Drug Abuse. (2015). Is marijuana a gateway drug? Retrieved from http://www.drugabuse.gov/publications/marijuana/marijuana-gateway-drug

149. Hasin, D.S., Wall, M., Keyes, K.M., et al. (2015). Medical marijuana laws and adolescent marijuana use in the USA from 1991 to 2014: Results from annual, repeated cross-sectional surveys. *The Lancet Psychiatry, 2*(7), 601–608.

150. Marijuana Resource Center: State Laws Related to Marijuana, Office of National Drug Control Policy, Retrieved Aug. 30, 2016, https://www.whitehouse.gov/ondcp/state-laws-related-to-marijuana

151. Firestone, D. (2014, July 27). Let states decide on marijuana. *The New York Times.* Retrieved from http://www.nytimes.com/2014/07/27/opinion/sunday/high-time-let-states-decide-on-marijuana.html

152. Ibid.

153. Ferner, M. (2014, November 5). Alaska becomes fourth state to legalize recreational marijuana. *The Huffington Post.* Retrieved from http://www.huffingtonpost.com/2014/11/05/alaska-marijuana-legalization_n_5947516.html

154. Remnick, D. (2014, January 27). Going the distance. *The New Yorker.* Retrieved from http://www.newyorker.com/magazine/2014/01/27/going-the-distance-2

155. Devaney, T. (2015, February 4). Surgeon General: Medical marijuana can be helpful. *The Hill.* Retrieved from https://www.google.com/?gws_rd=ssl#q="Surgeon+General:+Medical+marijuana+'can+be+helpful%2C'+"+The+Hill%2C+Feb.+4%2C+2015%2C

156. Halper, E. (2014, December 14). Congress quietly ends federal government's ban on medical marijuana. *Los Angeles Times.* Retrieved from http://www.latimes.com/nation/la-na-medical-pot-20141216-story.html

157. US Drug Enforcement Administration. (2015). Drug scheduling. Retrieved from http://www.dea.gov/druginfo/ds.shtml

158. Foreman, J. (2014). *A nation in pain* (pp. 201–210). New York: Oxford University Press.

159. Kovaleski, S.F. (2014, August 10). Medical marijuana research hits wall of U.S. law. *The New York Times.* Retrieved from http://www.nytimes.com/2014/08/10/us/politics/medical-marijuana-research-hits-the-wall-of-federal-law.html

160. Hampson, A.J., Axelrod, J., & Grimaldi, M. (n.d.). U.S Patent No. 6630507 Washington, DC: US Patent and Trademark Office.
161. Department of Health and Human Services. (2015). Developing the therapeutic potential of the endocannabinoid system for pain treatment (R01). Retrieved from http://grants.nih.gov/grants/guide/pa-files/PA-15-188.html
162. DrugScience.org. (n.d.). Coalition for rescheduling cannabis: Members. Retrieved from http://www.drugscience.org/coalition_members.html
163. DrugScience.org. (n.d.). Arguments supporting the cannabis rescheduling petition. Retrieved from http://www.drugscience.org/intro/arguments.html
164. Denial of Petition to Initiate Proceedings to Reschedule Marijuana, 76 Fed. Reg. 40552 (proposed July 8, 2011) (to be codified at 21 C.F.R. Chapter II). Retrieved from http://www.gpo.gov/fdsys/pkg/FR-2011-07-08/pdf/2011-16994.pdf
165. DrugScience.org. (n.d.). Arguments supporting the cannabis rescheduling petition. Retrieved from http://www.drugscience.org/intro/arguments.html
166. Global Commission on Drug Policy. (2011). *War on drugs: Report of the global commission on drug policy* (p. 3). Retrieved from http://www.globalcommissionondrugs.org/wp-content/themes/gcdp_v1/pdf/Global_Commission_Report_English.pdf
167. Smart Approaches to Marijuana. (2015). Rescheduling marijuana. Retrieved from http://learnaboutsam.org/the-issues/rescheduling-marijuana/
168. National Institute of Drug Abuse. (2012). Drug facts: K2/spice ("synthetic marijuana"). Retrieved from http://www.drugabuse.gov/publications/drugfacts/k2spice-synthetic-marijuana
169. Pierre, J.M. (2011). Cannabis, synthetic cannabinoids, and psychosis risk: What the evidence says. *Current Psychiatry, 10*(9), 49–57.
170. Goodnough, A., & Zezima, K. (2011, July 16). An alarming new stimulant, legal in many states. *The New York Times.* Retrieved from http://www.nytimes.com/2011/07/17/us/17salts.html?pagewanted=all
171. US Drug Enforcement Administration. (2011). Chemicals used in "Spice" and "K2" type products now under federal control and regulation [Press release]. Retrieved from http://www.justice.gov/dea/pubs/pressrel/pr030111.html
172. US Drug Enforcement Administration. (2010). DEA moves to emergency control synthetic marijuana [Press release]. Retrieved from http://www.justice.gov/dea/pubs/pressrel/pr112410.html

173. Russo, E., & Guy, G.W. (2006). A tale of two cannabinoids: The therapeutic rationale for combining tetrahydrocannabinol and cannabidiol. *Medical Hypotheses, 66,* 234–246.

174. E.A. Romero-Sandoval (personal communication, June 20, 2011).

175. Beltramo, M. (2009). Cannabinoid type 2 receptor as a target for chronic pain. *Mini-Reviews in Medicinal Chemistry, 9*(1), 11–25.

176. Vann, R.E., Cook, C.D., Martin, B.R., & Wiley, J.L. (2007). Cannabimimetic properties of ajulemic acid. *Journal of Pharmacology and Experimental Therapeutics, 320*(2), 678–686.

177. Burstein, S.H., Karst, M., Schneider, U., & Zurier, R.B. (2004). Ajulemic acid: A novel cannabinoid produces analgesia without a "high." *Life Sciences, 75*(12), 1513–1522.

178. Ware, M., Fitzcharles, M-A., Joseph, L., & Shir, Y. (2010). The effects of nabilone on sleep in fibromyalgia: Results of a randomized controlled trial. *Anesthesia & Analgesia, 110*(2), 604–610.

179. Narang, S., Gibson, D., Wasan, A.D., et al. (2008). Efficacy of dronabinol as an adjuvant treatment for chronic pain patients on opioid therapy. *The Journal of Pain, 9*(3), 254–264.

180. ProCon.org. (2015). 10 pharmaceutical drugs based on cannabis. Retrieved from http://medicalmarijuana.procon.org/view.resource.php?resourceID=000883

181. Frank, B., Serpell, M.G., Hughes, J., Matthews, J.N.S., & Kapur, D. (2008). Comparison of analgesic effects and patient tolerability of nabilone and dihydrocodeine for chronic neuropathic pain: Randomised, crossover, double blind study. *British Medical Journal, 336*(7637), 199.

182. Berlach, D.M., Shir, Y., & Ware, M. (2006). Experience with the synthetic cannabinoid nabilone in chronic noncancer pain. *Pain Medicine, 7*(1), 25–29.

183. Ware, M., & St. Arnaud-Trempe, E. (2010). The abuse potential of the synthetic cannabinoid nabilone. *Addiction, 105*(3), 494–503.

184. Grant, I. (2010, October 22). Medical marijuana: The science behind the smoke and fears. *San Diego Union Tribune.* Retrieved from http://www.utsandiego.com/news/2010/oct/22/medical-marijuana-science-behind-smoke-and-fears/

185. ProCon.org. (2015). 10 pharmaceutical drugs based on cannabis. Retrieved from http://medicalmarijuana.procon.org/view.resource.php?resourceID=000883

186. GW Pharmaceuticals. (2015). Press releases. Retrieved from http://www.gwpharm.com/news_2015.aspx

187. GW Pharmaceuticals. (2014). Sativex. Retrieved from http://www.gwpharm.com/Sativex.aspx
188. Abrams, D., Couey, P., Shade, S.B., Kelly, M.E. (2011). Cannabinoid–opioid interaction in chronic pain. *Clinical Pharmacology and Therapeutics, 90*(6), 844–851.
189. Bachhuber, M.A., Saloner, B., Cunningham, C.O., & Barry, C.L. (2014). Medical cannabis laws and opioid analgesic overdose mortality in the United States, 1999–2010. *Journal of the American Medical Association: Internal Medicine, 174*(10), 1668–1673.
190. McKinley, J. (2012, March 7). Pat Robertson says marijuana should be legal. *The New York Times.* Retrieved from http://www.nytimes.com/2012/03/08/us/pat-robertson-backs-legalizing-marijuana.html
191. Hotakainen, R. (2015, March 4). Marijuana gets lift as 2016 presidential race takes shape. *McClatchy DC.* Retrieved from http://www.mcclatchydc.com/2015/03/04/258623/marijuana-gets-lift-as-2016-presidential.html
192. Johnson, C. (2011, July 12). Obama cracks down on medical marijuana. National Public Radio. Retrieved from http://www.npr.org/2011/07/12/137791944/obama-cracks-down-on-medical-marijuana
193. Hutchison, C. (2011, July 12). Marijuana advocates sue feds after DEA rejects weed as medicine. *ABC News.* Retrieved from http://abcnews.go.com/Health/PainNews/marijuana-advocates-sue-feds-dea-rejects-weed-medicine/story?id=14046823#.T8V8uI6HpBI
194. Newport, F. (2011, October 17). Record-high 50% of Americans favor legalizing marijuana use. Gallup. Retrieved from http://www.gallup.com/poll/150149/record-high-americans-favor-legalizing-marijuana.aspx
195. Saad, L. (2014, November 6). Majority continues to support pot legalization in U.S. Gallup. Retrieved from http://www.gallup.com/poll/179195/majority-continues-support-pot-legalization.aspx
196. Editorial Board. (2014, July 27). Repeal prohibition, again. *The New York Times.* Retrieved from http://www.nytimes.com/interactive/2014/07/27/opinion/sunday/high-time-marijuana-legalization.html
197. American Society of Addiction Medicine. (2012, July 25). White paper on state-level proposals to legalize marijuana. Retrieved from http://www.asam.org/advocacy/find-a-policy-statement/view-policy-statement/public-policy-statements/2014/07/24/white-paper-on-state-level-proposals-to-legalize-marijuana

198. American Academy of Pediatrics. (2015). American Academy of Pediatrics reaffirms opposition to legalizing marijuana for recreational or medical use. Retrieved from http://www.aap.org/en-us/about-the-aap/aap-press-room/Pages/American-Academy-of-Pediatrics-Reaffirms-Opposition-to-Legalizing-Marijuana-for-Recreational-or-Medical-Use.aspx

199. American Academy of Pediatrics. (2015). The impact of marijuana policies on youth: Clinical, research, and legal update. Retrieved from http://pediatrics.aappublications.org/content/early/2015/01/20/peds.2014-4146

200. Caulkins, J.P., Hawken, A., Kilmer, B & Kleiman, M.R. (2012). *Marijuana legalization—what everyone needs to know now* (pp. 145–146). New York: Oxford University Press.

201. Miron, J.A. (2005). *The budgetary implications of marijuana prohibition.* Retrieved from http://www.prohibitioncosts.org/wp-content/uploads/2012/04/MironReport.pdf

202. Ibid.

203. Healy, J. (2015, May 9). Legal marijuana shops face another federal hurdle: Taxes. *The New York Times.* Retrieved from http://www.nytimes.com/2015/05/10/us/politics/legal-marijuana-faces-another-federal-hurdle-taxes.html?_r=0

204. Reichbach, G.L. (2012, May 16). A judge's plea for pot. *The New York Times.* Retrieved from http://www.nytimes.com/2012/05/17/opinion/a-judges-plea-for-medical-marijuana.html?_r=2&smid=tw-share

205. Dwyer, J. (2012, July 17). Gustin Reichbach, judge with a radical history, dies at 65. *The New York Times.* Retrieved from http://www.nytimes.com/2012/07/19/nyregion/gustin-reichbach-judge-with-a-radical-history-dies-at-65.html?_r=0

Chapter 6

1. S. Cohen (personal communication, July 12, 2015).

2. Institute of Medicine, Committee on Advancing Pain Research, Care, and Education. (2011). *Relieving pain in America: A blueprint for transforming prevention, care, education and research* (pp. 2–6). Washington, DC: National Academies Press.

3. S. Parazin (personal communication, December 21, 2011).

4. Haldeman, S., & Dagenais, S. (2008). What have we learned about the evidence-informed management of chronic low back pain? *The Spine Journal, 8*(1), 277.

5. Chou, R., Loeser, J.D., Owens, D.K., et al. (2009). Interventional therapies, surgery, and interdisciplinary rehabilitation for low back pain: An evidence-based clinical practice guideline from the American Pain Society. *Spine, 34(10),* 1066–1077.

6. Chou, R., Atlas, S.J., Stanos, S.P., & Rosenquist, R. (2009). Nonsurgical interventional therapies for low back pain: A review of the evidence for an American Pain Society clinical practice guideline. *Spine, 34(10),* 1078–1093.

7. J. Loeser (personal communication, October 24, 2011).

8. Melzack, R., & Wall, P.D. (1965). Pain mechanisms: A new theory. *Science, 150(699),* 971–979.

9. S. Fishman (personal communication, October 10, 2011).

10. S. Parazin (personal communication, December 21, 2011).

11. Smith, T.J., & Marineo, G. (2013). Treatment of postherpetic pain with Scrambler therapy, a patient-specific neurocutaneous electrical stimulation device [Abstract]. *American Journal of Hospice & Palliative Care* (Suppl.), e19564.

12. Moon, J.Y., Kurihara, C., Beckles, J.P., Williams, K.E., Jamison, D.E., & Cohen, S.P. Predictive factors associated with success and failure for Calmare (Scrambler) therapy: A multi-center analysis, *Clinical Journal of Pain, 31(8),* 750–756.

13. S. Cohen (personal communication, July 12, 2015).

14. J. Loeser (personal communication, October 24, 2011).

15. Johnson, M., & Martinson, M. (2007). Efficacy of electrical nerve stimulation for chronic musculoskeletal pain: A meta-analysis of randomized controlled trials [Abstract]. *PAIN, 130(1),* 157–165.

16. Haldeman, S., Carroll, L., Cassidy, J.D., Schubert, J., & Nygren, A. (2008). The Bone and Joint Decade 2000–2010 Task Force on Neck Pain and Its Associated Disorders: Executive summary. *Spine, 33*(Suppl. 4), S5–S7.

17. Haldeman, S., & Dagenais, S. (2008). What have we learned about the evidence-informed management of chronic low back pain? *The Spine Journal, 8*(1), 266–277.

18. Poitras, S., & Brosseau, L. (2008). Evidence-informed management of chronic low back pain with transcutaneous electrical nerve stimulation, interferential current, electrical muscle stimulation, ultrasound, and thermotherapy. *The Spine Journal, 8*(1), 226–233.

19. Dubinsky, R.M., & Miyasaki, J. (2010). Assessment: Efficacy of transcutaneous electric nerve stimulation in the treatment of pain in neurologic disorders (an evidence-based review) [Abstract]. *Neurology, 74*(2), 173–176.

20. Mulvey, M.R., Bagnall, A.M., Johnson, M.I., & Marchant, P.R. (2010). Transcutaneous electrical nerve stimulation (TENS) for phantom pain and stump pain following amputation in adults. *Cochrane Database of Systematic Reviews, 2010*(5), CD007264.

21. Centers for Medicare & Medicaid Services. (n.d.). Proposed decision memo for transcutaneous electrical nerve stimulation for chronic low back pain (CAG-00429N). Retrieved from http://www.cms.gov/medicare-coverage-database/details/nca-proposed-decision-memo.aspx?NCAId=256&ver=9&NcaName=Tras

22. Kloimstein, H., Likar, R., Kern, M., et al. (2014). Peripheral nerve field stimulation (PNFS) in chronic low back pain: A prospective multicenter trial. *Neuromodulation, 17*(2), 180–187.

23. Columbia University Medical Center. (n.d.). Peripheral nerve stimulation. Retrieved from http://www.cumc.columbia.edu/dept/peripheral-nerve/problems/pns.html

24. Raphael, J.H., Raheem, T.A., Southall, J.L., Bennett, A., Ashford, R L., & Williams, S. (2011). Randomized double-blind sham-controlled crossover study of short-term effect of percutaneous electrical nerve stimulation in neuropathic pain [Abstract]. *Pain Medicine, 12(10)*, 1515–1522.

25. Deyo, R.A., Mirza, S.K., Turner, J.A., & Martin, B.I. (2009). Overtreating chronic back pain: Time to back off? *The Journal of the American Board of Family Medicine, 22*(1), 62–68.

26. Guyer, R.D., Patterson, M., & Ohnmeiss, D.D. (2006). Failed back surgery syndrome: Diagnostic evaluation [Abstract]. *Journal of the American Academy of Orthopaedic Surgeons, 14*(9), 534–543.

27. Kumar, K., Taylor, R. S., Jacques, L., et al. (2008). The effects of spinal cord stimulation in neuropathic pain are sustained: A 24-month follow-up of the prospective randomized controlled multicenter trial of the effectiveness of spinal cord stimulation. *Neurosurgery, 63*(4), 762–770.

28. Mailis-Gagnon, A., Furlan, A., Sandoval, J., & Taylor, R. (2004). Spinal cord stimulation for chronic pain [Abstract]. *Cochrane Database of Systematic Reviews, 2004*(3), CD003783.

29. Kunnumpurath, S., Srinivasagopalan, R., & Vadivelu, N. (2009). Spinal cord stimulation: Principles of past, present and future practice: A review. *Journal of Clinical Monitoring and Computing, 23*(5), 333–339.

30. WebMD. (n.d). Spinal cord stimulation for chronic pain. Retrieved from http://www.webmd.com/back-pain/spinal-cord-stimulation-for-low-back-pain

31. de Vos, C.C., Meier, K., Zaalberg, P.B., et al. (2014). Spinal cord stimulation in patients with painful diabetic neuropathy: A multicenter randomized clinical trial. *PAIN, 155(11),* 2426–2431.

32. S. Cohen (personal communication, July 12, 2015).

33. Bittar, R.G., Kar-Purkayastha, I., Owen, S.L., et al. (2005). Deep brain stimulation for pain relief: A meta-analysis [Abstract]. *Journal of Clinical Neuroscience, 12*(5), 515–519.

34. S. Cohen (personal communication, July 12, 2015).

35. A. Pascual-Leone (personal communication, December 28, 2011).

36. Lefaucheur, J.P., Drouot, X., Keravel, Y., & Nguyen, J.P. (2001). Pain relief induced by repetitive transcranial magnetic stimulation of precentral cortex [Abstract]. *NeuroReport, 12(13),* 2963–2065.

37. Lefaucheur, J., Drouot, X., Menard-Lefaucheur, I., et al. (2004). Neurogenic pain relief by repetitive transcranial magnetic cortical stimulation depends on the origin and the site of pain. *Journal of Neurology, Neurosurgery & Psychiatry, 75*(4), 612–616.

38. Rosen, A.C., Ramkumar, M., Nguyen, T., & Hoeft, F. (2009). Noninvasive transcranial brain stimulation and pain. *Current Pain and Headache Reports, 13*(1), 12–17.

39. Leung, A., Donohue, M., Xu, R., et al. (2009). rTMS for suppressing neuropathic pain: A meta-analysis [Abstract]. *The Journal of Pain, 10(12),* 1205–1216.

40. Lipton, R.B., Dodick, D.W., Silberstein, S.D., et al. (2010). Single-pulse transcranial magnetic stimulation for acute treatment of migraine with aura: A randomised, double-blind, parallel-group, sham-controlled trial. *The Lancet Neurology, 9(4),* 373–380.

41. Soler, M.D., Kumru, H., Pelayo, R., et al. (2010). Effectiveness of transcranial direct current stimulation and visual illusion on neuropathic pain in spinal cord injury [Abstract]. *Brain, 133*(9), 2565–2577.

42. Mhalla, A., Baudic, S., De Andrade, D.C., et al. (2011). Long-term maintenance of the analgesic effects of transcranial magnetic stimulation in fibromyalgia [Abstract]. *PAIN, 152*(7), 1478–1485.

43. Fregni, F., Freedman, S., & Pascual-Leone, A. (2007). Recent advances in the treatment of chronic pain with non-invasive brain stimulation techniques. *The Lancet Neurology, 6*(2), 188–191.

44. Mylius, V., Borckardt, J.J., & Lefaucheur, J.P. (2012). Noninvasive cortical modulation of experimental pain, *PAIN, 153*(7), 1350–1363.

45. Sutherland, S. (2013, October 3). Transcranial magnetic stimulation: The next wave in pain treatment? Pain Research Forum. Retrieved from http://www.painresearchforum.org/news/32343-transcranial-magnetic-stimulation-next-wave-pain-treatment

46. O'Connell, N.E., Wand, B.M., Marston, L., Spencer, S., & DeSouza, L.H. (2010). Non-invasive brain stimulation techniques for chronic pain [Abstract]. *Cochrane Database of Systematic Reviews, 2010*(9), CD008208.

47. Sutherland, S. (2013, October 3). Transcranial magnetic stimulation: The next wave in pain treatment? Pain Research Forum. Retrieved from http://www.painresearchforum.org/news/32343-transcranial-magnetic-stimulation-next-wave-pain-treatment

48. Schabrun, S.M., Jones, E., Elgueta Cancino, E.L., & Hodges, P.W. (2014). Targeting chronic recurrent low back pain from the top-down and the bottom-up: A combined transcranial direct current stimulation and peripheral electrical stimulation intervention. *Brain Stimulation, 7*(3), 451–459.

49. Batuman, E. (2005, April 6). Electrified. *The New Yorker*. Retrieved from http://www.newyorker.com/magazine/2015/04/06/electrified

50. Fregni, F., Boggio, P.S., Lima, M.C., et al. (2006). A sham-controlled, phase II trial of transcranial direct current stimulation for the treatment of central pain in traumatic spinal cord injury. *PAIN 122*(1–2), 197–209.

51. Fregni, F., Gimenes, R., Valle, A.C., et al. (2006). A randomized, sham-controlled, proof of principle study of transcranial direct current stimulation for the treatment of pain in fibromyalgia. *Arthritis & Rheumatism, 54*(12), 3988–3998.

52. Antal, A., Terney, D., Kuhnl, S., & Paulus, W. (2010). Anodal transcranial direct current stimulation of the motor cortex ameliorates chronic pain and reduces short intracortical inhibition. *Journal of Pain and Symptom Management, 30*(5), 890–903.

53. Mori, F., Codeca, C., Kusayanagi, H., et al. (2010). Effects of anodal transcranial direct current stimulation on chronic neuropathic pain in patients with multiple sclerosis. *The Journal of Pain, 11*(5), 436–442.

54. Rutjes, A.W.S., Juni, P., da Costa, B.R., Trelle, S., Nuesch, E., & Reichenbach, S. (2012). Viscosupplementation for osteoarthritis of the knee: A systematic review and meta-analysis. *Annals of Internal Medicine, 157*(3), 180–191.

55. Dumais, R., Benoit, C., Dumais, A., et al. (2012). Effect of regenerative injection therapy on function and pain in patients with knee osteoarthritis: A randomized crossover study. *Pain Medicine, 13*(8), 990–999.

56. Nuensch, E., Trelle, S., Reichenbach, S., Rutjes, A.W.S., Tschannen, B., & Altman, D.G. (2012). Small study effects in meta-analyses of osteoarthritis trials: Meta-epidemiological study. *British Medical Journal, 341*, c3515.

57. Staal, J., De Bie, R., De Vet, H., Hildebrandt, J., & Nelemans, P. (2008). Injection therapy for subacute and chronic low-back pain [Abstract]. *Cochrane Database of Systematic Reviews, 2008*(3), CD001824.
58. Cohen, S.P. (2011). Epidural steroid injections for low back pain: Editorial. *British Medical Journal, 343*, d5301.
59. Iversen, T., Solberg, T.K., Romner, B., et al. (2011). Effect of caudal epidural steroid or saline injection in chronic lumbar radiculopathy: Multicentre, blinded, randomised controlled trial. *British Medical Journal, 343*, d5278.
60. Carette, S., Marcoux, S., Truchon, R., et al. (1991). A controlled trial of corticosteroid injections into facet joints for chronic low back pain [Abstract]. *The New England Journal of Medicine, 325(14)*, 1002–1007.
61. Carette, S., Leclaire, R., Marcoux, S., et al. (1997). Epidural corticosteroid injections for sciatica due to herniated nucleus pulposus [Abstract]. *The New England Journal of Medicine, 336(23)*, 1634–1640.
62. Peloso, P., Gross, A., Haines, T., Trinh, K., Goldsmith, C.H., & Aker, P. (2005). Medicinal and injection therapies for mechanical neck disorders. *Cochrane Database of Systematic Reviews, 2005*(3), CD000319.
63. Luijsterburg, P.A., Verhagen, A.P., Ostelo, R.W., Van Os, T.A., Peul, W.C., & Koes, B.W. (2007). Effectiveness of conservative treatments for the lumbosacral radicular syndrome: A systematic review. *European Spine Journal, 16(7)*, 881–899.
64. Haldeman, S., & Dagenais, S. (2008). What have we learned about the evidence-informed management of chronic low back pain? *The Spine Journal, 8(1)*, 266–277.
65. DePalma, M.J., & Slipman, C.W. (2008). Evidence-informed management of chronic low back pain with epidural steroid injections. *The Spine Journal, 8(1)*, 45–55.
66. Ghahreman, A., Ferch, R., & Bogduk, N. (2010). The efficacy of transforaminal injection of steroids for the treatment of lumbar radicular pain. *Pain Medicine, 11(8)*, 1149–1168.
67. Cohen, S. P., White, R.L., Kurihara, C., et al. (2012). Epidural steroids, etanercept, or saline in subacute sciatica. *Annals of Internal Medicine, 156(8)*, 551–559.
68. Radcliff, K., Kepler, C., Hilibrand, A., et al. (2013). Epidural steroid injections are associated with less improvement in patients with lumbar spinal stenosis: A subgroup analysis of the Spine Patient Outcomes Research Trial [Abstract]. *Spine, 38(4)*, 279–291.
69. Chou, R., Loeser, J.D., Owens, D.K., et al. (2009). Interventional therapies, surgery, and interdisciplinary rehabilitation for low

back pain: An evidence-based clinical practice guideline from the American Pain Society. *Spine, 34(10)*, 1066–1077.

70. Johnson, C.Y. (2012, October 10). Doctors split on value of low-back injections. *The Boston Globe*. Retrieved from https://www.bostonglobe.com/lifestyle/health-wellness/2012/10/09/contaminated-drug-draws-attention-steroid-injection-procedure-physicians-divided-value-low-back-steroid-injections/1cQdfBP0d-VidlJxNz2HogL/story.html

71. WebMD. (n.d.). Pain management and nerve blocks. Retrieved from http://www.webmd.com/pain-management/guide/nerve-blocks

72. Ilfeld, B.M. (2011). Continuous peripheral nerve blocks: A review of the published evidence [Abstract]. *Anesthesia & Analgesia, 113(4)*, 904–925.

73. WebMD. (n.d.). Nerve block for pain. Retrieved from http://www.webmd.com/sleep-disorders/nerve-block-for-pain-relief

74. Johns Hopkins Medicine. (n.d.). Sympathetic nerve blocks for pain. Retrieved from http://www.hopkinsmedicine.org/healthlibrary/printv.aspx?d=135,54

75. US Food and Drug Administration. (2015). Putting a patch on migraines. Retrieved from http://www.fda.gov/forconsumers/consumerupdates/ucm343935.htm?source=govdelivery

76. Jackson, J.L., Kuriyama, A., & Hayashino, Y. (2012). Botulinum toxin A for prophylactic treatment of migraine and tension headaches in adults. *The Journal of the American Medical Association, 307(16)*, 1736–1745.

77. National Institute of Dental and Craniofacial Research. (2014). TMJ disorders. Retrieved from http://www.nidcr.nih.gov/OralHealth/Topics/TMJ/TMJDisorders.htm?_ga=1.38186849.356205921.1410290835#treated

78. Chang-Miller, A. (2014, February 13). Can Botox injections relieve arthritis pain? Mayo Clinic. Retrieved from http://www.mayoclinic.org/diseases-conditions/arthritis/expert-answers/botox-injections/faq-20057967

79. Sutherland, S. (2014, May 1). Botulinum toxin targets mechanosensitive nociceptors. Pain Research Forum. Retrieved from http://www.painresearchforum.org/news/40155-botulinum-toxin-targets-mechanosensitive-nociceptors/

80. Paterson, K., Lolignier, S., Wood, J.N., McMahon, S.B., & Bennett, D.L. (2014). Botulinum toxin-A treatment reduces human mechanical pain sensitivity and mechanotransmission. *Annals of Neurology, 75(4)*, 591–596.

81. Malanga, G., & Wolff, E. (2008). Evidence-informed management of chronic low back pain with trigger point injections. *The Spine Journal, 8*(1), 243–252.

82. WebMD. (n.d.). Trigger point injection for pain management. Retrieved from http://www.webmd.com/pain-management/guide/trigger-point-injection

83. Dagenais, S., Yelland, M.J., Del Mar, C., & Schoene, M.L. (2007). Prolotherapy injections for chronic low back pain. *Cochrane Database of Systematic Reviews, 2007*(2), CD00409.

84. Dagenais, S., Mayer, J., Haldeman, S., & Borg-Stein, J. (2008). Evidence-informed management of low back pain with prolotherapy. *The Spine Journal, 8(1),* 203–212.

85. Chou, R., Loeser, J.D., Owens, D.K., et al. (2009). Interventional therapies, surgery, and interdisciplinary rehabilitation for low back pain: An evidence-based clinical practice guideline from the American Pain Society. *Spine, 34(10),* 1066–1077.

86. Distel, L.M., & Best, T.M. (2011). Prolotherapy: A critical review of its role in treating chronic musculoskeletal pain. *PM&R, 3*(6), S78–S81.

87. Cheng, O.T., Souzdalnitski, D., Vrooman, B., & Cheng, J. (2012). Evidence-based knee injections for the management of arthritis. *Pain Medicine, 13*(6), 740–753.

88. Rutjes, A.W.S., Juni, P., da Costa, B.R., Trelle, S., Nuesch, E., & Reichenbach, S. (2012). Viscosupplementation for osteoarthritis of the knee: A systematic review and meta-analysis. *Annals of Internal Medicine, 157*(3), 180–191.

89. Coombes, B.K., Bisset, L., Brooks, P., Khan, A., & Vicenzino, B. (2013). Effect of corticosteroid injection, physiotherapy, or both on clinical outcome in patients with unilateral lateral epicondylalgia: A randomized controlled trial [Abstract]. *The Journal of the American Medical Association, 309*(5), 461–469.

90. Patel, S., Dhillon, M.S., Aggarwal, S., Marwaha, N., & Jain, A. (2013). Treatment with platelet-rich plasma is more effective than placebo for knee osteoarthritis. *The American Journal of Sports Medicine, 41*(2), 356–364.

91. Halpern, B., Chaudhury, S., Rodeo, S., et al. (2013). Clinical and MRI outcomes after platelet-rich plasma treatment for knee osteoarthritis. *Clinical Journal of Sports Medicine, 23*(3), 238–239.

92. Vangsness, C.T., Farr, J. II, Boyd, J., Dellaero, D.T., Mills, R., & LeRoux-Williams, M. (2014). Adult human mesenchymal stem cells delivered via intra-articular injection to the knee following

partial medial miniscectomy. *Journal of Bone and Joint Surgery, 96*(2), 90–98.

93. Slear, T. (2014, April/May). 4 arthritis treatments to try now. *AARP: The Magazine.* Retrieved from http://www.aarp.org/health/conditions-treatments/info-2014/arthritis-treatments-to-try-now.html

94. Bhumiratana, S., Eton, R.E., Oungoulian, S.R., Wan, L.Q., Ateshian, G.A., & Vunjak-Novakovic, G. (2015). Large, stratified, and mechanically functional human cartilage grown in vitro by mesenchymal condensation. *Proceedings of the National Academy of Sciences, 111(19)*, 6940–6945.

95. Chen, G., Park, C., Xie, R., & Ji, R. (2015). Intrathecal bone marrow stromal cells inhibit neuropathic pain via TBF-*B* secretion. *The Journal of Clinical Investigation, 125*(8), 80883.

96. R. Ji (personal communication, July 13, 2015).

97. Pettine, K.A., Murphy, M.B., Suzuki, R. K., & Sand, T.T. (2015). Percutaneous injection of autologous bone marrow concentrate cells significantly reduces lumbar discogenic pan through 12 months. *Stem Cells, 33*(1), 146–156.

98. Straube, S., Derry, S., Moore, R.A., & McQuay, H.J. (2010). Cervicothoracic or lumbar sympathectomy for neuropathic pain and complex regional pain syndrome [Abstract]. *Cochrane Database of Systematic Reviews, 2010*(7), CD002918.

99. J. Loeser (personal communication, October 24, 2011).

100. S.P. Cohen (personal communication, November 21, 2011).

101. S.P. Cohen (personal communication, November 17, 2011).

102. J. Loeser (personal communication, November 22, 2011).

103. S.P. Cohen (personal communication, November 17, 2011).

104. J. Loeser (personal communication, November 22, 2011).

105. Cohen, S.P., Williams, K.A., Kurihara, C., et al. (2010). Multicenter, randomized, comparative cost-effectiveness study comparing 0, 1 and 2 diagnostic medial branch (facet joint nerve) block treatment paradigms before lumbar facet radiofrequency denervation. *Anesthesiology, 113*(2), 395–405.

106. Gupta, A. (2010). Evidence-based review of radiofrequency ablation techniques for chronic sacroiliac joint pain. *Pain Medicine News, 8(12)*, 69–77.

107. Niemisto, L., Kalso, E.A., Malmivaara, A., Seitsalo, S., & Hurri, H. (2003). Radiofrequency denervation for neck and back pain. *Cochrane Database of Systematic Reviews, 2003*(1), CD004058.

108. R. Chou (personal communication, April 3, 2012).

109. Ibid.
110. Don, A.S., & Carragee, E. (2008). A brief review of evidence-informed management of chronic low back pain with surgery. *The Spine Journal, 8*(1), 258–265.
111. Weinstein, J.N., Lurie, J.D., Olson, P., Bronner, K. K., Fisher, E.S., & Morgan, T.S. (2006). United States trends and regional variations in lumbar spine surgery: 1992–2003. *Spine, 31(23)*, 2707–2714.
112. S. Parazin (personal communication, December 21, 2011).
113. S. Cohen (personal communication, July 12, 2015).
114. Weinstein, J.N., Tosteson, T.D., Lurie, J.D., et al. (2006). Surgical vs. nonoperative treatment for lumbar disk herniation: The Spine Patient Outcomes Research Trial (SPORT): A randomized trial [Abstract]. *The Journal of the American Medical Association, 296(20)*, 2441–1450.
115. Chou, R., Loeser, J.D., Owens, D.K., et al. (2009). Interventional therapies, surgery, and interdisciplinary rehabilitation for low back pain: An evidence-based clinical practice guideline from the American Pain Society. *Spine, 34(10)*, 1066–1077.
116. R. Chou (personal communication, April 3, 2012).
117. Don, A.S., & Carragee, E. (2008). A brief review of evidence-informed management of chronic low back pain with surgery. *The Spine Journal, 8*(1), 258–265.
118. R. Chou (personal communication, April 3, 2012).
119. S. Parazin (personal communication, April 4, 2012).
120. Haldeman, S., & Dagenais, S. (2008). What have we learned about the evidence-informed management of chronic low back pain? *The Spine Journal, 8*(1), 266–277.
121. Don, A.S., & Carragee, E. (2008). A brief review of evidence-informed management of chronic low back pain with surgery. *The Spine Journal, 8*(1), 258–265.
122. S. Cohen (personal communication, July 12, 2015).
123. Wasan, A.D., Sullivan, M.D., & Clark, M.R. (2010). Psychiatric illness, depression, anxiety, and somatoform pain disorders. In *Bonica's management of pain* (4th ed.), ed. J.C. Ballantyne, J.P. Rathmell, & S.M. Fishman (pp. 393–417). Philadelphia: Lippincott Williams and Wilkins.
124. Berna, C., Leknes, S., Holmes, E.A., Edwards, R.R., Goodwin, G.M., & Tracey, I. (2010). Induction of depressed mood disrupts emotion regulation neurocircuitry and enhances pain unpleasantness. *Biological Psychiatry, 67(11)*, 1083–1090.
125. R. Jamison (personal communication, December 20, 2010).

126. Dersh, J., Mayer, T., Theodore, B.R., Polatin, P., & Gatchel, R.J. (2007). Do psychiatric disorders first appear preinjury or postinjury in chronic disabling occupational spinal disorders? [Abstract]. *Spine, 32*(9), 1045–1051.

127. American Academy of Neurology. (2012). Migraine linked to increased risk of depression in women [Press release]. Retrieved from http://www.aan.com/press/?fuseaction=release.view&release=1033

128. Wasan, A.D., Sullivan, M.D., & Clark, M.R. (2010). Psychiatric illness, depression, anxiety, and somatoform pain disorders. In *Bonica's management of pain* (4th ed.), ed. J.C. Ballantyne, J.P. Rathmell, & S.M. Fishman (pp. 393–417). Philadelphia: Lippincott Williams and Wilkins.

129. R. Jamison (personal communication, December 30, 2010).

130. Wasan, A.D., Sullivan, M.D., & Clark, M.R. (2010). Psychiatric illness, depression, anxiety, and somatoform pain disorders. In *Bonica's management of pain* (4th ed.), ed. J.C. Ballantyne, J.P. Rathmell, & S.M. Fishman (pp. 393–417). Philadelphia: Lippincott Williams and Wilkins.

131. Wasan, A.D., Davar, G., & Jamison, R. (2005). The association between negative affect and opioid analgesia in patients with discogenic low back pain [Abstract]. *PAIN, 117*(3), 450–461.

132. Kroenke, K. (2005). Somatic symptoms and depression: A double hurt. *Primary Care Companion to the Journal of Clinical Psychiatry, 7*(4), 148–149.

133. Kroenke, K. (2003). The interface between physical and psychological symptoms. *Primary Care Companion to the Journal of Clinical Psychiatry, 5*(Suppl. 7), 11–18.

134. Giesecke, T., Gracely, R.H., Williams, D.A., Geisser, M.E., Petzke, F.W., & Clauw, D.J. (2005). The relationship between depression, clinical pain, and experimental pain in a chronic pain cohort. *Arthritis & Rheumatism, 52*(5), 1577–1584.

135. Wasan, A.D., Sullivan, M.D., & Clark, M.R. (2010). Psychiatric illness, depression, anxiety, and somatoform pain disorders. In *Bonica's management of pain* (4th ed.), ed. J.C. Ballantyne, J.P. Rathmell, & S.M. Fishman (pp. 393–417). Philadelphia: Lippincott Williams and Wilkins.

136. Urquhart, D.M., Hoving, J.L., Assendelft, W.J., Roland, M., & van Tulder, M.W. (2008). Antidepressants for non-specific low back pain. *Cochrane Database of Systematic Reviews 2008*(1), CD001703.

137. Bair, M.J., Robinson, R.L., Katon, W., & Kroenke, K. (2003). Depression and pain comorbidity: A literature review. *Archives of Internal Medicine, 163(20)*, 2433–2445.

138. US Food and Drug Administration. (2010). FDA clears Cymbalta to treat chronic musculoskeletal pain [Press release]. Retrieved from http://www.fda.gov/NewsEvents/Newsroom/PressAnnouncements/ucm232708.htm

139. US National Library of Medicine. (n.d.). Venlafaxine. Retrieved from http://www.ncbi.nlm.nih.gov/pubmedhealth/PMH0000947/

140. US National Library of Medicine. (n.d.). Milnacipran. Retrieved from http://www.ncbi.nlm.nih.gov/pubmedhealth/PMH0000495/

141. US National Library of Medicine. (n.d.). Nortriptyline. Retrieved from http://www.ncbi.nlm.nih.gov/pubmedhealth/PMH0000732/

142. US National Library of Medicine. (n.d.). Amitriptyline. Retrieved from http://www.ncbi.nlm.nih.gov/pubmedhealth/PMH0000732/

143. US National Library of Medicine. (n.d.). Desipramine. Retrieved from http://www.ncbi.nlm.nih.gov/pubmedhealth/PMH0000665/

144. Urquhart, D.M., Hoving, J.L., Assendelft, W.J., Roland, M., & van Tulder, M.W. (2008). Antidepressants for non-specific low back pain. *Cochrane Database of Systematic Reviews, 2008(1)*, CD001703.

145. Seidel, S., Aigner, M., Ossege, M., Pernicka, E., Wildner, B., & Sycha, T. (2010). Antipsychotics for acute and chronic pain in adults [Abstract]. *Journal of Pain and Symptom Management, 39(4)*, 768–778.

146. US National Library of Medicine. (n.d.). Olanzapine. Retrieved from http://www.ncbi.nlm.nih.gov/pubmedhealth/PMH0000161/

147. US National Library of Medicine. (n.d.). Carisoprodol. Retrieved from http://www.ncbi.nlm.nih.gov/pubmedhealth/PMH0000717/

148. US National Library of Medicine. (n.d.). Cyclobenzaprine. Retrieved from http://www.ncbi.nlm.nih.gov/pubmedhealth/PMH0000699/

149. US National Library of Medicine. (n.d.). Diazepam. Retrieved from http://www.ncbi.nlm.nih.gov/pubmedhealth/PMH0000556/

150. Urquhart, D.M., Hoving, J.L., Assendelft, W.J., Roland, M., & van Tulder, M.W. (2008). Antidepressants for non-specific low back pain. *Cochrane Database of Systematic Reviews, 2008(1)*, CD001703.

151. Lunn, M.P., Hughes, R.A., & Wiffen, P.J. (2009). Duloxetine for treating painful neuropathy or chronic pain [Abstract]. *Cochrane Database of Systematic Reviews, 2009(4)*, CD007115.

152. Saarto, T., & Wiffen, P.J. (2005). Antidepressants for neuropathic pain [Abstract]. *Cochrane Database of Systematic Reviews, 2005(3)*, CD005454.

153. Jackson, J.L., O'Malley, P.G., & Kroenke, K. (2006). Antidepressants and cognitive-behavioral therapy for symptom syndromes. *CNS Spectrums, 11*(3), 212–222.

154. Kroenke, K., Bair, M.J., Damush, T.M., et al. (2009). Optimized antidepressant therapy and pain self-management in primary care patients with depression and musculoskeletal pain. *The Journal of the American Medical Association, 301(20)*, 2099–2110.

155. G. Bennett (personal communication, September 12, 2009).

156. Zheng, H., Xiao, W. H., & Bennett, G. J. (2011). Functional deficits in peripheral nerve mitochondria in rats with paclitaxel- and oxaliplatin-evoked painful peripheral neuropathy. *Experimental Neurology, 232*(2), 154–161.

157. Wilson, A.D., Hart, A., Brannstrom, T., Wiberg, M., & Terenghi, G. (2007). Delayed acetyl-l-carnitine administration and its effect on sensory neuronal rescue after peripheral nerve injury. *Journal of Plastic, Reconstructive and Aesthetic Surgery, 60*(2), 114–118.

158. US National Institutes of Health. (2013). Safety and efficacy of olesoxime (TRO19622) in 3–25 years SMA patients. Retrieved from http://clinicaltrials.gov/show/NCT01302600

159. Ward, S.J., Ramirez, M.D., Neelakantan, M.S., & Walker, E.A. (2011). Cannabidiol prevents the development of cold and mechanical allodynia in paclitaxel-treated female C57Bl6 mice. *Anesthesia & Analgesia, 113*(4), 947–950.

160. R. Ji (personal communication, July 13, 2015).

161. Ji, R., Xu, Z., & Gao, Y. (2014). Emerging targets in neuroinflammation-driven chronic pain. *Nature Reviews Drug Discovery, 13*, 533–548.

162. Xu, Z., Zhang, L., Liu, T., et al. (2010). Resolvins RvE1 and RvD1 attenuate inflammatory pain via central and peripheral actions. *Nature Medicine, 16*(5), 592–597.

163. Xu, Z., Liu, X., Berta, T., et al. (2013). Neuroprotectin/protectin D1 protects against neuropathic pain in mice after nerve trauma. *Annals of Neurology, 74*(3), 490–495.

164. Serhan, C.N. (2014). Pro-resolving lipid mediators are leads for resolution physiology. *Nature, 510*, 92–101.

165. Ji, R., Xu, Z., Strichartz, G., & Serhan, C.N. (2011). Emerging roles of resolvins in the resolution of inflammation and pain. *Trends in Neuroscience, 34(11)*, 599–609.

166. Ibid.

167. R. Ji (personal communication, July 13, 2015).

168. Goldman, N., Chen, M., Fujita, T., et al. (2010). Adenosine A1 receptors mediate local anti-nociceptive effects of acupuncture. *Nature Neuroscience, 13*, 883–888.

169. M. Zylka (personal communication, November 2, 2011).

170. Zylka, M.J., Sowa, N.A., Taylor-Blake, B., et al. (2008). Prostatic acid phosphatase is an ectonucleotidase and suppresses pain by generating adenosine. *Neuron, 60*(1), 111–122.

171. Street, S.E., & Zylka, M.J. (2011). Emerging roles for ectonucleotidases in pain-sensing neurons. *Neuropsychopharmacology, 36*(1), 358.

172. Zylka, M.J. (2011). Pain-relieving properties for adenosine receptors and ectonucleotidases [Abstract]. *Trends in Molecular Medicine, 17*(4), 188–196.

173. Sowa, N.A., Street, S.E., Vihko, P., & Zylka, M.J. (2010). Prostatic acid phosphatase reduces thermal sensitivity and chronic pain sensitization by depleting phosphatidylinositol 4,5-bisphosphate [Abstract]. *Journal of Neuroscience, 30*(31), 10282–10293.

174. Sowa, N.A., Taylor-Blake, B., & Zylka, M.J. (2010). Ecto-5'-nucleotidase (CD73) inhibits nociception by hydrolyzing AMP to adenosine in nociceptive circuits [Abstract]. *Journal of Neuroscience, 30*(6), 2235–2244.

175. Hurt, J.K., & Zylka, M.J. (2012). PAPupuncture has localized and long-lasting antinociceptive effects in mouse models of acute and chronic pain. *Molecular Pain, 8*(1), 28.

176. Zylka, M.J. (2011). Pain-relieving prospects for adenosine receptors and ectonucleotidases. *Trends in Molecular Medicine, 17*(4), 188–196.

177. Schnabel, J. (2011, January14). Drug for chronic pain shows promise in preclinical tests. Retrieved from http://www.dana.org/news/features/detail.aspx?id=29760

178. Sharif-Naeini, R., & Basbaum, A.I. (2011). Targeting pain where it resides . . . in the brain. *Science Translational Medicine, 3(65)*, 65ps1.

179. Wang, H., Xu, H., Wu, L.J., et al. (2011). Identification of an adenylyl cyclase inhibitor for treating neuropathic and inflammatory pain [Abstract]. *Science Translational Medicine, 3(65)*, 65ra3.

180. Jimenez-Andrade, J.M., Martin, C.D., Koewler, N.J., et al. (2001). Nerve growth factor sequestering therapy attenuates non-malignant skeletal pain following fracture [Abstract]. *PAIN, 133*(1–3), 183–196.

181. Watson, J.J., Allen, S.J., & Dawbarn, D. (2008). Targeting nerve growth factor in pain: What is the therapeutic potential? [Abstract]. *BioDrugs, 22*(6), 349–359.

182. Woolf, C.J. (1996). Phenotypic modification of primary sensory neurons: The role of nerve growth factor in the production of persistent pain. *Philosophical Transactions: Biological Sciences, 351*(1338), 441–448.
183. US National Institutes of Health. (2008, August 11). Tanezumab in osteoarthritis of the knee. Retrieved from http://www.clinicaltrials.gov/show/NCT00733902
184. US National Institutes of Health. (2008, August 29). Tanezumab in osteoarthritis of the hip. Retrieved from http://www.clinicaltrials.gov/show/NCT00744471
185. Ko, J. (2011, May). Efficacy and safety of IV tanezumab in osteoarthritis hip and knee pain. Paper presented at the American Pain Society's annual scientific meeting, Austin, TX.
186. Lane, N.E., Schnitzer, T.J., Birbara, C.A., et al. (2010). Tanezumab for the treatment of pain from osteoarthritis of the knee. *The New England Journal of Medicine, 363*, 1521–1531.
187. Wood, J.N. (2010). Nerve growth factor and pain. *The New England Journal of Medicine, 363*, 1572–1573.
188. Allen, J.E. (2010, September 30). "Game-changing" arthritis drug blocks pain too well in some. *ABC News.* Retrieved from http://abcnews.go.com/Health/PainArthritis/pfizer-arthritis-drug-blocks-pain/story?id=11758493
189. McCaffrey, P. (2012, October 2). NGF update: Antibodies get a second chance and small molecules zero in on TrkA. Pain Research Forum. Retrieved from http://www.painresearchforum.org/news/20470-ngf-update-antibodies-get-second-chance-and-small-molecules-zero-trka?search_term=antibodies%20get%20second%20chance
190. Pfizer. (2010, June 23). Pfizer suspends chronic pain studies in tanezumab clinical trial [Press release]. Retrieved from http://www.pfizer.com/news/press_releases/pfizer_press_release_archive.jsp#guid=tanezumab_clinical_hold_062310&source=RSS_2010&page=6
191. M. Brown (personal communication, October 11, 2012).
192. Brown, M.T., Murphy, F.T., Radin, D.M., Davignon, I., Smith, M.D., & West, C.R. (2013). Tanezumab reduces osteoarthritic hip pain: Results of a randomized, double-blind, placebo-controlled phase III trial. *Arthritis & Rheumatology, 65*(7), 1795–1803.
193. Lee, J., Park, C., Chen, G., et al. (2014). A monoclonal antibody that targets a NaV1.7 channel voltage sensor for pain and itch. *Cell, 157*(6), 1393–1404.

194. US National Library of Medicine. (n.d.). Gabapentin. Retrieved from http://www.ncbi.nlm.nih.gov/pubmedhealth/PMH0000940

195. US National Library of Medicine. (n.d.). Pregabalin. Retrieved from http://www.ncbi.nlm.nih.gov/pubmedhealth/PMH0000327/

196. Moore, R.A., Straube, S., Wiffen, P.J., Derry, S., & McQuay, H.J. (2009). Pregabalin for acute and chronic pain in adults. *Cochrane Database of Systematic Reviews, 2009*(3), CD007076.

197. S. Cohen (personal communication, July 12, 2015).

198. Schofferman, J., & Mazanec, D. (2008). Evidence-informed management of chronic low back pain with opioid analgesics. *The Spine Journal, 8*(1), 185–194.

199. P. Fine (personal communication, October 27, 2011).

200. Woodcock, J. (2009). A difficult balance: Pain management, drug safety and the FDA. *The New England Journal of Medicine, 361*(22), 2105–2107.

201. US Food and Drug Administration. (2011). FDA drug safety communication: Prescription acetaminophen products to be limited to 325 mg per dosage unit; boxed warning will highlight potential for severe liver failure. Retrieved from http://www.fda.gov/Drugs/DrugSafety/ucm239821.htm

202. Gerth, J., & Miller, T.C. (2013, September 20). Use only as directed. ProPublica. Retrieved from http://www.propublica.org/article/tylenol-mcneil-fda-use-only-as-directed

203. Foreman, J. (2014, April 14). Opinion: Why Zohydro ban is a tough call. Judyforeman.com. Retrieved from http://judyforeman.com/2014/04/opinion-zohydro-ban-tough-call/

204. Forster, C. (2015, March 12). Analysts weigh in on Zogenix in light of selling Zohydro. Seeking Alpha. Retrieved from http://seekingalpha.com/article/2996866-analysts-weigh-in-on-zogenix-in-light-of-selling-zohydro

205. US National Library of Medicine. (n.d.). Ibuprofen—important warning. Retrieved from http://www.ncbi.nlm.nih.gov/pubmedhealth/PMH0000598

206. Lanza, F.L., Chan, F., Quigley, E.M., & the Practice Parameters Committee of the American College of Gastroenterology. (2009). Guidelines for prevention of NSAID-related ulcer complications. *American Journal of Gastroenterology, 104*, 728–738.

207. American Geriatrics Society Panel on the Pharmacological Management of Persistent Pain in Older Persons. (2009). Pharmacological management of persistent pain in older persons. *Journal of the American Geriatrics Society, 57*(8), 1331–1346.

208. Agency for Healthcare Research and Quality, US Department of Health and Human Services. (2009). Choosing non-opioid analgesics for osteoarthritis: Clinician summary guide. *Journal of Pain & Palliative Care Pharmacotherapy, 23*(4), 433–457.

209. Fauber, J., & Gabler, E. (2012, May 29). Experts linked to drug firms tout benefits but downplay chance of addiction, other risks. *The Milwaukee-Wisconsin Journal Sentinel.* Retrieved from http://search.jsonline.com/Search.aspx?k=John%20Fauber,%20experts%20linked

210. Schmidt, M., Christiansen, C.F., Mehnert, F., Rothman, K.J., & Sorensen, H.T. (2011). Non-steroidal anti-inflammatory drug use and risk of atrial fibrillation or flutter: Population based case-control study. *British Medical Journal, 343,* d3450.

211. Fosbel, E.L., Folke, F., Jacobsen, S., et al. (2010). Cause-specific cardiovascular risk associated with nonsteroidal anti-inflammatory drugs among healthy individuals. *Circulation: Cardiovascular Quality and Outcomes, 3,* 395–405.

212. Trelle, S., Reichenbach, S., Wandel, S., et al. (2011). Cardiovascular safety of non-steroidal anti-inflammatory drugs: Network meta-analysis. *British Medical Journal, 342,* c7086.

213. McGettigan, P., & Henry, D. (2011). Cardiovascular risk with non-steroidal anti-inflammatory drugs: Systematic review of population-based controlled observational studies. *PLoS Medicine, 8*(9), e1001098.

214. Coxib and Traditional NSAID Trialists' (CNT) Collaboration. (2013). Vascular and upper gastrointestinal effects of non-steroidal anti-inflammatory drugs: Meta-analyses of individual participant data from randomised trials. *The Lancet, 382*(9894), 769–779.

215. US Food and Drug Administration. (2015). FDA strengthens warning of heart attack and stroke risk for non-steroidal anti-inflammatory drugs. Retrieved from http://www.fda.gov/ForConsumers/ConsumerUpdates/ucm453610.htm

216. S. Parazin (personal communication, December 21, 2011).

217. Mayo Clinic Staff. (2013, August 1). Arthritis pain: Treatments absorbed through your skin. Mayo Clinic. Retrieved from http://www.mayoclinic.org/diseases-conditions/osteoarthritis/in-depth/pain-medications/art-20045899

218. Hayman, M., & Kam, P.C. (2008). Capsaicin: A review of its pharmacology and clinical applications [Abstract]. *Current Anaesthesia & Critical Care, 19*(5), 338–343.

219. Caterina, M.J., Schumacher, M.A., Tominaga, M., Rosen, T.A., Levine, J.D., & Julius, D. (1997). The capsaicin receptor: A heat-activated ion channel in the pain pathway. *Nature, 389*(6653), 816–824.
220. Patwardhan, A.M., Akopian, A.N., Ruparel, N.B., et al. (2010). Heat generates oxidized linoleic acid metabolites that activate TRPV1 and produce pain in rodents. *The Journal of Clinical Investigation, 120*(5), 1617–1626.
221. Agency for Healthcare Research and Quality, US Department of Health and Human Services. (2009). Choosing non-opioid analgesics for osteoarthritis: Clinician summary guide. *Journal of Pain & Palliative Care Pharmacotherapy, 23*(4), 433–457.
222. De Silva, V., El-Metwally, A., Ernst, E., Lewith, G., & Macfarlane, G.J. (2011). Evidence for the efficacy of complementary and alternative medicines in the management of osteoarthritis: A systematic review. *Rheumatology, 50*(5), 911–920.
223. R. Ji (personal communication, July 13, 2015).
224. Medline Plus. (n.d.). Lidocaine transdermal patches. Retrieved from http://www.nlm.nih.gov/medlineplus/druginfo/meds/a603026.html
225. Agency for Healthcare Research and Quality, US Department of Health and Human Services. (2009). Choosing non-opioid analgesics for osteoarthritis: Clinician summary guide. *Journal of Pain & Palliative Care Pharmacotherapy, 23*(4), 433–457.
226. Prabhakar, S., Taherian, M., Gianni, D., et al. (2013). Regression of Schwannomas induced by adeno-associated virus-mediated delivery of caspase-1. *Human Gene Therapy, 24*(2), 152–162.
227. Andrews, N. (2012, July 9). Moving pain treatments forward: NIH Pain Consortium Symposium. Pain Research Forum. Retrieved from http://www.painresearchforum.org/news/17877-moving-pain-treatments-forward-nih-pain-consortium-symposium
228. Iyer, S.M., Montgomery, K.L., Towne, C., et al. (2014). Virally mediated optogenetic excitation and inhibition of pain in freely moving nontransgenic mice. *Nature Biotechnology, 32*, 274–278.

Chapter 7

1. National Center for Complementary and Integrative Health. (2014). NIH complementary and integrative health agency gets new name [Press release]. Retrieved from https://nccih.nih.gov/news/press/12172014

2. National Center for Complementary and Alternative Medicine. (2008). Health conditions prompting CAM use. Retrieved from http://nccam.nih.gov/news/camstats/2007/camsurvey_fs1.htm

3. Barnes, P.M., Bloom, B., & Nahin, R.L. (2008). *Complementary and alternative medicine use among adults and children: United States, 2007* (National Health Statistics Reports No. 12). Atlanta, GA: Centers for Disease Control and Prevention. Retrieved from http://www.cdc. gov/nchs/data/nhsr/nhsr012.pdf

4. Cohen, S.P., Argoff, C.E., & Carragee, E.J. (2009). Management of low back pain [Clinical review]. *British Journal of Medicine, 338,* 100–106.

5. Nally, K. (2014, September 21). Chronic pain is the most common reason for dietary supplement use. HCPLive. Retrieved from http:// www.hcplive.com/conferences/2014-aapmgmt/Chronic-Pain-Is-the-Most-Common-Reason-for-Dietary-Supplement-Use

6. National Center for Complementary and Alternative Medicine. (2014). NIH and VA address pain and related conditions in U.S. military personnel, veterans and their families: Research will focus on nondrug approaches [Press release]. Retrieved from http://www. hcplive.com/conferences/2014-aapmgmt/Chronic-Pain-Is-the-Most-Common-Reason-for-Dietary-Supplement-Use

7. National Center for Complementary and Alternative Medicine. (2015). The use of complementary and alternative medicine in the United States [Press release]. Retrieved from https://nccih.nih.gov/ news/camstats/2007/camsurvey_fs1.htm

8. National Center for Complementary and Alternative Medicine. (2015). National survey reveals widespread use of mind and body practices, shifts in use of natural products. Retrieved from http:// www.nih.gov/news/health/feb2015/nccih-10a.htm

9. Barnes, P.M., Bloom, B., & Nahin, R.L. (2008). *Complementary and alternative medicine use among adults and children: United States, 2007* (National Health Statistics Reports No. 12). Atlanta, GA: Centers for Disease Control and Prevention. Retrieved from http://www.cdc. gov/nchs/data/nhsr/nhsr012.pdf

10. ConsumerReports.org. (2011). Natural health: Alternative treatments. Retrieved from http://www.consumerreports.org/health/ natural-health/alternative-treatments/overview/index.htm

11. Wax-Thibodeaux, E. (2014, September 26). Federal research seeks alternatives to addictive opioids for veterans in pain. *The Washington*

Post. Retrieved from http://www.washingtonpost.com/blogs/ federal-eye/wp/2014/09/25/federal-research-seeks-alternatives-to-addictive-opioids-for-veterans-in-pain/

12. Nally, K. (2014). NIH and VA address pain and related conditions in U.S. military personnel, veterans and their families: Research will focus on nondrug approaches [Press release]. Retrieved from http:// www.hcplive.com/conferences/2014-aapmgmt/Chronic-Pain-Is-the-Most-Common-Reason-for-Dietary-Supplement-Use

13. Sheftick, G. (2014, May 14). Acupuncture helping reduce use of pain killers. Military.com. Retrieved from http://www.military.com/ daily-news/2014/05/05/acupuncture-helping-reduce-use-of-pain-killers-in-army.html

14. Brennan, T. (2014, April 3). Naval hospital adds acupuncture to list of available services. JDNews.com. Retrieved from http://www. jdnews.com/article/20140403/News/304039906

15. Department of the Navy of Bureau of Medicine and Surgery. (2013*). BUMED Instruction 6320.100 (Medical, Chiropractic, and Licensed Acupuncture).* Retrieved from http://www.med.navy.mil/direc-tives/ExternalDirectives/6320.100.pdf

16. National Center for Complementary and Integrative Health (2014). Complementary health approaches for chronic pain: What the science says. Retrieved from https://nccih.nih.gov/health/providers/ digest/chronic-pain-science

17. Ibid.

18. Ibid.

19. Ibid.

20. Ibid.

21. MacPherson, H., & Asghar, A. (2006). Acupuncture needle sensations associated with *de qi:* A classification based on experts' ratings. *Journal of Alternative and Complementary Medicine, 12*(7), 633–637.

22. Hui, K.K., Liu, J., Marina, O., et al. (2005). The integrated response of the human cerebro-cerebellar and limbic systems to acupuncture stimulation at ST 36 as evidenced by fMRI. *NeuroImage, 27*(3), 479–496.

23. Singh, S., & Ernst, E. (2008). *Trick or treatment—The undeniable facts about alternative medicine* (p. 77). New York: W.W. Norton.

24. Ernst, E. (2006). Acupuncture—A critical analysis. *Journal of Internal Medicine, 259*(2), 125–137.

25. National Center for Complementary and Integrative Health. (2015). Acupuncture: What you need to know. Retrieved from https:// nccih.nih.gov/health/acupuncture/introduction

26. Langevin, H.M., Wayne, P.M., MacPherson, H., et al. (2011). Paradoxes in acupuncture research: Strategies for moving forward [Review article]. *Evidence-Based Complementary and Alternative Medicine*, 180805. Retrieved from http://www.hindawi.com/journals/ecam/2011/180805/

27. Derry, C.J., Derry, S., McQuay, H.J., & Moore, R.A. (2006). Systematic review of systematic reviews of acupuncture published 1996–2005. *Clinical Medicine*, 6(4), 381–386.

28. Johnson, M.I. (2006). The clinical effectiveness of acupuncture for pain relief—You can be certain of uncertainty. *Acupuncture in Medicine*, 24, 71–79.

29. Cherkin, D.C., Sherman, K.J., Deyo, R.A., & Shekelle, P.G. (2003). A review of the evidence for the effectiveness, safety, and cost of acupuncture, massage therapy, and spinal manipulation for back pain. *Annals of Internal Medicine*, 138(11), 898–906.

30. V. Napadow (personal communication, November 29, 2011).

31. Sun, Y., Gan, T.J., Dubose, J.W., & Habib, A.S. (2008). Acupuncture and related techniques for postoperative pain: A systematic review of randomized clinical trials. *British Journal of Anesthesia*, 101(2), 151–160.

32. Berman, B.M., Lao, L., Langenberg, P., Lee, W.L., Gilpin, A.M.K., & Hochberg, M.C. (2004). Effectiveness of acupuncture as adjunctive therapy in osteoarthritis of the knee: A randomized, controlled trial. *Annals of Internal Medicine*, 141(12), 901–910.

33. Jubb, R.W., Tukmachi, E.S., Jones, P.W., Dempsey, E., Waterhouse, L., & Brailsford, S. (2008). A blinded randomised trial of acupuncture (manual and electroacupuncture) compared with a non-penetrating sham for the symptoms of osteoarthritis of the knee. *Acupuncture in Medicine*, 26, 69–78.

34. P. Wayne (personal communication, November 28, 2011).

35. Manheimer, E., White, A., Berman, B., Forys, K., & Ernst, E. (2005). Meta-analysis: acupuncture for low back pain. *Annals of Internal Medicine*, 142(8), 651–663.

36. Shen, Y.F., Younger, J., Goddard, G., & Mackey, S. (2009). Randomized clinical trial of acupuncture for myofascial pain of the jaw muscles. *Journal of Oral & Facial Pain and Headache*, 23(4), 353–359.

37. Berman, B.M., Langevin, H.M., Witt, C.M., & Dubner, R. (2010). Acupuncture for chronic low back pain. *The New England Journal of Medicine*, 363(5), 454–461.

38. Ammendolia, C., Furlan, A.D., Imamura, M., Irvin, E., & van Tulder, M. (2008). Evidence-informed management of chronic low back pain with needle acupuncture. *The Spine Journal*, 8(1), 160–172.

39. Cherkin, D.C., Sherman, K.J., Avins, A.L., et al. (2009). A randomized trial comparing acupuncture, simulated acupuncture and usual care for chronic low back pain. *Archives of Internal Medicine, 169*(9), 858–866.
40. Singh, S., & Ernst, E. (2008). *Trick or treatment—The undeniable facts about alternative medicine* (p. 87). New York: W.W. Norton.
41. Foreman, J. (2005, March 22). Acupuncture has won medical acceptance. *The Boston Globe.* Retrieved from http://www.boston.com/news/globe/health_science/articles/2005/03/22/acupuncture_has_won_medical_acceptance/
42. National Institutes of Health Consensus Development Program. (1997). Acupuncture. NIH Consensus Development Conference Statement, November 3–5. Retrieved from http://consensus.nih.gov/1997/1997Acupuncture107html.htm
43. MedlinePlus. (n.d.). Acupuncture. Retrieved from http://vsearch.nlm.nih.gov/vivisimo/cgi-bin/query-meta?v%3Aproject=medlineplus&query=acupuncture&x=21&y=17
44. Foreman, J. (2005, March 22). Acupuncture has won medical acceptance. *The Boston Globe.* Retrieved from http://www.boston.com/news/globe/health_science/articles/2005/03/22/acupuncture_has_won_medical_acceptance/
45. National Institutes of Health Consensus Development Program. (1997). Acupuncture. NIH Consensus Development Conference Statement, November 3–5. Retrieved from http://consensus.nih.gov/1997/1997Acupuncture107html.htm
46. Harris, R.E., Zubieta, J., Scott, D.J., Napadow, V., Gracely, R.J., & Clauw, D.J. (2009). Traditional Chinese acupuncture and placebo (sham) acupuncture are differentiated by their effects on mu-opioid receptors (MORs). *NeuroImage, 47*(3), 1077–1085.
47. Goldman, N., Chen, M., Fujita, T., et al. (2010). Adenosine A1 receptors mediate local anti-nociceptive effects of acupuncture. *Nature Neuroscience, 13,* 883–888.
48. Takano, T., Chen, X., Luo, F., et al. (2012). Traditional acupuncture triggers a local increase in adenosine in human subjects. *The Journal of Pain, 12*(13), 1213–1223.
49. More, A.O., Cidral-Filho, F.J., Mazzardo-Martins, L., et al. (2013). Caffeine at moderate doses can inhibit acupuncture-induced analgesia in a mouse model of postoperative pain. *Journal of Caffeine Research, 3*(3), 143–148.
50. US National Library of Medicine. (2011). Carpal tunnel syndrome. Retrieved from http://www.ncbi.nlm.nih.gov/pubmedhealth/PMH0001469

51. Napadow, V., Kettner, N., Ryan, A., Kwong, K.K., Audette, J., & Hui, K.K. (2006). Somatosensory cortical plasticity in carpal tunnel syndrome—A cross-sectional fMRI evaluation. *NeuroImage, 31*(2), 520–530.

52. Napadow, V., Kettner, N., Liu, J., et al. (2007). Hypothalamus and amygdala response to acupuncture stimuli in carpal tunnel syndrome. *PAIN, 130*(2), 254–266.

53. Napadow, V., Liu, J., Li, M., et al. (2007). Somatosensory cortical plasticity in carpal tunnel syndrome treated by acupuncture. *Human Brain Mapping, 28*(3), 159–171.

54. Dhond, R.P., Yeh, C, Park, K., Kettner, N., & Napadow, V. (2008). Acupuncture modulates resting state connectivity in default and sensorimotor brain networks. *PAIN, 136*(3), 407–418.

55. Napadow, V., Lacount, L., Park, K., As-Sanie, S., Clauw, D.J., & Harris, R.E. (2010, November). Intrinsic brain connectivity in fibromyalgia is associated with chronic pain intensity and modulated by acupuncture. Paper presented at the 40th annual meeting of the Society for Neuroscience, San Diego, CA.

56. V. Napadow (personal communication, January 27, 2012).

57. Kong, J., Kaptchuk, T.J., Polich, G., et al. (2009). Expectancy and treatment interactions: A dissociation between acupuncture analgesia and expectancy evoked placebo analgesia. *NeuroImage, 45*(3), 940–949.

58. Chou, R., & Huffman, L.H. (2007). Nonpharmacologic therapies for acute and chronic low back pain: A review of the evidence for an American Pain Society/American College of Physicians clinical practice guideline. *Annals of Internal Medicine, 147*(7), 492–504.

59. Hinman, R.S., McCrory, P., Pirotta, M., et al. (2014). Acupuncture for chronic knee pain: a randomized clinical trial. *The Journal of the American Medical Association, 312*(13), 1313–1322.

60. Trinh, K., Graham, N., Gross, A., et al. (2010). Acupuncture for neck disorders. *Cochrane Database of Systematic Reviews, 2010*(3), CD004870.

61. Furlan, A.D., van Tulder, M.W., Cherkin, D., et al. (2008). Acupuncture and dry-needling for low back pain. *Cochrane Database of Systematic Reviews, 2008*(4), CD001351.

62. Sun, Y., Gan, J., Dubose, W., & Habib, A.S. (2008). Acupuncture and related techniques for postoperative pain: a systematic review of randomized controlled trials. *British Journal of Anaesthesia, 101*(2), 151–160.

63. Vickers, A.J., Cronin, A.M., Maschino, A.C., et al. (2012). Acupuncture for chronic pain. *Archives of Internal Medicine, 172*(19), 1444–1453.

64. Vickers, A.J., & Linde, K. (2014). Acupuncture for chronic pain. *The Journal of the American Medical Association, 311*(9), 955–956.

65. Berman, B.M., Langevin, H.M., Witt, C.M., & Dubner, R. (2010). Acupuncture for chronic low back pain. *The New England Journal of Medicine, 363*(5), 454–461.

66. National Institutes of Health Consensus Development Program. (1997). Acupuncture. NIH Consensus Development Conference Statement November 3–5. Retrieved from http://consensus.nih.gov/1997/1997Acupuncture107html.htm

67. Ernst, E., Lee, M.S., & Choi, T-Y. (2011). Acupuncture: Does it alleviate pain and are there serious risks? A review of reviews. *PAIN, 152*(4), 755–64.

68. Calabro, S. (2013, February 20). 7 Acupuncture side effects that you should know about. *The Huffington Post.* Retrieved from http://www.huffingtonpost.com/sara-calabro/acupuncture-side-effects_b_2719101.html

69. Rapaport, M.H., Schettler, P., & Bresee, C. (2010). A preliminary study of the effects of a single session of Swedish massage on hypothalamic-pituitary-adrenal and immune function of normal individuals. *Journal of Alternative and Complementary Medicine, 16*(10), 1–10.

70. Barnes, P.M., Bloom, B., & Nahin, R.L. (2008). *Complementary and alternative medicine use among adults and children: United States, 2007* (National Health Statistics Reports No. 12). Atlanta, GA: Centers for Disease Control and Prevention. Retrieved from http://www.cdc.gov/nchs/data/nhsr/nhsr012.pdf

71. Chou, R., & Huffman, L.H. (2007). Nonpharmacologic therapies for acute and chronic low back pain: A review of the evidence for an American Pain Society/American College of Physicians clinical practice guideline. *Annals of Internal Medicine, 147*(7), 492–504.

72. Haldeman, S., & Dagenais, S. (2008). What have we learned about the evidence-informed management of chronic low back pain? *The Spine Journal, 8,* 266–277.

73. Imamura, M., Furlan, A.D., Dryden, T., & Irvin, E. (2008). Evidence-informed management of chronic low back pain with massage. *The Spine Journal, 8,* 121–133.

74. Leavitt, S.B. (2011, October 21). More people turning to clinical massage for pain. Pain Treatment Topics. Retrieved from http://updates.pain-topics.org/2011/10/more-people-turning-to-clinical-massage.html

75. Cherkin, D.C., Sherman, K.J., Deyo, R.A., & Shekelle, P.G. (2003). A review of the evidence for the effectiveness, safety, and cost of acupuncture, massage therapy, and spinal manipulation for back pain. *Annals of Internal Medicine, 138*(11), 898–906.

76. Furlan, A., Imamura, M., Dryden, T., & Irvin, E. (2008). Massage for low back pain: An updated systematic review within the framework of the Cochrane Back Review Group. *Spine, 34*(16), 1669–1684.

77. National Center for Complementary and Integrative Health. (2015). Massage therapy for health purposes: What you need to know. Retrieved from https://nccih.nih.gov/health/massage/massageintroduction.htm

78. Chou, R., & Huffman, L.H. (2007). Nonpharmacologic therapies for acute and chronic low back pain: A review of the evidence for an American Pain Society/American College of Physicians clinical practice guideline. *Annals of Internal Medicine, 147*(7), 492–504.

79. Deyo, R. (2014, September 29). Massage studies: Reviews/guidelines for therapy [Video file]. Retrieved from https://www.youtube.com/watch?v=gngqEcLIuW8&feature=youtube_gdata

80. Cherkin, D.C., Sherman, K.J., Kahn, J., et al. (2011). A comparison of the effects of 2 types of massage and usual care on chronic low back pain. *Annals of Internal Medicine, 155*, 1–9.

81. Rapaport, M.H., Schettler, P., & Bresee, C. (2010). A preliminary study of the effects of a single session of Swedish massage on hypothalamic-pituitary-adrenal and immune function in normal individuals. *Journal of Alternative and Complementary Medicine, 16*(10), 1079–1088.

82. Kutner, J.S., Smith, M.C., Corbin, L., et al. (2008). Massage therapy versus simple touch to improve pain and mood in patients with advanced cancer: A randomized trial. *Annals of Internal Medicine, 149*(6), 369–379.

83. Sherman, K.J., Cook, A.J., Wellman, R.D., et al. (2014). Five-week outcomes from a dosing trial of therapeutic massage for chronic neck pain. *American Family Medicine, 12*(2), 112–120.

84. Perlman, A. I., Ali, A., Njike, V.Y., et al. (2012, February 8). Massage therapy for osteoarthritis of the knee: a randomized dose-finding trial. *PLoS ONE 7*(2), e30248. Retrieved from http://journals.plos.org/plosone/article?id=10.1371/journal.pone.0030248

85. ConsumerReports.org. (n.d.). Alternative treatments. Retrieved from http://www.consumerreports.org/health/natural-health/alternative-treatments/overview/index.htm

86. Jain, S., & Mills, P.J. (2010). Biofield therapies: Helpful or full of hype? A best evidence synthesis. *International Journal of Behavioral Medicine, 17*, 1–16.

87. So, P.S., Jiang, Y., & Qin, Y. (2008). Touch therapies for pain relief in adults. *Cochrane Database of Systematic Reviews, 2008*(4), CD006535.

88. Leavitt, S.B. (2009, November 7). Biofield therapies for pain: Help or hype. Pain Research Forum. Retrieved from http://updates. pain-topics.org/2009/11/biofield-therapies-for-pain-help-or.html

89. Singh, S., & Ernst, E. (2008). *Trick or treatment—The undeniable facts about alternative medicine* (p. 327). New York: W.W. Norton.

90. Rosa, L., Rosa, E., Sarner, L., & Barrett, S. (1998). A close look at therapeutic touch. *The Journal of the American Medical Association, 279*(13), 1005–1010.

91. National Center for Complementary and Alternative Medicine. (2008). Spinal manipulation for low-back pain. Retrieved from http://nccam.nih.gov/health/pain/spinemanipulation.htm

92. American Chiropractic Association. (2015). What is chiropractic? Retrieved from http://www.acatoday.org/level2_css.cfm?T1ID=13 &T2ID=61

93. Ibid.

94. National Center for Complementary and Alternative Medicine. (2015). Chiropractic: An introduction. Retrieved from https:// nccih.nih.gov/health/chiropractic/introduction.htm?lang=en

95. Consumer Reports. (2009). Relief for aching backs. Retrieved from http://www.consumerreports.org/cro/magazine-archive/may-2009/health/back-pain/overview/back-pain-ov.htm

96. J. Kornfeld (personal communication, December 7, 2011).

97. Liliedahl, R.L., Finch, M.D., Axene, D.V., & Goertz, C.M. (2010). Cost of care for common back pain conditions initiated with chiropractic doctor vs. medical doctor/doctor of osteopathy as first physician: Experience of one Tennessee-based general health insurer. *Journal of Manipulative and Physiological Therapeutics, 33*(9), 640–643.

98. Chou, R., Qaseem, A., Snow, V., et al. (2007). Diagnosis and treatment of low back pain: A joint clinical practice guideline from the American College of Physicians and the American Pain Society. *Annals of Internal Medicine, 147*(7), 478–491.

99. National Center for Complementary and Alternative Medicine. (2008). Spinal manipulation for low-back pain. Retrieved from http://nccam.nih.gov/health/pain/spinemanipulation.htm

100. Chou, R., & Huffman, L.H. (2007). Nonpharmacologic therapies for acute and chronic low back pain: A review of the evidence for an American Pain Society/American College of Physicians clinical practice guideline. *Annals of Internal Medicine, 147*(7), 492–504.

101. Bronfort, G., Haas, M., Evans, R.L., Kawchuk, G., & Dagenais, S. (2008). Evidence-informed management of chronic low back

pain with spinal manipulation and mobilization. *The Spine Journal,* *8,* 213–225.

102. Bronfort, G., Hass, M., Evans, R.L., & Bouter, L.M. (2004). Efficacy of spinal manipulation and mobilization for low back pain and neck pain: A systematic review and best evidence synthesis. *The Spine Journal, 4*(3), 335–356.

103. Senna, M., & Machaly, S. (2011). Does maintained spinal manipulation therapy for chronic nonspecific low back pain result in better long-term outcome? *Spine, 36*(18), 1427–1437.

104. Muller, R., & Giles, L.G. (2005). Long-term follow-up of a randomized clinical trial assessing the efficacy of medication, acupuncture, and spinal manipulation for chronic mechanical spinal pain syndromes. *Journal of Manipulative and Physiological Therapeutics, 28*(1), 3–11.

105. Clinical Guideline Subcommittee on Low Back Pain. (2010). American Osteopathic Association Guidelines for osteopathic manipulative treatment (OMT) for patients with low back pain. *Journal of the American Osteopathic Association, 110*(11), 653–666.

106. Hurwitz, E.L., Morgenstern, H., Kominski, G.F., Yu, F., & Chiang, L. (2006). A randomized trial of chiropractic and medical care for patients with low back pain: Eighteen-month follow-up outcomes from the UCLA low back pain study. *Spine, 31*(6), 611–621.

107. Cherkin, D.C., Sherman, K.J., Deyo, R.A., & Shekelle, P.G. (2003). A review of the evidence for the effectiveness, safety, and cost of acupuncture, massage therapy, and spinal manipulation for back pain. *Annals of Internal Medicine, 138*(11), 898–906.

108. UK BEAM Trial Team. (2004). United Kingdom Back Pain Exercise and Manipulation (UK BEAM) randomised trial: Effectiveness of physical treatments for back pain in primary care. *British Medical Journal, 329*(7479), 1377.

109. Ferreira, M.L., Ferreira, P.H., Latimer, J., et al. (2007). Comparison of general exercise, motor control exercise and spinal manipulative therapy for chronic low back pain: A randomized trial. *PAIN, 131*(1–2), 31–37.

110. Hoving, J.L., Koes, B.W., de Vet, H.C., et al. (2002). Manual therapy, physical therapy, or continued care by a general practitioner for patients with neck pain: A randomized, controlled trial. *Archives of Internal Medicine, 136*(10), 713–722.

111. Vernon, H., Humphreys, K., & Hagino, C. (2007). Chronic mechanical neck pain in adults treated by manual therapy: A systematic

review of change scores in randomized clinical trials. *Journal of Manipulative and Physiological Therapeutics, 30*(3), 215–227.

112. Bronfort, G., Evans, R., Anderson, A.V., Svendsen, K.H., Bracha, Y., & Grimm, R.H. (2012). Spinal manipulation, medication, or home exercise with advice for acute and subacute neck pain. *Annals of Internal Medicine, 156*, 1–10.

113. Gross, A., Miller, J., D'Sylva, J., et al. (2010). Manipulation or mobilisation for neck pain. *Cochrane Database of Systematic Reviews, 2010*(1), CD004249.

114. Ernst, E. (2010). Deaths after chiropractic: A review of published cases. *International Journal of Clinical Practice, 64*(8), 1162–1165.

115. Haldeman, S., Carey, P., Townsend, M., & Papadopoulos, C. (2001). Arterial dissections following cervical manipulation: The chiropractic experience. *Canadian Medical Association Journal, 165*(7), 905–906.

116. Haldeman, S., Kohlbeck, F.J., & McGregor, M. (2002). Stroke, cerebral artery dissection, and cervical spine manipulation therapy. *Journal of Neurology, 249*(8), 1098–1104.

117. Haldeman, S., Carroll, L., Cassidy, J.D., Schubert, J., & Nygren, A. (2008). The Bone and Joint Decade 2000–2010 Task Force on Neck Pain and Its Associated Disorders. *European Spine Journal, 17*(Suppl. 1), S5–S7.

118. S. Haldeman (personal communication, December 8, 2011).

119. Rubenstein, S.M., Leboeuf-Yde, C., Knol, D.L., de Koekkoek, T.E., Pfeifle, C.E., & van Tulder, M.W. (2007). The benefits outweigh the risks for patients undergoing chiropractic care for neck pain: A prospective, multicenter, cohort study [Abstract]. *Journal of Manipulative and Physiological Therapeutics, 30*(6), 408–418.

120. Gouveia, L.O., Castanho, P., & Ferreira, J.J. (2009). Safety of chiropractic interventions: A systematic review. *Spine, 34*(11), E405–E413.

121. Wand, B.M., Heine, P.J., & O'Connell, N.E. (2012). Should we abandon cervical spine manipulation for mechanical neck pain? Yes. *British Medical Journal, 344*, e3679.

122. Cassidy, J.D., Bronfort, G., & Hartvigsen, J. (2012). Should we abandon cervical spine manipulation for mechanical neck pain? No. *British Medical Journal, 344*, e3680.

123. Marziali, M., Venza, M., Lazzaro, S., Lazzaro, A., Micossi, C., & Stolfi, V.M. (2012). Gluten-free diet: A new strategy for management of painful endometriosis-related symptoms? *Minerva Chirurgica, 6*(67), 499–504.

124. Ruskin, D.N., Kawamura., M. Jr., & Masino, S.A. (2009). Reduced pain and inflammation in juvenile and adult rats fed a ketogenic diet. *PLoS ONE, 12*(4), e8349.
125. Masino, S.A., & Ruskin, D.N. (2013). Ketogenic diets and pain. *Journal of Child Neurology, 8*(28), 993–1001.
126. Weil, A. (2005). *Healthy aging* (pp. 141–160). New York: Alfred A. Knopf.
127. Galland, L. (2010). Diet and inflammation. *Nutrition in Clinical Practice, 6*(25), 634–640.
128. Foreman, J. (2004, February 10). Fatty acid imbalance hurts our health. *The Boston Globe.* Retrieved from http://www.boston.com/news/globe/health_science/articles/2004/02/10/fatty_acid_imbalance_hurts_our_health/
129. Maroon, J.C., & Bost, J.W. (2006). Omega-3 fatty acids (fish oil) as an anti-inflammatory: An alternative to non-steroidal anti-inflammatory drugs for discogenic pain. *Surgical Neurology, 65*(4), 326–331.
130. ConsumerLab.com. (n.d.). Product review: Fish oil and omega-3 fatty acid supplements (EPA and DHA from fish, algae and krill). Retrieved from https://www.consumerlab.com/list.asp
131. University of Maryland Medical System. (2013). Omega-3 fatty acids. Retrieved from http://umm.edu/health/medical/altmed/supplement/omega3-fatty-acids
132. Wynn, R. (n.d.). I'll have the fish, with an aspirin on the side: Attacking inflammation with combined aspirin and omega-3s. Lexicomp. Retrieved from https://www.lexi.com/individuals/dentistry/newsletters.jsp?id=april-13.
133. Zhang, M.J., & Spite, M. (2012). Resolvins: Anti-inflammatory and proresolving mediators derived from omega-3 polyunsaturated fatty acids. *Annual Review of Nutrition, 32,* 203–227.
134. Weylandt, K. H., Chiu, C., Gomolka, B., Waechter, S.F., & Wiedenmann, B. (2012). Omega-3 fatty acids and their lipid mediators: Towards an understanding of resolving and protectin formation. *Prostaglandins & Other Lipid Mediators, 97*(3–4), 73–82.
135. US National Library of Medicine. (2011). Osteomalacia. Retrieved from http://www.ncbi.nlm.nih.gov/pubmedhealth/PMH0001414/
136. National Institutes of Health, Office of Dietary Supplements. (2014). Vitamin D. Retrieved from http://ods.od.nih.gov/factsheets/VitaminD-HealthProfessional.
137. Institute of Medicine. (2010). Dietary reference intakes for calcium and vitamin D. Retrieved from http://www.iom.edu/

Reports/2010/Dietary-Reference-Intakes-for-Calcium-and-Vitamin-D.aspx

138. Holick, M.F., Binkley, N.C., Bischoff-Ferrari, H.A., et al. (2011). Evaluation, treatment, and prevention of vitamin D deficiency: An endocrine society clinical practice guideline. *Journal of Clinical Endocrinology & Metabolism, 96*(7), 1911–1930.

139. R. Chou (personal communication, January 3, 2012).

140. McBeth, J., Pye, S.R., O'Neill, T.W., et al. (2010). Musculoskeletal pain is associated with very low levels of vitamin D in men: Results from the European male aging study. *Annals of Rheumatic Diseases, 69*, 1448–1452.

141. Straube, S., Derry, S., & McQuay, H.J. (2010). Vitamin D for the treatment of chronic painful conditions in adults. *Cochrane Database of Systematic Reviews, 2010*(1), CD007771.

142. Rastelli, A.L., Taylor, M.E., Gao, F., et al. (2011). Vitamin D and aromatase inhibitor-induced musculoskeletal symptoms (AIMSS): A phase II, double-blind, placebo-controlled, randomized trial. *Breast Cancer Research and Treatment, 129*(1), 107–116.

143. Gopinath, K. & Danda, D. (2011). Supplementation of 1,25 dihydroxy vitamin D3 in patients with treatment naïve early rheumatoid arthritis: A randomised controlled trial. *International Journal of Rheumatic Diseases, 14*(4), 332–339.

144. Sakalli, H., Arslan, D., & Yucel, A.E. (2011). The effect of oral and parenteral vitamin D supplementation in the elderly: A prospective, double-blinded, randomized, placebo-controlled study. *Rheumatology International, 32*(8), 2279–2283.

145. Song, G.G., Bae, S.C., & Lee, Y.H. (2012). Association between vitamin D intake and the risk of rheumatoid arthritis: A meta-analysis. *Clinical Rheumatology, 31*(12), 1733–1739.

146. Lasco, A., Catalano, A., & Benvenga, S. (2012). Improvement of primary dysmenorrhea caused by a single oral dose of vitamin D: Results of a randomized, double-blind, placebo-controlled trial. *Archives of Internal Medicine, 172*(4), 366–367.

147. Huang, W., Shah, S., Long, Q., Crankshaw, A.K., & Tangpricha, V. (2012). Improvement of pain, sleep, and quality of life in chronic pain patients with vitamin D supplementation. *The Clinical Journal of Pain, 29*(4), 341–347.

148. Mowry, E.M., Waubant, E., McCulloch, C.E., et al. (2012). Vitamin D status predicts new brain magnetic resonance imaging activity in multiple sclerosis. *Annals of Neurology, 72*(2), 234–240.

149. Bischoff-Ferrari, H.A., Willett, W.C., Orav, E.J., et al. (2012). A pooled analysis of Vitamin D dose requirements for fracture prevention. *The New England Journal of Medicine, 367*, 40–49.

150. Leavitt, S. B. (2012, July 6). Vitamin D—Current research roundup. Pain Treatment Topics. Retrieved from http://updates.pain-topics. org/2012/07/vitamin-d-current-research-roundup.html

151. McCabe, P. (2014). New research suggests that vitamin D deficiency is associated with the development of chronic widespread pain [Press release]. British Society for Rheumatology. Retrieved from http://www.rheumatology.org.uk/about_bsr/press_releases/vitamind_cwp.aspx

152. Bjelakovic, G., Gluud, L.L., Nikolova, D., et al. (2011). Vitamin D supplementation for prevention of mortality in adults. *Cochrane Database of Systematic Reviews, 2011*(7), CD007470.

153. Holick, M.F., Biancuzzo, R.M., Chen, T.C., et al. (2008). Vitamin D2 is as effective as vitamin D3 in maintaining circulating concentrations of 25-hydroxyvitamin D. *The Journal of Clinical Endocrinology & Metabolism, 93*(3), 677–681.

154. Biancuzzo, R.M., Young, A., Bibuld, D., et al. (2010). Fortification of orange juice with vitamin D2 or vitamin D3 is as effective as an oral supplement in maintaining vitamin D status in adults. *The American Journal of Clinical Nutrition, 91*, 1621–1626.

155. Holmes, E.W., Garbincius, J., & McKenna, K.M. (2012, June). Analytical performance characteristics of two new automated immunoassays for 25 hydroxy Vitamin D. Paper presented at the Endocrine Society's 94th annual meeting, Houston, TX.

156. Sanders, K.M., Stuart, A.L., Williamson, E.J., et al. (2010). Annual high-dose oral vitamin D and falls and fractures in older women. *The Journal of the American Medical Association, 303*(18), 1815–1822.

157. Dawson-Hughes, B., & Harris, S.S. (2010). High dose vitamin D supplementation: Too much of a good thing? *The Journal of the American Medical Association, 303*(18), 1861–1862.

158. Clegg, D.O., Reda, D.J., Harris, C.L., et al. (2006). Glucosamine, chondroitin sulfate, and the two in combination for painful knee osteoarthritis. *The New England Journal of Medicine, 354*, 795–808.

159. Sawitzke, A.D., Shi, H., Finco, M.F., et al. (2008). The effect of glucosamine and/or chondroitin sulfate on the progression of knee osteoarthritis: A report from the glucosamine/chondroitin arthritis intervention trial. *Arthritis & Rheumatism, 58*(10), 3183–3191.

160. Sawitzke, A.D., Shi, H., Finco, M.F., et al. (2010). Clinical efficacy and safety of glucosamine/chondroitin sulphate, their combination, celecoxib or placebo taken to treat osteoarthritis of the knee: 2-year results from GAIT. *Annals of the Rheumatic Diseases, 69,* 1459–1464.

161. Agency for Healthcare Research and Quality. (2009). Choosing nonopioid analgesics for osteoarthritis (Pub. No. 06[07]-EHC009-3). Retrieved from http://www.sciencedirect.com/science/article/pii/S0965229911001063

162. Altman, R.D., & Marcussen, K.C. (2001). Effects of a ginger extract on knee pain in patients with osteoarthritis. *Arthritis & Rheumatism,* 44(11), 2531–2538.

163. Terry, R., Posadzki, P., Watson, L.K., & Ernst, E. (2011). The use of ginger (*Zingiber officinale*) for the treatment of pain: A systematic review of clinical trials. *Pain Medicine, 12*(12), 1808–1818.

164. Sepahvand, R., Esmaeili-Mahani, S., Arzi, A., Rasoulian, B., & Abbasnejad, M. (2010). Ginger (Zingiber officinale Roscoe) elicits antinociceptive properties and potentiates morphine-induced analgesia in the rat radiant heat tail-flick test. *Journal of Medicine and Food, 13*(6), 1397–1401.

165. Black, C., Herring, M.P., Hurley, D.J., & O'Connor, P.J. (2010). Ginger (Zingiber officinale) reduces muscle pain caused by eccentric exercise. *The Journal of Pain, 11*(9), 894–903.

166. National Center for Complementary and Integrative Medicine. (2012). Ginger. Retrieved from https://nccih.nih.gov/health/ginger

167. Zhao, C., Wacnik, P.W., Tall, J.M., et al. (2004). Analgesic effects of a soy-containing diet in three murine bone cancer pain models. *The Journal of Pain, 5*(2), 104–110.

168. Valsecchi, A.E., Franchi, S., Panerai, A.E., Sacerdote, P., Trovato, A.E., & Colleoni, M. (2008). Genistein, a natural phytoestrogen from soy, relieves neuropathic pain following chronic constriction sciatic nerve injury in mice: Anti-inflammatory and antioxidant activity. *Journal of Neurochemistry, 107*(1), 230–240.

169. Johns Hopkins Medicine. (2002). Dietary soy reduces pain, inflammation in rats [Press release]. Retrieved from http://www.hopkinsmedicine.org/press/2002/MARCH/020315.htm

170. Arjmandi, B.H., Khalil, D.A., Lucas, E.A., et al. (2004). Soy protein may alleviate osteoarthritis symptoms [Abstract]. *Phytomedicine, 11*(7–8), 567–575.

171. National Center for Complementary and Integrative Health. (2014). Complementary health approaches for chronic pain.

Retrieved   from   https://nccih.nih.gov/health/providers/digest/ chronic-pain-science

172. Funk, J.L., Frye, J.B., Oyarzo, J.N., et al. (2006). Efficacy and mechanism of action of turmeric supplements in the treatment of experimental arthritis. *Arthritis & Rheumatism, 54*(11), 3452–3464.

173. University of Arizona. (n.d.). Tapping the power of turmeric. Retrieved from http://www.arizona.edu/features/tapping-power-turmeric

174. Harrington, A.N., Hughes, P.A., Martin, C.M., et al. (2011). A novel role for TRPM8 in visceral afferent function. *PAIN, 152*(7), 1459–1468.

175. Gagnier, J.J., van Tulder, M.W., Berman, B.M., & Bombardier, C. (2006). Herbal medicine for low back pain. *Cochrane Database of Systematic Reviews, 2006*(2), CD004504.

176. Haldeman, S., & Dagenais, S. (2008). What have we learned about the evidence-informed management of chronic low back pain? *The Spine Journal, 8,* 266–277.

177. Gagnier, J.J. (2008). Evidence-informed management of chronic low back pain with herbal, vitamin, mineral, and homeopathic supplements. *The Spine Journal, 8,* 70–79.

178. National Center for Complementary and Integrative Health. (2015). Magnets for pain relief. Retrieved from https://nccih.nih. gov/health/magnet/magnetsforpain.htm.

179. Cepeda, M.S., Carr, D.B., Sarquis, T., Miranda, N., Garcia, R.J., & Zarate, C. (2007). Static magnetic therapy does not decrease pain or opioid requirements: A randomized double-blind trial. *Anesthesia & Analgesia, 104*(2), 290–294.

180. Federal Trade Commission. (1999). "Operation Cure.all" targets Internet health fraud [Press release]. Retrieved from http://www. ftc.gov/opa/1999/06/opcureall.shtm

181. Richmond, S.J., Brown, S.R., Campion, P.D., et al. (2009). Therapeutic effects of magnetic and copper bracelets in osteoarthritis: A randomized   placebo-controlled   crossover   trial.   *Complementary Therapies in Medicine, 17*(5–6), 249–256.

182. A. Pascual-Leone (personal communication, December 29, 2011).

183. Inoue, S., Ohashi, T., Yasuda, I., & Fukada, E. (1977). Electret induced callus formation in the rat. *Clinical Orthopaedics and Related Research, 124,* 57–58.

184. Morone, M.A., & Feuer, H. (2002). The use of electrical stimulation to enhance spinal fusion. *Neurosurgical Focus, 13*(6), 1–7.

185. Bassett, C.A., Mitchell, S.N., Norton, L., & Pilla, A. (1978). Repair of non-unions by pulsing electromagnetic fields. *Acta Orthopaedica Belgica, 44*(5), 706–724.

186. Bassett, C.A., Pawluk, R.J., & Pilla, A.A. (1974). Augmentation of bone repair by inductively coupled electromagnetic fields. *Science, 184*(136), 575–577.

187. Bassett, C.A. (1989). Fundamental and practical aspects of therapeutic uses of pulsed electromagnetic fields (PEMFs) [Abstract]. *Critical Reviews in Biomedical Engineering, 17*(5), 451–529.

188. Colson, D.J., Browett, J.P., Fiddian, N.J., & Watson, B. (1988). Treatment of delayed- and non-union of fractures using pulsed electromagnetic fields. *Journal of Biomedical Engineering, 10*(4), 301–304.

189. Satter, S.A., Islam, M.S., Rabbani, K.S., & Talukder, M.S. (1999). Pulsed electromagnetic fields for the treatment of bone fractures. *Bangladesh Medical Research Council Bulletin, 25*(1), 6–10.

190. Mackenzie, D., & Veninga, F.D. (2004). Reversal of delayed union of anterior cervical fusion treated with pulsed electromagnetic field stimulation: Case report. *Southern Medical Journal, 97*(5), 519–524.

191. McCarthy, C.J., Callaghan, M.J., & Oldham, J.A. (2006). Pulsed electromagnetic energy treatment offers no clinical benefit in reducing the pain of knee osteoarthritis: A systematic review. *BMC Musculoskeletal Disorders, 7*, 51.

192. National Center for Complementary and Integrative Health. (2015). Magnets for pain relief. Retrieved from https://nccih.nih.gov/health/magnet/magnetsforpain.htm

193. Harreby, M., Hesselsøe, G., Kjer, J., & Neergaard, K. (1997). Low back pain and physical exercise in leisure time in 38-year-old men and women: A 25-year prospective cohort study of 640 school children. *European Spine Journal, 6*(3), 181–186.

194. Suni, J.H., Oja, P., Miilunpalo, S.I., Pasanen, M.E., Vuori, I.M., & Bös, K. (1998). Health-related fitness test battery for adults: Associations with perceived health, mobility, and back function and symptoms. *Archives of Physical Medicine and Rehabilitation, 79*(5), 559–569.

195. Croft, P.R., Papageorgiou, A.C., Thomas, E., Macfarlane, G.J., & Silman, A.J. (1999). Short-term physical risk factors for new episodes of low back pain: Prospective evidence from the South Manchester Back Pain Study. *Spine, 24*(15), 1556.

196. Landmark, T., Romundstad, P., Borchgrevink, P.C., Kaasa, S., & Dale, O. (2011). Associations between recreational exercise and chronic pain in the general population: Evidence from the HUNT 3 study. *PAIN, 152*(10), 2241–2247.

197. Cohen, I., & Rainville, J. (2002). Aggressive exercise as treatment for chronic low back pain. *Sports Medicine, 32*(1), 75–82.

198. Rainville, J. (2003, December). Exercise for low back pain: What it can and cannot do for your patients. PowerPoint presented at New England College of Occupational and Environmental Medicine annual conference, Newton, MA. Retrieved from http://www.necoem.org/documents/0312Rainville.PDF

199. Ibid.

200. Rainville, J., Hartigan, C., Martinez, E., Limke, J., Jouve, C., & Finno, M. (2004). Exercise as a treatment for chronic low back pain. *The Spine Journal, 4*(1), 106–115.

201. Maher, C., Latimer, J., & Refshauge, K. (1999). Prescription of activity for low back pain: What works? *Australian Journal of Physiotherapy, 45,* 121–132.

202. Hagen, K.B., Jamtvedt, G., Hilde, G., & Winnem, M.F. (2005). The updated Cochrane review of bed rest for low back pain and sciatica [Abstract]. *Spine, 30*(5), 542–546.

203. Lindström, I., Öhlund, C., Eek, C., et al. (1992). The effect of graded activity on patients with subacute low back pain: A randomized prospective clinical study with an operant-conditioning behavioral approach [Abstract]. *Physical Therapy, 72*(4), 279–290.

204. Taimela, S., Diederich, C., Hubsch, M., & Heinricy, M. (2000). The role of physical exercise and inactivity in pain recurrence and absenteeism from work after active outpatient rehabilitation for recurrent or chronic low back pain: A follow-up study. *Spine, 25*(14), 1809–1816.

205. Kool, J., de Bie, R., Oesch, P., Knusel, O., van den Brandt, P., & Bachman, S. (2004). Exercise reduces sick leave in patients with non-acute non-specific low back pain: A meta-analysis. *Journal of Rehabilitation Medicine, 36*(2), 49–62.

206. Maul, I., Laubli, T., Oliveri, M., & Krueger, H, (2005). Long-term effects of supervised physical training in secondary prevention of low back pain. *European Spine Journal, 14*(6), 599–611.

207. Choi, B.K., Verbeek, J.H., Tam, W.W., & Jiang, J.Y. (2010). Exercises for the prevention of recurrences of low-back pain. *Occupational and Environmental Medicine, 67,* 795–796.

208. Hayden, J., van Tulder, M.W., Malmivaara, A., & Koes, B.W. (2005). Exercise therapy for treatment of non-specific low back pain. *Cochrane Database of Systematic Reviews, 2005*(3), CD000335.

209. Sofi, F., Molino, L.R., Nucida, V., et al. (2011). Adaptive physical therapy and back pain: A non-randomised community-based intervention trial. *European Journal of Physical and Rehabilitation Medicine, 47*(4), 543–549.

210. Lin, C.C., McAuley, J.H., Macedo, L., Barnett, D.C., Smeets, R.J., & Verbunt, J.A. (2011). Relationship between physical activity and disability in low back pain: A systematic review and meta-analysis [Abstract]. *PAIN, 152*(3), 607–613.

211. Rainville, J., Sobel, J., Hartigan, C., Monlux, G., & Bean, J. (1997). Decreasing disability in chronic back pain through aggressive spine rehabilitation. *Journal of Rehabilitation Research and Development, 34*(4), 383–393.

212. Hartigan, C., Rainville, J., Sobel, J.B., & Hipona, M. (2000). Long-term exercise adherence after intensive rehabilitation for chronic low back pain. *Medicine & Science in Sports and Exercise, 32*(3), 551–557.

213. Kernan, T., & Rainville, J. (2007). Observed outcomes associated with a quota-based exercise approach on measures of kinesiophobia in patients with chronic low back pain. *The Journal of Orthopaedic and Sports Physical Therapy, 37*(11), 679–687.

214. Rainville, J., Hartigan, C., Jouve, C., & Martinez, E. (2004). The influence of intense exercise-based physical therapy program on back pain anticipated before and induced by physical activities. *The Spine Journal, 4*(2), 176–183.

215. Mailloux, J., Finno, M., & Rainville, J. (2006). Long-term exercise adherence in the elderly with chronic low back pain. *American Journal of Physical Medicine & Rehabilitation, 85*(2), 120–126.

216. Moffett, J.K., Torgerson, D., Bell-Syer, S., et al. (1999). Randomised controlled trial of exercise for low back pain: Clinical outcomes, costs, and preferences. *British Medical Journal, 319*(7205), 279–283.

217. Chou, R., & Huffman, L.H. (2007). Nonpharmacologic therapies for acute and chronic low back pain: A review of the evidence for an American Pain Society/American College of Physicians clinical practice guideline. *Annals of Internal Medicine, 147*(7), 492–504.

218. Rainville, J., Ahern, D.K., Phalen, L., Childs, L.A., & Sutherland, R. (1992). The association of pain with physical activities in chronic low back pain. *Spine, 17*(9), 1060–1064.

219. Rainville, J., Ahern, D.K., & Phalen, L. (1993). Altering beliefs about pain and impairment in a functionally oriented treatment program for chronic low back pain. *The Clinical Journal of Pain, 9,* 196–201.

220. Roelofs, J., Goubert, L., Peters, M.L., Vlaeyen, J.W., & Crombez, G. (2004). The Tampa Scale for Kinesiophobia: Further examination of psychometric properties in patients with chronic low back pain and fibromyalgia [Abstract]. *European Journal of Pain, 8*(5), 495–502.

221. Waddell, G., Newton, M., Henderson, K., Somerville, D., & Main, C.J. (1993). A Fear-Avoidance Beliefs Questionnaire (FABQ) and the role of fear-avoidance beliefs in chronic low back pain and disability [Abstract]. *PAIN, 52*(2), 157–168.

222. Damsgard, E., Thrane, G., Anke, A., Fors, T., & Roe, C. (2010). Activity-related pain in patients with chronic musculoskeletal disorders [Abstract]. *Disability and Rehabilitation, 32*(17), 1428–1437.

223. Vlaeyen, J., & Linton, S.J. (2000). Fear-avoidance and its consequences in chronic musculo-skeletal pain [Abstract]. *PAIN, 85*(3), 317–332.

224. Wilson, A.C., Lewandowski, A.S., & Palermo, T.M. (2011). Fear-avoidance beliefs and parental responses to pain in adolescents with chronic pain [Abstract]. *Pain Research Management, 16*(3), 178–182.

225. Picavet, H.S., Vlaeyen, J.W., & Schouten, J.S. (2002). Pain catastrophizing and kinesiophobia: Predictors of chronic low back pain [Abstract]. *American Journal of Epidemiology, 156*(11), 1028–1034.

226. Brox, J.I., Storheim, K., Grotle, M., Tveito, T.H., Indahl, A., & Eriksen, H.R. (2008). Evidence-informed management of chronic low back pain with back schools, brief education, and fear-avoidance training. *The Spine Journal, 8,* 28–39.

227. Buchbinder, R., & Jolley, D. (2005). Effects of a media campaign on back beliefs is sustained 3 years after its cessation [Abstract]. *Spine, 30*(11), 1323–1330.

228. Consumer Reports. (2011). Special report: Working out your back pain. *Consumer Reports on Health, 23*(9), 8–9.

229. Liddle, S.D., Baxter, G.D., & Gracey, J.H. (2004). Exercise and chronic low back pain: What works [Abstract]? *PAIN, 107*(1), 176–190.

230. Mayer, J., Mooney, V., & Dagenais, S. (2008). Evidence-informed management of chronic low back pain with lumbar extensor strengthening exercises. *The Spine Journal, 8,* 96–113.

231. Standaert, C.J., Weinstein, S.M., & Rumpeltes, J. (2008). Evidence-informed management of chronic low back pain with lumbar stabilization exercises. *The Spine Journal, 8,* 114–120.

232. Hayden, J.A., van Tulder, M.W., Malmivaara, A., & Koes, B.W. (2005). Meta-analysis: Exercise therapy for nonspecific low back pain [Abstract]. *Annals of Internal Medicine, 142*(9), 765–775.

233. Hayden, J.A., van Tulder, M.W., & Tomlinson, G. (2005). Systematic review: Strategies for using exercise therapy to improve outcomes in chronic low back pain. *Annals of Internal Medicine, 142*(9), 776–785.

234. Murtezani, A., Hundozi, H., Orovanec, N., Silamniku, S., & Osmani, T. (2011). A comparison of high intensity aerobic exercise

and passive modalities for the treatment of workers with chronic low back pain: A randomized, controlled trial. *European Journal of Physical and Rehabilitation Medicine, 47*(3), 359–366.

235. van der Velde, G., & Mierau, D. (2000). The effect of exercise on percentile rank aerobic capacity, pain, and self-rated disability in patients with chronic low back pain: A retrospective chart review. *Archives of Physical Medicine and Rehabilitation, 81*(11), 1457–1463.

236. Chan, C.W., Mok, N.W., & Yeung, E.W. (2011). Aerobic exercise training in addition to conventional physiotherapy for chronic low back pain: A randomized controlled trial. *Archives of Physical Medicine and Rehabilitation, 92*(10), 1681–1685.

237. Bentsen, H., Lindgarde, F., & Manthorpe, R. (1997). The effect of dynamic strength back exercise and/or a home training program in 57-year-old women with chronic low back pain: Results of a prospective randomized study with a 3-year follow-up period. *Spine, 22*(13), 1494–1500.

238. Bronfort, G., Maiera, M.J., Evans, R.L., et al. (2011). Supervised exercise, spinal manipulation, and home exercise for chronic low back pain: A randomized clinical trial [Abstract]. *The Spine Journal, 11*(7), 585–598.

239. Jordan, J.L., Holden, M.A., Mason, E.E., & Foster, N.E. (2010). Interventions to improve adherence to exercise for chronic musculoskeletal pain in adults. *Cochrane Database of Systematic Reviews, 2010*(1), CD005956.

240. Waller, B., Lambeck, J., & Daly, D. (2009). Therapeutic aquatic exercise in the treatment of low back pain: A systematic review. *Clinical Rehabilitation, 23*(1), 3–14.

241. National Center for Complementary and Integrative Health. (2015). National survey reveals widespread use of mind and body practices. Retrieved from http://www.nih.gov/news/health/feb2015/nccih-10a.htm

242. National Center for Complementary and Alternative Medicine. (n.d.). Yoga. Retrieved from http://nccam.nih.gov/health/yoga

243. Posadzki, P., & Ernst, E. (2011). Yoga for low back pain: A systematic review of randomized clinical trials. *Clinical Rheumatology, 30*(9), 1257–1262.

244. Posadzki, P., Ernst, E., Terry, R., & Lee, M. S. (2011). Is yoga effective for pain? A systematic review of randomized clinical trials [Abstract]. *Complementary Therapies in Medicine, 19*(5), 281–287.

245. Williams, K.A., Petronis, J., Smith, D., et al. (2005). Effect of Iyengar yoga therapy for chronic low back pain [Abstract]. *PAIN, 115*(1–2), 107–117.

246. Williams, K., Abildso, C., Steinberg, L., et al. (2009). Evaluation of the effectiveness and efficacy of Iyengar yoga therapy on chronic low back pain. *Spine, 34*(19), 2066–2076.

247. Chou, R., & Huffman, L.H. (2007). Nonpharmacologic therapies for acute and chronic low back pain: A review of the evidence for an American Pain Society/American College of Physicians clinical practice guideline. *Annals of Internal Medicine, 147*(7), 492–504.

248. Tilbrook, H.E., Cox, H., Hewitt, C.E., et al. (2011). Yoga for chronic low back pain: A randomized trial. *Annals of Internal Medicine, 115*, 569–573.

249. Sherman, K.J., Cherkin, D.C., Wellman, R.D., et al. (2011). A randomized trial comparing yoga, stretching, and a self-care book for chronic low back pain [Abstract]. *Archives of Internal Medicine, 171*(22), 2019–2026.

250. Broad, W.J. (2012, January 8). All bent out of shape. *The New York Times Magazine*, p. 16.

251. Lim, E.C., Poh, R.L., Low, A.Y., & Wong, W.P. (2011). Effects of Pilates-based exercises on pain and disability in individuals with persistent nonspecific low back pain: A systematic review with meta-analysis. *Journal of Orthopaedic and Sports Physical Therapy, 41*(2), 70–80.

252. Faas, A., Chavannes, A.W., van Eijk, J.T., & Gubbels, J.W. (1993). A randomized, placebo-controlled trial of exercise therapy in patients with acute low back pain. *Spine, 18, 1388*–1395.

253. Schaafsma, F., Schonstein, E., Whelan, K.M., Ulvestad, E., Kenny, D.T., & Verbeek, J.H. (2010). Physical conditioning programs for improving work outcomes in workers with back pain. *Cochrane Database of Systematic Reviews, 2010*(1), CD001822.

254. Soukup, M.G., Glomsrod, B., Lonn, J.H., Bo, K., & Larsen, S. (199). The effect of a Mensendieck exercise program as a secondary prophylaxis for recurrent low back pain: A randomized, controlled trial with 12-month follow-up [Abstract]. *Spine, 24*(15), 1585.

255. Hides, J.A., Jull, G.A., & Richardson, C.A. (2001). Long-term effects of specific stabilizing exercises for first-episode low back pain [Abstract]. *Spine, 26*(11), e243–e248.

256. Centers for Disease Control and Prevention. (n.d.). Arthritis: The nation's most common cause of disability. Retrieved from http://

www.cdc.gov/chronicdisease/resources/publications/AAG/ar-thritis.htm

257. Arthritis Foundation. (n.d.). Osteoarthritis, rheumatoid arthritis. Retrieved from http://www.arthritis.org

258. Poirot, L. (2012). High-intensity exercise and arthritis. *Arthritis Today.* Retrieved from http://www.arthritistoday.org/conditions/rheumatoid-arthritis/staying-active/high-intensity-exercise.php

259. Munneke, M., de Jong, Z., Zwinderman, A.H., et al. (2004). High intensity exercise or conventional exercise for patients with rheumatoid arthritis? Outcome expectations of patients, rheumatologists, and physiotherapists. *Annals of the Rheumatic Diseases, 63,* 804–804.

260. de Jong, Z., Munneke, M., Jansen, L.M., et al. (2004). Differences between participants and nonparticipants in an exercise trial for adults with rheumatoid arthritis. *Arthritis Care & Research, 51*(4), 593–600.

261. Munneke, M., de Jong, Z., Zwinderman, A.H., et al. (2005). Effect of a high-intensity weight-bearing exercise program on radiologic damage progression of the large joints in subgroups of patients with rheumatoid arthritis. *Arthritis Care & Research, 53*(3), 410–417.

262. de Jong, Z., Vlieland, V., & Theodora, P.M. (2005). Safety of exercise in patients with rheumatoid arthritis [Abstract]. *Current Opinion in Rheumatology, 17*(2), 177–182.

263. de Jong, Z., Munneke, M., Zwinderman, A.H., et al. (2003). Is a long-term high-intensity exercise program effective and safe in patients with rheumatoid arthritis? Results of a randomized controlled trial. *Arthritis & Rheumatism, 48*(9), 2415–2424.

264. Munneke, M., de Jong, Z., Zwinderman, A.H., et al. (2003). Adherence and satisfaction of rheumatoid arthritis patients with a long-term intensive dynamic exercise program (RAPIT program). *Arthritis Care & Research, 49*(5), 665–672.

265. de Jong, Z., Munneke, M., Kroon, H.M., et al. (2009). Long-term follow-up of a high-intensity exercise program in patients with rheumatoid arthritis. *Clinical Rheumatology, 28,* 663–671.

266. de Jong, Z., Munneke, M., Lems, W.F., et al. (2004). Slowing of bone loss in patients with rheumatoid arthritis by long-term high-intensity exercise: Results of a randomized, controlled trial. *Arthritis & Rheumatism, 50*(4), 1066–1076.

267. de Jong, Z., Munneke, M., Zwinderman, A.H., et al. (2004). Long term high intensity exercise and damage of small joints in rheumatoid arthritis. *Annals of the Rheumatic Diseases, 63,* 1399–1405.

268. Hurkmans, E., van der Giesen, F.J., Vliet Vlieland, T.P., Schoones, J., & Van den Ende, E.C. (2009). Dynamic exercise programs (aerobic capacity and/or muscle strength training) in patients with rheumatoid arthritis. *Cochrane Database of Systematic Reviews, 2009*(4), CD006853.

269. Bailet, A., Zeboulon, N., Gossec, L., et al. (2010). Efficacy of cardiorespiratory aerobic exercise in rheumatoid arthritis: Meta-analysis of randomized controlled trials. *Arthritis Care & Research, 62*(7), 984–992.

270. Cooney, J.K., Law, R.J., Matschke, V., et al. (2011). Benefits of exercise in rheumatoid arthritis. *Journal of Aging Research, 2011*(681640), 1–14.

271. Bartels, E.M., Lund, H., Hagen, K.B., Dagfinrud, H., Christensen, R., & Danneskiold-Samsoe, B. (2007). Aquatic exercise for the treatment of knee and hip osteoarthritis [Abstract]. *Cochrane Database of Systematic Reviews, 2007*(4), CD005523.

272. Cadmus, L., Patrick, M.B., Maciejewski, M.L., Topolski, T., Belza, B., & Patrick, D.L. (2010). Community-based aquatic exercise and quality of life in persons with osteoarthritis [Abstract]. *Medicine & Science in Sports & Exercise, 42*(1), 8–15.

273. Lim, J.Y., Tchai, E., & Jang, S.N. (2010). Effectiveness of aquatic exercise for obese patients with knee osteoarthritis: A randomized controlled trial [Abstract]. *PM&R, 2*(8), 723–731.

274. Ettinger, W.H., Burns, R., Messier, S.P., et al. (1997). A randomized trial comparing aerobic exercise and resistance training exercise with a health education program in older adults with knee osteoarthritis. The Fitness Arthritis and Seniors Trial (FAST). *The Journal of the American Medical Association, 277*(1), 25–31.

275. Messier, S.P., Loeser, R.F., Miller, G.D., et al. (2004). Exercise and dietary weight loss in overweight and obese older adults with knee osteoarthritis: The Arthritis, Diet, and Activity Promotion Trial [Abstract]. *Arthritis & Rheumatism, 50*(5), 1501–1510.

276. Pisters, M.F., Veenhof, C., Schellevis, F.G., Twisk, J.W., Dekker, J., & De Bakker, D.H. (0210). Exercise adherence improving long-term patient outcome in patients with osteoarthritis of the hip and/or knee. *Arthritis Care & Research, 62*(8), 1087–1094.

277. Sommer, C. (2010). Fibromyalgia: A clinical update. *PAIN, 18*(4), 1–4.

278. Wolf, F., Smythe, H.A., Yunus, M.B., et al. (1990). The American College of Rheumatology 1990 criteria for the classification of fibromyalgia. *Arthritis & Rheumatism, 33*(2), 160–172.

279. Yeh, G.Y., Kaptchuk, T.J., & Shmerling, R.H. (2010). Prescribing tai chi for fibromyalgia—Are we there yet? *The New England Journal of Medicine, 363*(8), 783–784.
280. Spaeth, M. (2009). Editorial: Epidemiology, costs, and the economic burden of fibromyalgia. *Arthritis Research & Therapy, 11*(3), 117.
281. Sommer, C. (2010). Fibromyalgia: A clinical update. *PAIN, 18*(4), 1–4.
282. Schweinhardt, P., Sauro, K.M., & Bushnell, M.C. (2008). Fibromyalgia: A disorder of the brain? *Neuroscientist, 14*(5), 415–421.
283. Kuchinad, A., Schweinhardt, P., Seminowicz, D.A., Wood, P.B., Chizh, B.A., & Bushnell, M.C. (2007). Accelerated brain gray matter loss in fibromyalgia patients: Premature aging of the brain? *Journal of Neuroscience, 27*(15), 4004–4007.
284. D.L. Goldenberg (personal communication, August 26, 2011).
285. Ortega, E., Garcia, J.J., Bote, M.E., et al. (2009). Exercise in fibromyalgia and related inflammatory disorders: Known effects and unknown chances. *Exercise Immunology Review, 15*, 42–65.
286. McBeth, J., Nicholl, B.I., Cordingley, L., Davies, K.A., & Macfarlane, G.J. (2010). Chronic widespread pain predicts physical inactivity: Results from the prospective EPIFUND study [Abstract]. *European Journal of Pain, 14*(9), 972–979.
287. Goldenberg, D. (2011). *Fibromyalgia: The final chapter* [Kindle version]. Retrieved from Amazon.com.
288. Rooks, D.S., Gautam, S., Romeling, M., et al. (2007). Group exercise, education, and combination self-management in women with fibromyalgia [Abstract]. *Archives of Internal Medicine, 167*(20), 2192–2200.
289. Kayo, A.H., Peccin, M.S., Sanches, C.M., & Trevisani, V.F. (2010). Effectiveness of physical activity in reducing pain in patients with fibromyalgia: A blinded randomized clinical trial [Abstract]. *Rheumatology International, 32*(8), 2285–2292.
290. Fontaine, K.R., Conn, L., & Claw, D.J. (2010). Effects of lifestyle physical activity on perceived symptoms and physical function in adults with fibromyalgia: Results of a randomized trial. *Arthritis Research & Therapy, 12*(2), R55.
291. Jones, K.D., Adams, D., Winters-Stone, K., & Burckhardt, C.S. (2006). A comprehensive review of 46 exercise treatment studies in fibromyalgia (1988–2005). *Health and Quality of Life Outcomes, 4*, 67.
292. Busch, A.J., Barber, K.A., Overend, T.J., Peloso, P.M., & Schachter, C.L. (2007). Exercise for treating fibromyalgia syndrome. *Cochrane Database of Systematic Reviews, 2007*(4), CD003786.

293. Busch, A.J., Schachter, C.L., Overend, T.J., Peloso, P.M., & Barber, K.A. (2008). Exercise for fibromyalgia: A systematic review. *The Journal of Rheumatology, 35*(6), 1130–1144.
294. Busch, A.J., Barber, K.A., Overend, T.J., Peloso, P.M., & Schachter, C.L. (2006). Exercise for treating fibromyalgia (Review). *Cochrane Database System Review, 2006*(3), 1–35.
295. Hauser, W., Klose, P., Langhorst, J., et al. (2010). Efficacy of different types of aerobic exercise in fibromyalgia syndrome: A systematic review and meta-analysis of randomised controlled trials. *Arthritis Research & Therapy, 12*(3), R79.
296. Hauser, W., Thieme, K., & Turk, D.C. (2010). Guidelines on the management of fibromyalgia syndrome—A systematic review [Abstract]. *European Journal of Pain, 14*(1), 5–10.
297. Gusi, N., Tomas-Carus, P., Hakkinen, A., Hakkinen, K., & Ortega-Alonso, A. (2006). Exercise in waist-high warm water decreases pain and improves health-related quality of life and strength in the lower extremities in women with fibromyalgia [Abstract]. *Arthritis & Rheumatology, 55*(1), 66–73.
298. Mannerkorpi, K., Nordeman, L., Ericsson, A., & Arndorw, M. (2009). Pool exercise for patients with fibromyalgia or chronic widespread pain: A randomized controlled trial and subgroup analyses [Abstract]. *Journal of Rehabilitation Medicine, 41*(9), 751–760.
299. Langhorst, J., Musial, F., Klose, P., & Hauser, W. (2009). Efficacy of hydrotherapy in fibromyalgia syndrome - A meta-analysis of randomized controlled trials [Abstract]. *Rheumatology, 48*(9), 1155–1159.
300. Wang, C., Schmid, C.H., Rones, R., et al. (2010). A randomized trial of tai chi for fibromyalgia. *The New England Journal of Medicine, 363*(8), 743–754.
301. National Center for Complementary and Alternative Medicine. (2006). Tai chi: An introduction. Retrieved from http://nccam.nih.gov/health/taichi/introduction.htm
302. Ibid.
303. P. Wayne (personal communication, March 18, 2012).
304. Taggart, H.M., Arslanian, C.L., Bae, S., & Singh, K. (2003). Effects of tai chi exercise on fibromyalgia symptoms and health-related quality of life [Abstract]. *Orthopaedic Nursing, 22*(5), 353–360.
305. Wang, C., Schmid, C.H., Rones, R., et al. (2010). A randomized trial of tai chi for fibromyalgia. *The New England Journal of Medicine, 363*(8), 743–754.

306. Yeh, G.Y., Kaptchuk, T.J., & Shmerling, R.H. (2010). Prescribing tai chi for fibromyalgia—Are we there yet? *The New England Journal of Medicine, 363*(8), 783–784.

307. Bingel, U., Wanigasekera, V., Wiech, K., et al. (2011). The effect of treatment expectation on drug efficacy: Imaging the analgesic benefit of the opioid remifentanil [Abstract]. *Science Translational Medicine, 3*(70), 70ra14.

308. Gollub, R.L., & Kong, J. (2011). For placebo effects in medicine, seeing is believing [Abstract]. *Science Translational Medicine, 3*(70), 70ps5.

309. Kaptchuk, T.J., Friedlander, E., Kelley, J.M., et al. (2010). Placebos without deception: A randomized controlled trial in irritable bowel syndrome. *PloS ONE, 5*(12), e15591.

310. T. Kaptchuk (personal communication, December 29, 2010).

311. Finniss, D. G., Kaptchuk, T. J., Miller, F., & Benedetti, F. (2010). Biological, clinical, and ethical advances of placebo effects. *The Lancet, 375*(9715), 686–695.

312. Jensen, K.B., Kaptchuk, T.J., Kirsch, I., et al. (2012). Nonconscious activation of placebo and nocebo pain responses. *Proceedings of the National Academy of Sciences, 109*(39), 15959–15964.

313. Kong, J., Kaptchuk, T.J., Polich, G., Kirsch, I., & Gollub, R.L. (2007). Placebo analgesia: Findings from brain imaging studies and emerging hypotheses. *Reviews in the Neurosciences, 18*(3–4), 173–190.

314. Wager, T.D., Rilling, J.K., Smith, E.E., et al. (2004). Placebo-induced changes in fMRI in the anticipation and experience of pain [Abstract]. *Science, 303*(5661), 1162–1167.

315. Price, D.D., Craggs, J., Verne, G.N., Perlstein, W.M., & Robinson, M.E. (2007). Placebo analgesia is accompanied by large reductions in pain-related activity in irritable bowel syndrome patients [Abstract]. *PAIN, 127*(1), 63–72.

316. R. Gollub (personal communication, January 5, 2011).

317. Levine, J.D., Gordon, N.C., & Fields, H.L. (1978). The mechanism of placebo analgesia. *The Lancet, 312*(8091), 654–657.

318. Petrovic, P., Kalso, E., Petersson, K.M., & Ingvar, M. (2002). Placebo and opioid analgesia--imaging a shared neuronal network [Abstract]. *Science, 295*(5560), 1737–1740.

319. Zubieta, J., Yau, W.Y., Scott, D.J., & Stohler, C.S. (2006). Belief or need? Accounting for individual variations in the neurochemistry of the placebo effect [Abstract]. *Brain, Behavior, and Immunity, 20*(1), 15–26.

320. Benedetti, F., Arduino, C., & Amanzio, M. (1999). Somatotopic activation of opioid systems by target-directed expectations of analgesia [Abstract]. *The Journal of Neuroscience, 19*(9), 3639–3648.

321. Benedetti, F., Amanzio, M., Rosato, R., & Blanchard, C. (2011). Nonopioid placebo analgesia is mediated by CB1 cannabinoid receptors. *Nature Medicine, 17*(10), 1228–1230.

322. L. Zeltzer (personal communication, August 31, 2010).

323. Keefe, F.J., Lefebvre, J.C., Egert, J.R., Affleck, G., Sullivan, M.J., & Caldwell, D.S. (2000). The relationship of gender to pain, pain behavior, and disability in osteoarthritis patients: The role of catastrophizing. *PAIN, 87*(3), 325–334.

324. Edwards, R.R., Haythornthwaite, J.A., Sullivan, M.J., & Fillingim, R.B. (2004). Catastrophizing as a mediator of sex differences in pain: Differential effects for daily pain versus laboratory-induced pain. *PAIN, 111*(3), 335–341.

325. Sullivan, M.J., Bishop, S.R., & Pivik, J. (1995). The Pain Catastrophizing Scale: Development and validation. *Psychological Assessment, 7*(4), 524–532.

326. Edwards, R.R., Bingham, C.O. III, Bathon, J., & Haythornthwaite, J.A. (2006). Catastrophizing and pain in arthritis, fibromyalgia, and other rheumatic diseases. *Arthritis Care & Research, 55*(2), 325–332.

327. Edwards, R.R., Kronfli, T., Haythornthwaite, J.A., Smith, M.T., McGuire, L., & Page, G.G. (2008). Association of catastrophizing with interleukin-6 responses to acute pain. *PAIN, 140*(1), 135–144.

328. Seminowicz, D.A., & Davis, K.D. (2006). Cortical responses to pain in healthy individuals depends on pain catastrophizing. *PAIN, 120*(3), 297–306.

329. Chou, R., & Huffman, L. (2007). Nonpharmacologic therapies for acute and chronic low back pain: A review of the evidence for an American Pain Society/American College of Physicians clinical practice guideline. *Annals of Internal Medicine, 147*(7), 492–504.

330. Gatchel, R.J., & Rollings, K.H. (2008). Evidence-informed management of chronic low back pain with cognitive behavioral therapy. *The Spine Journal, 8*, 40–44.

331. Ehde, D.M., Dillworth, T.M., & Turner, J.A. (2014). Cognitive-behavioral therapy for individuals with chronic pain. *American Psychologist, 69*(2), 153–166.

332. Keefe, F.J., Abernethy, A.P., & Campbell, L.C. (2005). Psychological approaches to understanding and treating disease-related pain. *Annual Review of Psychology, 56*, 601–630.

333. Turner, J.A., Mancl, L., & Aaron, L.A. (2006). Short-and long-term efficacy of brief cognitive-behavioral therapy for patients with chronic temporomandibular disorder pain: A randomized, controlled trial [Abstract]. *PAIN, 121*(3), 181–194.

334. Jackson, J.L., O'Malley, P.G., & Kroenke, K. (2006). Antidepressants and cognitive-behavioral therapy for symptom syndromes. *CNS Spectrums, 11*(3), 212–222.

335. Butler, A.C., Chapman, J.E., Forman, E.M., & Beck, A.T. (2006). The empirical status of cognitive-behavioral therapy: A review of meta-analyses [Abstract]. *Clinical Psychology Review, 26*(1), 17–31.

336. Morley, S., Eccleston, C., & Williams, A. (1999). Systematic review and meta-analysis of randomized controlled trials of cognitive behaviour therapy and behaviour therapy for chronic pain in adults, excluding headache. *PAIN, 80*(1–2), 1–13.

337. Morley, S., Williams, A., & Hussain, S. (2008). Estimating the clinical effectiveness of cognitive behavioural therapy in the clinic: Evaluation of a CBT informed pain management programme. *PAIN, 137*(3), 670–680.

338. S. Morley (personal communication, February 3, 2011).

339. Morley, S. (2011). Efficacy and effectiveness of cognitive behaviour therapy for chronic pain: Progress and some challenges. *PAIN, 152*(3), S99–S106.

340. Eccleston, C., Palermo, T.M., de C Williams, A. C., Lewandowski, A., & Morley, S. (2009). Psychological therapies for the management of chronic and recurrent pain in children and adolescents [Abstract]. *Cochrane Database of Systematic Reviews, 2009*(2), CD003968.

341. Macea, D.D., Gajos, K., Daglia Calil, Y.A., & Fregni, F. (2010). The efficacy of web-based cognitive behavioral interventions for chronic pain: A systematic review and meta-analysis [Abstract]. *The Journal of Pain, 11*(10), 917–929.

342. Jensen, M.P., Turner, J.A., & Romano, J.M. (2001). Changes in beliefs, catastrophizing, and coping are associated with improvement in multidisciplinary pain treatment. *Journal of Consulting and Clinical Psychology, 69*(4), 655–662.

343. Edwards, R.R., Bingham, C.O. III, Bathon, J., & Haythornthwaite, J.A. (2006). Catastrophizing and pain in arthritis, fibromyalgia, and other rheumatic diseases. *Arthritis Care & Research, 55*(2), 325–332.

344. Cepeda, M.S., Carr, D.B., Lau, J., & Alvarez, H. (2006). Music for pain relief [Abstract]. *Cochrane Database of Systematic Reviews, 2006*(2), CD004843.

345. M. Jensen & D. Patterson (personal communication, February 2, 2010).

346. Hoffman, H.G., Patterson, D.R., Magula, J., et al. (2004). Water-friendly virtual reality pain control during wound care [Abstract]. *Journal of Clinical Psychology, 60*(2), 189–195.

347. Hoffman, H.G., Patterson, D.R., & Carrougher, G.J. (2000). Use of virtual reality for adjunctive treatment of adult burn pain during physical therapy: A controlled study [Abstract]. *The Clinical Journal of Pain, 16*(3), 244–250.

348. Hoffman, H.G., Seibel, E.J., Richards, T.L., Furness, T.A., Patterson, D.R., & Sharar, S.R. (2006). Virtual reality helmet display quality influences the magnitude of virtual reality analgesia [Abstract]. *The Journal of Pain, 7*(11), 843–850.

349. Sprenger, C., Elppert, F., Finsterbusch, J., Bingel, U., Rose, M., & Buchel, C. (2012). Attention modulates spinal cord responses to pain. *Current Biology, 22*(11), 1019–1022.

350. Association for Applied Psychophysiology and Biofeedback. (n.d.). About biofeedback. Retrieved from http://www.aapb.org/i4a/pages/index.cfm?pageid=3463

351. Nestoriuc, Y., & Martin, A. (2007). Efficacy of biofeedback for migraine: A meta-analysis. *PAIN, 128*(1), 111–27.

352. Nestoriuc, Y., Martin, A., Rief, W., & Andrasik, F. (2008). Biofeedback treatment for headache disorders: A comprehensive efficacy review. *Applied Psychophysiology and Biofeedback, 33*(3), 125–140.

353. Frank, D.L., Khorshid, L., Kiffer, J.F., Moravec, C.S., & McKee, M.G. (2010). Biofeedback in medicine: Who, when, why and how? *Mental Health in Family Medicine, 7*(2), 85–91.

354. Jensen, M.P., Hakimian, S., Sherlin, L.H., & Fregni, F. (2009). New insights into neuromodulatory approaches for the treatment of pain. *The Journal of Pain, 9*(3), 193–199.

355. DeCharms, R.C., Maeda, F., Glover, G.H., et al. (2005). Control over brain activation and pain learned by using real-time functional MRI. *Proceedings of the National Academy of Sciences, 102*(51), 18626–18631.

356. S. Mackey (personal communication, April 14, 2012).

357. Foreman, J. (2003, April 22). Meditation and the brain. *The Boston Globe.* Retrieved from www.judyforeman.com

358. Kabat-Zinn, J. (1990). *Full catastrophe living: Using the wisdom of your body and mind to face stress, pain, and illness.* New York: Bantam Dell.

359. Goleman, D. (1988). *The meditative mind: The varieties of meditative experience.* New York: J.P. Tarcher.

360. Goldsmith, J.S. (1990). *The art of meditation*. New York: HarperCollins.

361. Gardner-Nix, J., & Costin-Hall, L. (2009). *The mindfulness solution to pain: Step-by-step techniques for chronic pain management*. Oakland, CA: New Harbinger.

362. Vowles, K.E., McCracken, L.M., & Dahl, J.C. (2010, May 7). Acceptance and commitment therapy and chronic pain. PowerPoint presented at the American Pain Society's 29th annual meeting, Baltimore, MD.

363. Davidson, R.J., Kabat-Zinn, J., Schumacher, J., et al. (2003). Alterations in brain and immune function produced by mindfulness meditation. *Psychosomatic Medicine, 65(4)*, 564–570.

364. Lazar, S.W., Kerr, C.E., Wasserman, R.H., et al. (2005). Meditation experience is associated with increased cortical thickness. *Neuroreport, 16(17)*, 1893–1897.

365. Grant, J.A., Courtemanche, J., Duerden, E.G., Duncan, G.H., & Rainville, P. (2010). Cortical thickness and pain sensitivity in Zen meditators [Abstract]. *Emotion, 10(1)*, 43–53.

366. Grant, J.A., Courtemanche, J., & Rainville, P. (2010). A non-elaborative mental stance and decoupling of executive and pain-related cortices predicts low pain sensitivity in Zen meditators [Abstract]. *PAIN, 152(1)*, 150–156.

367. Lush, E., Salmon, P., Floyd, A., Studts, J.L., Weissbecker, I., & Sephton, S.E. (2009). Mindfulness meditation for symptom reduction in fibromyalgia: Psychophysiological correlates [Abstract]. *Journal of Clinical Psychology in Medical Settings, 16(2)*, 200–207.

368. Grossman, P., Tiefenthaler-Gilmer, U., Raysz, A., & Kesper, U. (2007). Mindfulness training as an intervention for fibromyalgia: Evidence of postintervention and 3-year follow-up benefits in well-being [Abstract]. *Psychotherapy and Psychosomatics, 76(4)*, 226–233.

369. Vago, D.R., & Nakamura, Y. (2011). Selective attentional bias towards pain-related threat in fibromyalgia: Preliminary evidence for effects of mindfulness meditation training. *Cognitive Therapy and Research, 35(6)*, 581–594.

370. Schmidt, S., Grossman, P., Schwarzer, B., Jena, S., Naumann, J., & Walach, H. (2011). Treating fibromyalgia with mindfulness-based stress reduction: Results from a 3-armed randomized controlled trial [Abstract]. *PAIN, 152(2)*, 361–369.

371. Zeidan, F., Martucci, K.T., Kraft, R.A., Gordon, N.S., McHaffie, J.G., & Coghill, R.C. (2011). Brain mechanisms supporting the

modulation of pain by mindfulness meditation. *The Journal of Neuroscience, 31*(14), 5540–5548.

372. Zeidan, F., Gordon, N.S., Merchant, J., & Goolkasian, P. (2010). The effects of brief mindfulness meditation training on experimentally induced pain [Abstract]. *The Journal of Pain, 11*(3), 199–209.

373. Rosenzweig, S., Greeson, J.M., Reibel, D.K., Green, J.S., Jasser, S.A., & Beasley, D. (2010). Mindfulness-based stress reduction for chronic pain conditions: Variation in treatment outcomes and role of home meditation practice [Abstract]. *Journal of Psychosomatic Research, 68*(1), 29–36.

374. Brown, C.A., & Jones, A.K. (2010). Meditation experience predicts less negative appraisal of pain: Electrophysiological evidence for the involvement of anticipatory neural responses [Abstract]. *PAIN, 150*(3), 428–438.

375. Hölzel, B.K., Carmody, J., Vangel, M., et al. (2011). Mindfulness practice leads to increases in regional brain gray matter density. *Psychiatry Research: Neuroimaging, 191*(1), 36–43.

376. Gard, T., Holzel, B.K., Sack, A.T., et al. (2011). Pain attenuation through mindfulness is associated with decreased cognitive control and increased sensory processing in the brain. *Cerebral Cortex, 22*(11), 2692–2702.

377. S. Lazar (personal communication, April 10, 2012).

378. Patterson, D.R., & Jensen, M.P. (2003). Hypnosis and clinical pain. *Psychological Bulletin, 129*(4), 495–521.

379. Jensen, M.P. & Patterson, D.R. (2014). Hypnotic approaches for chronic pain management. *American Psychologist, 69*(2), 167–177.

380. Jensen, M.P., Ehde, D.M., Gertz, K.J., et al. (2011). Effects of self-hypnosis training and cognitive restructuring on daily pain intensity and catastrophizing in individuals with multiple sclerosis and chronic pain. *International Journal of Clinical and Experimental Hypnosis, 59*(1), 45–63.

381. Jensen, M.P., Barber, J., Romano, J.M., et al. (2009). Effects of self-hypnosis training and EMG biofeedback relaxation training on chronic pain in persons with spinal-cord injury. *International Journal of Clinical and Experimental Hypnosis, 57*(3), 239–268.

382. Zeltzer, L., & LeBaron, S. (1982). Hypnosis and nonhypnotic techniques for reduction of pain and anxiety during painful procedures in children and adolescents with cancer. *Journal of Pediatrics, 101*(6), 1032–1035.

383. Patterson, D.R., & Jensen, M.P. (2003). Hypnosis and clinical pain. *Psychological Bulletin, 129*(4), 495–521.

384. M. Jensen & D. Patterson (personal communication, February 2, 2010).

385. Jensen, M., McArthur, K., Barber, J., et al. (2006). Satisfaction with, and the beneficial side effects of, hypnotic analgesia. *International Journal of Clinical and Experimental Hypnosis, 54*(4), 432–447.

Chapter 8

1. Americans with Disabilities Act of 1990. (n.d.). Wikipedia. Retrieved from https://en.wikipedia.org/wiki/Americans_with_Disabilities_Act_of_1990

2. Gereau, R.W. IV, Sluka, K.A., Maixner, W., et al. (2014). A pain research agenda for the 21st century. *The Journal of Pain, 15*, 1203–1214.

3. M.R. Rajagopal (personal communication, June 17, 2015).

4. Pallium India. (2015). About Pallium India. Retrieved from http://palliumindia.org/about/about-pallium-india

5. Express News Service. (2012, March 2). TIPS declared as a WHO Collaborating Centre. *The New Indian Express.* Retrieved from http://www.newindianexpress.com/cities/thiruvananthapuram/article339480.ece

6. M.R. Rajagopal (personal communication, June 17, 2015).

7. ET Bureau. (2014, February 24). M.R. Rajagopal: The man who spearheaded efforts to improve access to morphine. *The Economic Times.* Retrieved from http://articles.economictimes.indiatimes.com/2014-02-24/news/47635745_1_morphine-ngo-cankids-cancer-patients

8. Vishnu, U. (2009, October 30). A fight for life and death with dignity. *The Indian Express.* Retrieved from http://archive.indianexpress.com/news/a-fight-for-life-and-death-with-dignity/534982/

9. M.R. Rajagopal (personal communication, June 17, 2015).

10. Cherny, N.I., Cleary, J., Scholten, W., Radbruch, L., & Torode, J. (2013). The Global Opioid Policy Initiative (GOPI) to evaluate the availability and accessibility of opioids for the management of cancer pain in Africa, Asia, Latin America and the Caribbean, and the Middle East: Introduction and Methodology. *Annals of Oncology, 24*(11), xi7–xi13.

11. McNeil, D.G. (2007, September 11). In India, a quest to ease the pain of the dying. *The New York Times.* Retrieved from http://www.nytimes.com/2007/09/11/health/11pain.html?pagewanted=all

12. M.R. Rajagopal (personal communication, June 17, 2015).

13. M.R. Rajagopal. (2015, March 3). How do you treat pain when most of the world's population can't get opioids? *Los Angeles Times*. Retrieved from http://www.latimes.com/opinion/op-ed/la-oe-rajagopal-pain-opioids-20150304-story.html

14. M.R. Rajagopal (personal communication, June 17, 2015).

15. Ibid.

16. Ibid.

17. McNeil, D.G. (2007, September 11). In India, a quest to ease the pain of the dying. *The New York Times*. Retrieved from http://www.nytimes.com/2007/09/11/health/11pain.html?pagewanted=all

18. M.R. Rajagopal. (2015, March 3). How do you treat pain when most of the world's population can't get opioids? *Los Angeles Times*. Retrieved from http://www.latimes.com/opinion/op-ed/la-oe-rajagopal-pain-opioids-20150304-story.html

19. ET Bureau. (2014, February 24). M.R. Rajagopal: The man who spearheaded efforts to improve access to morphine. *The Economic Times*. Retrieved from http://articles.economictimes.indiatimes.com/2014-02-24/news/47635745_1_morphine-ngo-cankids-cancer-patients

20. Johari, A. (2014, March 4). Why cancer patients are cheering a recent change in the narcotics law. Scroll.in. Retrieved from http://scroll.in/article/657603/one-achievement-of-indias-least-productive-parliament-amending-narcotics-act-to-help-cancer-patients

21. M.R. Rajagopal (personal communication, June 17, 2015).

22. ET Bureau. (2014, February 24). M.R. Rajagopal: The man who spearheaded efforts to improve access to morphine. *The Economic Times*. Retrieved from http://articles.economictimes.indiatimes.com/2014-02-24/news/47635745_1_morphine-ngo-cankids-cancer-patients

23. Ibid.

24. Ibid.

25. M.R. Rajagopal (personal communication, June 17, 2015).

26. Human Rights Watch. (2009). *Unbearable pain—India's obligation to ensure palliative care* (p. 33). Retrieved from http://www.hrw.org/reports/2009/10/28/unbearable-pain-0

27. M.R. Rajagopal (personal communication, June 17, 2015).

28. Ibid.

29. World Health Organization. (2015). Palliative care for HIV and cancer patients in Africa. Retrieved from http://www.who.int/cancer/palliative/projectproposal/en

30. Dr. Anne Merriman, Leader of Palliative Care in Africa, UCD School of Medicine and Medical Science. (n.d.). Retrieved from http://

www.ucd.ie/medicine/ourcommunity/ouralumni/alumnipro-filesinterviews/drannemerriman

31. University College Dublin School of Medicine & Medical Science. (2012). Dr. Anne Merriman: Leader of palliative care in Africa. Retrieved from http://www.ucd.ie/medicine/ourcommunity/ouralumni/alumniprofilesinterviews/drannemerriman

32. Merriman, A., & Harding, R. (2010). Pain control in the African context: The Ugandan introduction of affordable morphine to relieve suffering at the end of life. *Philosophy, Ethics and Humanities in Medicine, 5,* 10.

33. University College Dublin School of Medicine & Medical Science. (2012). Dr. Anne Merriman: Leader of palliative care in Africa. Retrieved from http://www.ucd.ie/medicine/ourcommunity/ouralumni/alumniprofilesinterviews/drannemerriman

34. Pastrana, T., Torres-Vigil, I., & De Lima, L. (2014). Palliative care development in Latin America: An analysis using macro indicators. *Palliative Medicine, 28,* 1–8.

35. Knaul, F.M., Farmer, P.E., & Bhadelia, A. (2015). Closing the divide: The Harvard Global Equity Initiative–Lancet Commission on global access to pain control and palliative care, Comment, *The Lancet, 386*(9995), 722–744.

36. Steedman, M. R., Hughes-Hallett, T., Knaul, F.M., Knuth, A., Shamieh, O. & Darzi, A. (2014). Innovation can improve and expand aspects of end-of-life care in low and middle-income countries. *Health Affairs, 33*(9), 1612–1619.

37. Human Rights Watch. (2011). *Global palliative care* (p. 3). Retrieved from http://www.hrw.org/reports/2011/06/02/global-state-pain-treatment-0

38. Paudel, B.D., Ryan, K.M., Brown, M.S., et al. (2014). Opioid availability and palliative care in Nepal: influence of an international pain policy fellowship. *Journal of Pain and Symptom Management, 49,* 110–116.

39. Cleary, J., Radbruch, L., Torode, J. & Cherny, N.I. (2013). Next steps in access and availability of opioids for the treatment of cancer pain: Reaching the tipping point? *Annals of Oncology, 24*(11), xi60–xi64.

40. Ibid.

41. Krakauer, E.L., Cham, N.T., Husain, S.A., et al. (2015). Toward safe accessibility of opioid medicines in Vietnam and other developing countries: A balanced policy model. *Journal of Pain and Symptom Management, 49*(5), 916–922.

42. Cleary, J., Radbruch, L., Torode, J. & Cherny, N.I. (2013). Next steps in access and availability of opioids for the treatment of cancer pain: Reaching the tipping point? *Annals of Oncology, 24*(11), xi60–xi64.

43. Powell, R.A., Mwangi-Powell, F., Radbruch, L., et al. (2015). Putting palliative care on the global health agenda. *The Lancet Oncology, 16*, 131–133.

44. J. Cleary (personal communication, June 5, 2015).

45. World Health Organization. (2011). *Ensuring balance in national policies on controlled substances.* Retrieved from http://www.atome-project.eu/documents/gls_ens_balance_eng.pdf

46. World Health Assembly. (2014). *Strengthening of palliative care as a component of integrated treatment within the continuum of care* (Agenda item 9.4). Retrieved from http://apps.who.int/gb/ebwha/pdf_files/EB134/B134_R7-en.pdf

47. Knaul, F.M., Farmer, P.E., & Bhadelia, A. (2015). Closing the divide: The Harvard Global Equity Initiative–Lancet Commission on global access to pain control and palliative care, Comment. *The Lancet, 386*(9995), 722–744.

48. Harvard Global Equity Initiative. (2015). Commission members. Retrieved from http://hgei.harvard.edu/icb/icb.do?keyword=k62597&pageid=icb.page704147

49. Gereau, R.W. IV, Sluka, K.A., Maixner, W., et al. (2014). A pain research agenda for the 21st century. *The Journal of Pain, 15*, 1203–1214.

50. Ibid.

51. Ibid.

52. Ibid.

53. National Institutes of Health. (2014). *Pathways to Prevention workshop: The role of opioids in the treatment of chronic pain* (p. 34). Retrieved from https://prevention.nih.gov/docs/programs/p2p/ODPPainPanelStatementFinal_10-02-14.pdf

54. Ibid.

55. M. Christopher (personal communication, June 22, 2015).

56. National Pain Strategy, March 18, 2016 https://iprcc.nih.gov/National_Pain_Strategy/NPS_Main.htm

57. Interagency Pain Research Coordinating Committee. (n.d.). National Pain Strategy: A comprehensive population health level strategy for pain. Retrieved from http://iprcc.nih.gov/National_Pain_Strategy/NPS_Main.htm

58. Ibid.
59. Ibid., p. 13.
60. Ibid., p. 26.
61. Ibid., p. 30.
62. Ibid., p. 36
63. Pain Action Alliance to Implement a National Strategy. (2015). Our vision. Retrieved from http://www.painsproject.org
64. Consumer Pain Advocacy Task Force. (2015). What we believe. Retrieved fromhttp://consumerpainadvocacy.org
65. M. Christopher (personal communication, July 22, 2015).
66. American Chronic Pain Association. (2015). About us. Retrieved from http://theacpa.org/About-Us
67. Patient-Centered Outcomes Research Institute. (2015). Penney Cowan. Retrieved from http://www.pcori.org/people/penney-cowan
68. Champeau, R. (2013, October 16). UCLA to house worldwide database of brain images for chronic pain conditions. UCLA Newsroom. Retrieved from http://newsroom.ucla.edu/releases/nih-funding-helps-launch-worldwide-24881
69. Stanford Medicine. (2015). Collaborative health outcomes information registry. Retrieved from http://snapl.stanford.edu/choir/
70. Tufts University School of Medicine. (2015). Faculty. Retrieved from http://publichealth.tufts.edu/Academics/MS-Pain-Research-Education-and-Policy/People/Faculty/Daniel-Carr
71. Tufts University School of Medicine. (2015). Master of science in pain research, education and policy. Retrieved from http://publichealth.tufts.edu/Academics/MS-Pain-Research-Education-and-Policy/MS-PREP
72. National Institutes of Health. (2014). Federal pain research database launched. Retrieved from http://www.nih.gov/news/health/may2014/ninds-27.htm
73. National Institutes of Health. (2015). Pain Consortium Centers of Excellence in Pain Education. Retrieved from http://painconsortium.nih.gov/NIH_Pain_Programs/CoEPES.html
74. D. Thomas (personal communication, April 20, 2015).
75. Gereau, R.W. IV, Sluka, K.A., Maixner, W., et al. (2014). A pain research agenda for the 21st century. *The Journal of Pain, 15*, 1203–1214.
76. Ibid.
77. C. Steinberg (personal communication, September 22, 2011).
78. C. Steinberg (personal communication, June 28, 2015).

79. Massachusetts Pain Initiative. (2015). *Health Professions Licensing Boards issue rulings on the management of pain*. Retrieved from http://mi.gov/documents/mdch/MassPI_Board_Ruling_Press_Release_5-1-09_278782_7.pdf

80. C. Steinberg (personal communication, July 2, 2015).

81. Steinberg, S. (2014, November 17). Memo to Gov.-Elect: Include pain sufferers as you seek opiate solution. *CommonHealth*. Retrieved from http://commonhealth.wbur.org/2014/11/chronic-pain-opiate-solution

82. Commonwealth of Massachusetts. (2015). *Recommendations of the Governor's Opioid Working Group*. Retrieved from http://www.mass.gov/eohhs/images/dph/stop-addiction/recommendations-of-the-governors-opioid-working-group.pdf

83. Mass.gov. (2015). Governor Baker releases Opioid Working Group recommendations. Retrieved from http://www.mass.gov/governor/press-office/press-releases/fy2015/governor-releases-opioid-working-group-recommendations.html

84. Commonwealth of Massachusetts. (2015). *Recommendations of the Governor's Opioid Working Group* (p. 2). Retrieved from http://www.mass.gov/eohhs/images/dph/stop-addiction/recommendations-of-the-governors-opioid-working-group.pdf

Appendix II

1. D. Carr (personal communication, December 4, 2014).

INDEX